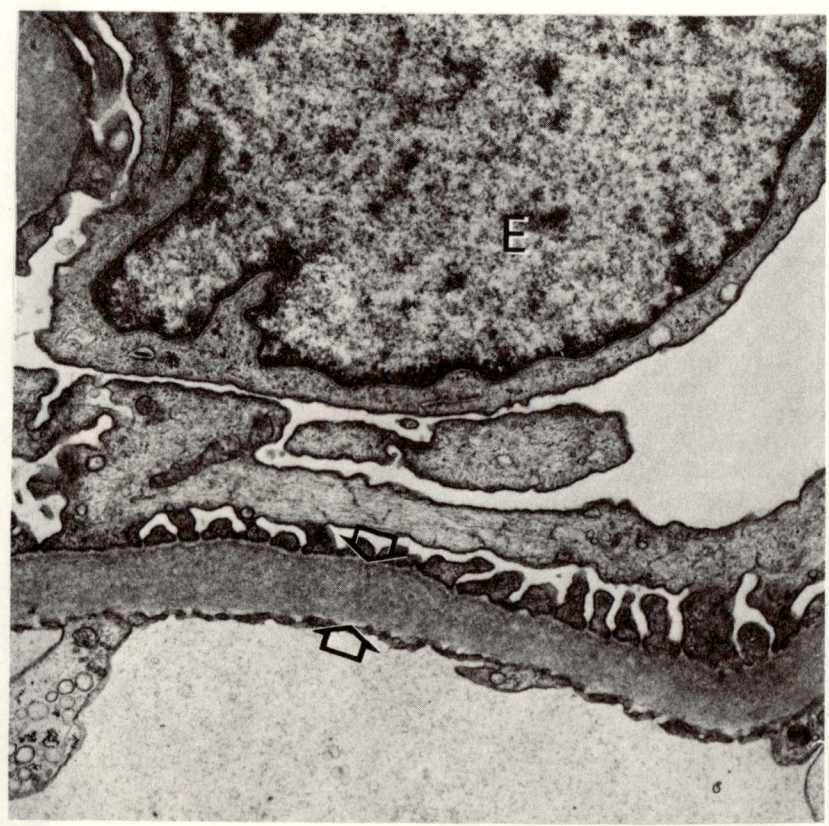

The hallmark of diabetes in the tissues. Glomerular capillary basement membrane thickening (between arrows) as a result of excess glycoprotein synthesis in epithelium **E**. Electron micrograph of renal tissue obtained by percutaneous biopsy from a diabetic patient

× 12,000

Diabetes Today

A HANDBOOK
FOR THE CLINICAL TEAM

J T IRELAND MD FRCPEdin
*Consultant Physician, Southern General
Hospital, Glasgow; Honorary Clinical Lecturer
in Medicine, University of Glasgow*

**W S T THOMSON PhD FRCPGlas
FRCPath**
*Consultant Biochemist, Southern
General Hospital, Glasgow;
Honorary Lecturer in Pathological Biochemistry,
University of Glasgow*

**J WILLIAMSON MD FRCSGlas
DOEng**
*Consultant Ophthalmologist, Victoria
and Southern General Hospitals, Glasgow;
Honorary Clinical Lecturer in Ophthalmology,
University of Glasgow*

With 10 colour illustrations

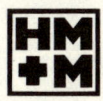

HM+M PUBLISHERS

First published in 1980
by HM + M Publishers Ltd
Milton Road, Aylesbury, Buckinghamshire, England

ISBN 0 85602 053 2

Filmset in 'Monophoto' Plantin by
Servis Filmsetting Ltd, Manchester

Printed in Great Britain by A. Wheaton & Co. Ltd., Exeter

Contents

Colour plates I and II between pages 192, 193
Colour plates III and IV between pages 208, 209

Preface

Many traditional ideas about diabetic management with diet, insulin or oral hypoglycaemic agents have been challenged in recent years by enlightened clinicians and researchers who have brought a new clarity to our understanding of the disorder. This text is not for these experts. Instead, it is addressed to a new generation of students and doctors in training, as well as to general practitioners and hospital specialists who may not have had the time or opportunity to bring themselves up to date about new approaches to diabetes or its various complications.

We now believe that improved control of the metabolic disorder is an essential aspect of delaying the onset of certain specific complications. Too often in the past strict or rigid control has been advocated without thought for the practical implications or for patient compliance. Improved and more flexible control obtained through better understanding of self regulation by diabetics and those responsible for their care is a central theme of this text. The alternative of ignorance about the disorder often breeds unnecessary fear in both patient and doctor.

Many fundamental problems concerning diabetes remain to be solved. Nevertheless we have attempted to examine the issues and highlight the more controversial aspects of diabetic care in the hope that, with better understanding, patients may be given advice most appropriate to their individual circumstances. If as a result more diabetics are encouraged to go about their business and enjoy life to the full, without fear of the disorder or of its complications, so much the the better.

We are indebted to Mr. J. Paterson, Medical Photography Department, Southern General Hospital, for the artwork and to Miss M.I.F. Bethel, SRD, Chief Dietician, Southern General Hospital, for the diets in the Appendices.

J.T. IRELAND
W.S.T. THOMSON
J. WILLIAMSON
Glasgow
September 1979

Glossary of Abbreviations

ADH	antidiuretic hormone
ADP	adenosine diphosphate
ATP	adenosine triphosphate
BMT	basement membrane thickening
CSG	chronic simple glaucoma
DCA	dichloroacetic acid
DIC	diffuse intravascular coagulation
DIDMOAD	diabetes insipidus, diabetes mellitus, optic atrophy and deafness
DNA	deoxyribonucleic acid
ECF	extracellular fluid
FFA	free fatty acid
GFR	glomerular filtration rate
GH-RIH	growth hormone – release inhibiting hormone (somatostatin)
GIP	gastric inhibitory polypeptide (also known as glucose-dependent insulin-releasing polypeptide)
GTT	glucose tolerance test
Hb A_1	haemoglobin A_1
HDL	high density lipoprotein
HLA	human leucocyte antigen (histocompatibility antigen)
HPL	human placental lactogen
ICA	islet cell antibody
IDL	intermediate density lipoprotein
IRMA	intraretinal microvascular abnormalities
JOD	juvenile-onset diabetes
kcal	kilocalorie
LCAT	lecithin: cholesterol acyltransferase
LDL	low density lipoprotein
MC	monocomponent
MOD	maturity-onset diabetes
MODY	maturity-onset diabetes of youth
MJ	megajoule
RDS	respiratory distress syndrome
RNA	ribonucleic acid
TSH	thyroid stimulating hormone (thyrotrophin)
TCA	tricarboxylic acid
UGDP	University Group Diabetes Programme
VLDL	very low density lipoprotein

CHAPTER 1

Introduction: Diabetes the Enigma

The thirst and copious sweet urine of diabetes mellitus have been known from the dawning of medical history – yet the disorder remains an enigma. Although relatively simple to detect and diagnose, we still do not understand why about one per cent. of the population become so afflicted – nor why the other ninety and nine drawn from the same environment do not – and we remain virtually unable to prevent the disorder. We know that it tends to cluster in some families, especially amongst those who develop mild diabetes in later life. But many have no family history and despite recent advances in histocompatibility antigen (HLA) typing suggestive of immune deficiency in juvenile-onset diabetes, geneticists still have no reliable method of predicting who will, or will not, develop the clinical syndrome. Nevertheless, studies of the HLA system have not only confirmed genetic heterogeneity in diabetes, but also given the scientist further encouragement to search for those infections or other insults which, in the susceptible youngster, may damage the pancreatic beta cell.

The isolation of insulin in 1921 was heralded as the ultimate answer to a serious and life-threatening problem. Certainly, diabetes is no longer a death sentence. But many of those in whom the sentence has been commuted to a life of insulin injections still run a significant risk of developing renal damage, or becoming blind through retinopathy, both as a result of capillary and small-blood-vessel disease specific to diabetes. These patients are also likely to develop peripheral and autonomic neuropathy which, in combination with lower-limb digital capillary disease, leads to an ever present risk of gangrene. None of these insults can be regarded as side effects of insulin therapy because even the mildest of diabetics who have escaped insulin injections also may be similarly afflicted. And as if these horrible complications were not enough, diabetics (especially if female) are more likely than non-diabetics to have their larger blood vessels corroded by atheroma, arteriosclerosis and other degenerative disease.

The central issue facing those concerned with diabetic care is whether these various complications are an inevitable part of the diabetic syndrome or are alternatively due to our inability fully to

9

return the metabolic upset to normal. If the discovery of insulin has been to date the medical world's most conspicuous success in overcoming the immediate dangers of diabetes, this has not always been matched by our ability to put it to effective use especially in the long term. Thus, evidence accumulated recently from various sources now implicates the abnormally high blood glucose of poorly or badly controlled diabetes as a major factor causing small blood vessel disease by altering the structure and function of the basement membrane ground substance of capillaries. Unfortunately, this does not mean that good control of the blood glucose will cure all the diabetic's problems. As will become increasingly apparent, nothing concerning diabetes mellitus can be expressed in such simple terms. Good control may prevent small-blood-vessel pathology, but the corrosive effects of atheroma and large-vessel disease are probably accelerated by altered blood lipids, abnormal platelet behaviour, fibrin deposition and other factors.

In wrestling with the problems of intermediary and vessel wall metabolism, the medical scientist has learned that insulin is a key hormone of storage and cell growth, regulating protein and fat turn-over besides that of carboyhydrate. We know that acute lack of insulin may be fatal; we know also that insulin will restore to normal the biochemical and hormonal changes of diabetes, but we are just beginning to realise that excess of insulin ultimately may be as harmful as too little. Too rich a diet in the non-diabetic may stimulate hyperinsulinism causing excessive nutrient storage with stock-piling of lipids in adipose tissue depôts, besides seeding dangerously as atheromatous plaques in vessel walls. Too often the poorly controlled diabetic is subjected to erratic swings between insulin lack and insulin excess. Indeed, these wide swings are probably particularly harmful because they upset the normal ebb and flow of nutrient storage and release, exaggerating the worst elements of plasma lipid abnormality and hormonal imbalance which play havoc with vessel wall metabolism in particular and the cardio-vascular system in general. If all this appears too complex, too confusing (or too confused), the various elements involved in the complicated jig-saw of intermediary metabolism are examined and unfolded step by step in subsequent chapters.

When the patient first presents with thirst, polyuria and other symptoms of diabetes, absolute or relative deficiency of insulin due to pancreatic beta cell failure lies at the heart and soul of the immediate problem. Understanding insulin secretion and its hormonal function is fundamental, not only to the clinician, but also to the researcher who seeks to unravel the diabetic enigma and to explore new ways of preventing the onset of the disorder.

With the possibility of so many appalling difficulties besetting diabetics and their families, this book aims at doing the best for our patients within the limits of present knowledge. All too often the traditional approach to management has advocated shackling the patient to rigid dietary and insulin regimens, allowing the doctor to blame poor diabetic control on the patient's failure to comply. Despite a long clinical experience with insulin, besides an ever increasing variety of preparations available to us, we remain incredibly clumsy in their use. The achievement of good diabetic control in the artificial circumstances of a hospital ward or diabetic clinic is of little practical value. On the other hand the diabetic requires education and guidance in the use of insulin or oral hypoglycaemic agents in order to lead as normal and unrestricted a life as possible. This text attempts to provide practical suggestions on various aspects of management with the aim of taking good diabetic care into the home, the workplace and the leisure-ground. Because many diabetics present as emergencies or create management problems in any general practice or in various hospital wards, guidance is given which may be of value to those managing patients at home or in hospital and which also may be helpful to students or postgraduates who tend to see diabetic patients in the hospital environment. Nevertheless, it is hoped that they too will learn that diabetes is not just a bedside problem, but something that the patient must be taught and encouraged to live with – successfully – outwith the sheltered hospital environment.

Some readers may find the approach too elementary or hampered by frequent simplistic analogies. But many aspects of diabetes have to be explained to patients or to members of the diabetic clinical team who have not had the luxury of a lengthy medical training. And some who have may no longer remember how glucose is metabolised to CO_2 and water, or the subtle steps by which it switches into various intermediates or is re-cycled from amino-acids, lactate or glycerol. Perhaps for them and others the diagrams and biochemical shorthand may be useful.

Some readers may feel that the spotlight concentrates too depressingly on the more serious diabetic complications, yet these often create clinical problems requiring the greatest skill in management. Perhaps, as a consequence of realising the possible ravages of diabetes, some of those who read this introduction to the disorder may be encouraged to set their enquiring minds to these problems. Challenging questions which remain unanswered are scattered through the text. Finding one or more of the answers to the enigma would be a worthy and rewarding pursuit.

Further Reading

References to up-to-date reviews, leading articles or textbooks by recognised authorities appear at the end of subsequent chapters, and are intended for wider reading, although occasionally particular points of reference are indicated in the text.

CHAPTER 2

A Melting Down of Flesh and Limbs into Urine

An account of the nature of diabetes mellitus and the function of insulin

To the physicians of ancient Greece diabetes meant a 'syphoning of water through the body'. Centuries earlier, Indian and Egyptian writings included remedies for sweet urine, but the expression mellitus – sweet as honey – was not added to medical literature until the 18th century. Aretaeus the Cappadocian, writing in the second century AD, saw diabetes as a mysterious disease yet described its features with dramatic clarity:

> 'Diabetes is a wonderful affection, not very frequent among men, being a melting down of the flesh and limbs into urine ... life is short, disgusting and painful, thirst unquenchable, death is inevitable'.

Today, with the most sophisticated means of metabolic study at our disposal, we remain unable to pin-point with certainty the cause of diabetes mellitus or the exact locus of the defect, but we are getting much closer to the heart of the problem. Thus it is of value for the student of diabetes to examine the progress made; at least we can now give a rational explanation for the melting down of the flesh and limbs into the urine ...

The key is *insulin*. Before examining the function and purpose of this pancreatic hormone, however, some of the steps in its discovery are worth retracing.

In the *London Medical Journal* of 1788 Thomas Cawley published the sad account of a jovial, rotund alcohol imbiber whose fondness for rich eating and the good life was suddenly interrupted when he was struck down by ghastly abdominal pains. Simultaneously, the poor fellow developed the features of diabetes mellitus and gradually wasted away. Pancreatic calcification was found at post-mortem examination leading Cawley to speculate that the pancreas might be the source of diabetes (today, alcoholic pancreatitis associated with diabetes, although relatively uncommon, is well recognised; see Chapter 19).

Paul Langerhans, while still a final-year medical student, took us

13

a stage further in understanding the importance of the pancreas when in 1869 he wrote his thesis identifying small islands of specialised cells which every medical student now recognises as the islets of Langerhans and the source of insulin. But the significance of the pancreas in diabetes was not fully appreciated until in 1889 a scrupulously clean laboratory attendant was upset by a house-trained dog which was repeatedly urinating on his normally spotless laboratory floor. The unfortunate animal had had its pancreas removed surgically in a study of the exocrine function of the gland. Oscar Minkowski, who was studying pancreatic function, investigated the animal's problem and, as any well trained observer of polyuria should do, he tested the urine and on finding sugar established that pancreatectomy caused diabetes.

The final step – the isolation of insulin – was one of the major medical triumphs of all time. Research workers in several countries were attempting to extract insulin from the pancreatic islets, amongst them Paulesco of Roumania and Zuelzer in Germany. But it was the Canadian surgeon Frederick Banting, working with an honours physiology student in the Toronto medical school Charles Best, who in 1921 caught the imagination of the world. Their extract of 'Isletin' was successfully injected into a pancreatectomised (diabetic) dog. Not only were the dog's symptoms of diabetes relieved, but Best was simultaneously able to show a fall in the animal's blood sugar. A third collaborator James Collip then concentrated on the difficult chemical problem of further isolating the active principle by preparing an alcohol-precipitated pancreatic extract which was almost entirely free of harmful proteins likely to provoke allergic reactions. After further successful trials of this extract in dogs Banting and Best were ready in January 1922 to give it to a young diabetic patient Leonard Thomson, and then to a diabetic nurse, with dramatic results in both cases. But a word of caution to any zealous student with a potential prize-winning discovery up his sleeve. In 1923 the Nobel Prize was awarded to Professor MacLeod who provided the laboratories for the research and to Frederick Banting. Charles Best, the medical student who had made the crucial blood sugar estimations for Banting, was not included in the Nobel Prize citation because he had not completed his medical studies and was still unqualified. History, however, has put the record straight: the names of Banting and Best remain synonymous with the discovery of insulin.

Today, insulin is widely available and constantly being improved in efficiency and purity, but the tantalizing problem of pancreatic failure in diabetes remains to be solved. The difficulties can best be understood by examining in detail the function of insulin and the various anti-insulin hormones.

The function of insulin

Insulin is secreted in response to feeding and, as Figure 2.1 shows, the blood glucose normally rises in the hour following a meal. This is due to the absorption from the gut into the blood of glucose derived from its precursor carbohydrates –

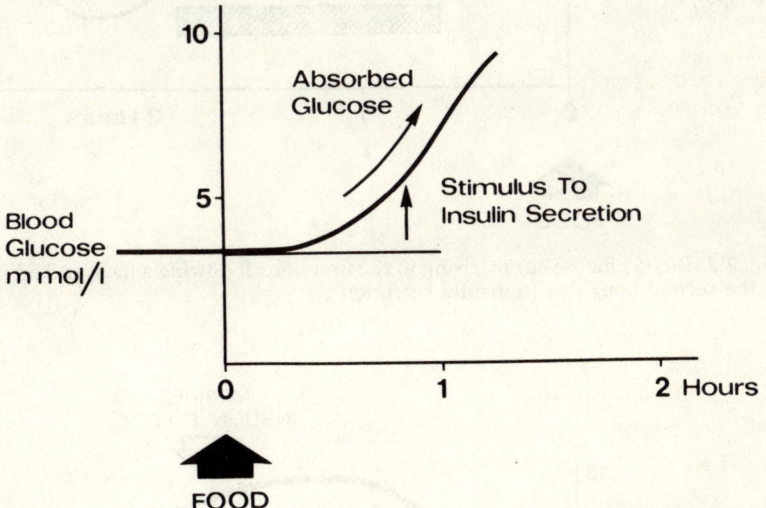

Fig. 2.1 Blood glucose rise in response to feeding stimulating pancreatic insulin release

starch and other sugars – contained in the meal. The rise in blood glucose is the main stimulus to the pancreas to release insulin into the circulation, but it takes time for the liberated insulin to become effective. Thus, as Figure 2.2 shows, although the blood sugar falls in the second hour, the insulin release has occurred much earlier. This curve of the blood sugar with its rise and fall – like the ebb and flow of the tide – occurs with every meal and forms the basis of the *glucose tolerance curve* (Chapter 5) upon which the diagnosis of diabetes still rests. Thus diabetes as it is currently arbitrarily defined implies a failure in the insulin response to a meal, a failure to control the blood sugar rise (Fig. 2.3), in a word – hyperglycaemia.

But what is the purpose of insulin? Insulin is the hormone of fuel storage and of cell growth. We have just seen how it is normally

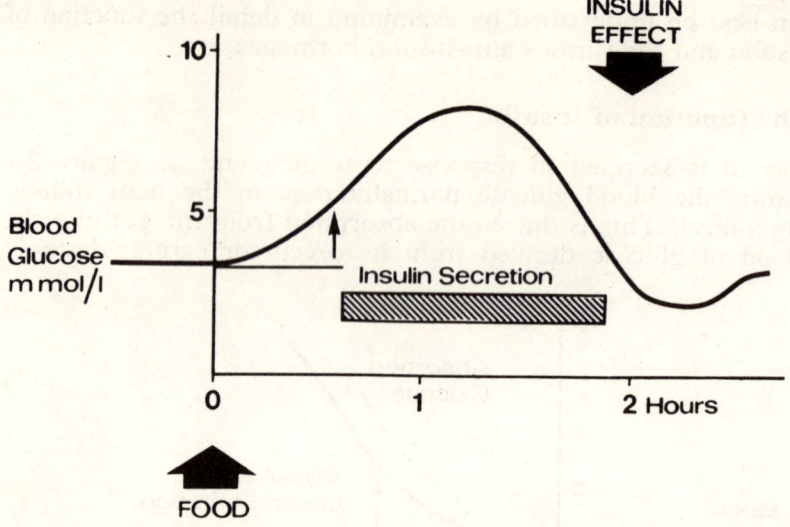

Fig. 2.2 Blood glucose curve, rising in the first hour following a meal and falling in the second hour due to insulin secretion

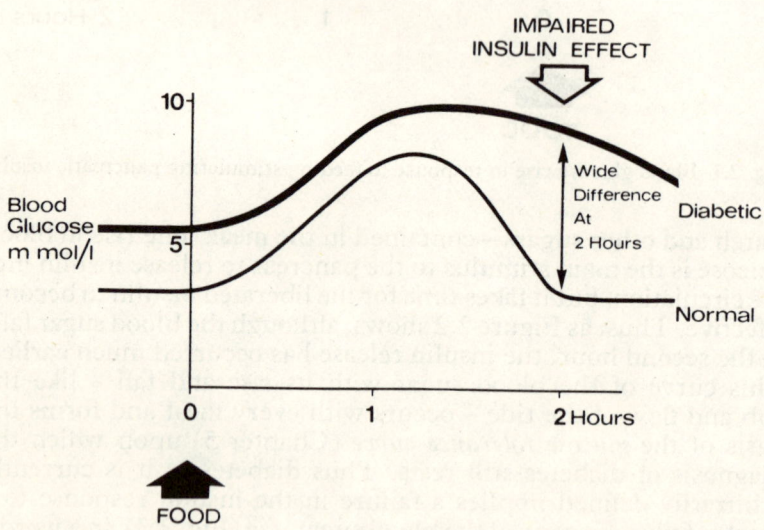

Fig. 2.3 Normal blood glucose curve compared with mild diabetes showing greatest deviation at two hours

secreted in response to feeding. Its function in terms of storage promotes the uptake of glucose into cells for energy and stimulates the key enzymes in growth-promoting pathways of metabolism. Expressed another way, insulin prevents cell breakdown. Insulin is anti-lipolytic: it prevents the breakdown of fat; it also promotes protein synthesis and is anti-proteolytic, but its storage function in relation to glucose is fundamental and is worth examining in greater detail.

We could imagine the blood in which sugar circulates as a reservoir similar to a water conservation system, with well-defined points at which it will either overflow or be so low that efficient flow to provide essential fuel to the brain will stop. At times of feeding, sugar flows into the system (Fig. 2.4). The sugar level rises and triggers insulin release. Insulin controls the outflow from the reservoir by switching the flow of sugar into muscle for energy (Fig. 2.5), or into adipose tissue (fat) where the sugar is metabolised to glycerol and acetyl-CoA, both participating in fat synthesis to make neutral fat as storage energy.

Insulin has another important action related to the function of the blood-sugar reservoir in times of fasting. In fact we've been designed to exist, if necessary, for extended periods and remain

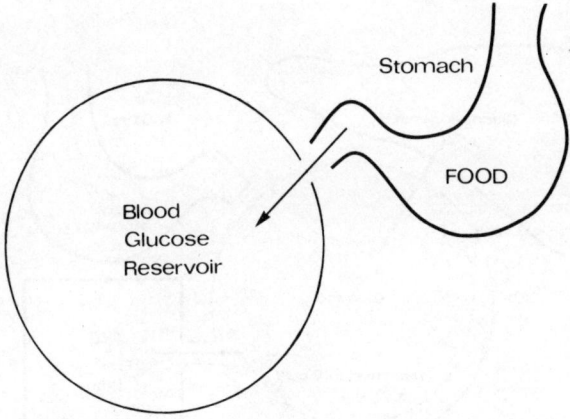

Fig. 2.4 Effect of feeding on the blood glucose reservoir

active without any food. In this respect, however, we are no match for migratory birds which travel extraordinary distances on stored energy: thus the tiny humming bird migrates 500 miles across the Gulf of Mexico without refuelling or splashdown. During fasting

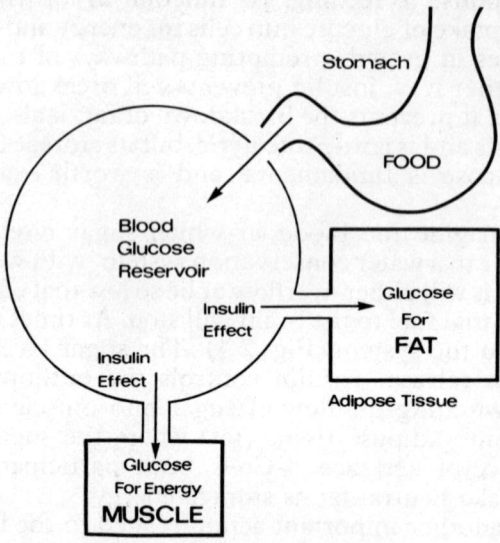

Fig. 2.5 Effect of insulin secretion on glucose uptake into muscle and fat

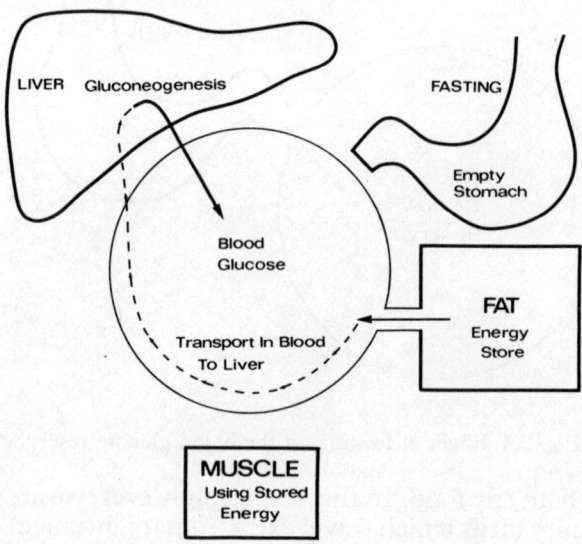

Fig. 2.6 Hepatic glucose production in fasting

the liver takes over from the stomach the function of putting sugar into the reservoir (Fig. 2.6). Two systems in the liver's sophisticated metabolic pathways are available:

emergency: glycogen breakdown – glycogenolysis, and
routine and long-term: gluconeogenesis.

In an emergency catecholamines stimulate the liver to release its stored sugar normally packaged as glycogen. However, relatively little fuel is stock-piled in this form and if you skip breakfast in the morning the liver preferentially switches to its second and main system, gluconeogenesis. You have the choice – cornflakes or gluconeogenesis for breakfast. Gluconeogenesis involves making sugar using fat as the energy source and tissue protein as the nuts and bolts of the sugar structure (see Chapter 4). Lack of food means that insulin levels will be low – in these circumstances the key enzymes of hepatic gluconeogenesis are stimulated. And whenever the fast is broken insulin will be secreted: insulin feedback to the liver will switch off gluconeogenesis (and prevent glycogenolysis) (Fig. 2.7).

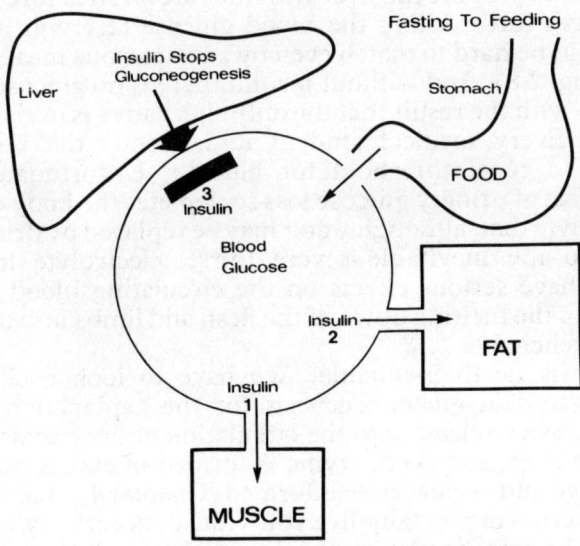

Fig. 2.7 Effect of insulin on muscle uptake **1**, fat uptake **2** and inhibition of hepatic glucose release **3**

So far we can identify three actions of insulin, all of which will lower the blood glucose:

uptake of glucose into muscle,
uptake of glucose into fat, and
switch off hepatic sugar release.

Thus gluconeogenesis is a clever adaptive process designed to allow us to skip meals or go on hunger strike without ill effects. Moreover, in normal circumstances gluconeogenesis never gets out of hand – it simply prevents the blood-glucose reservoir from falling low during fasting. If it caused a rise in blood glucose, insulin release would be triggered, the key enzymes of gluconeogenesis would then be depressed and the process would grind to a halt.

But not so in severe diabetes: when insulin is missing the gluconeogenesis feedback is foiled and the normal adaptive process of starvation roars into top gear. Mild inflation goes on to hyperinflation with disastrous consequences. Without insulin to restrain lipolysis, stored fat is rapidly melted into the circulation and carried to the liver. Likewise the tissue proteins – normally preserved with great care – are wasted down into circulating amino-acids to provide the liver with the carbon structure of sugar which surges forth, filling the blood glucose reservoir at a rate which would be hard to match even by an enormous meal of sugar goodies (Fig. 2.8). And without insulin there is no glucose uptake into tissues with the result that the only alternative is overflow into the urine. Every medical student understands the imaginary concept of a renal threshold for glucose. Unfortunately, the osmotic effect of urinary glucose loss so depletes the body of water and electrolyte that, although water may be replaced by drinking in response to the inevitable severe thirst, electrolyte loss will ultimately have serious effects on the circulating blood volume (Fig. 2.9) . . . the melting down of the flesh and limbs into urine . . . thirst unquenchable . . .

But why is death inevitable? We have to look back to the metabolic steps in gluconeogenesis for the explanation. When there is excessive release into the circulation of fatty acids, which flood to the liver, acetyl coenzyme A formed in excess cannot be fully oxidised and acetoacetate is formed (Chapter 4). Acetoacetate can be converted into betahydroxybutyrate or decarboxylated into acetone – the trio known as the *ketone bodies*. In other words gluconeogenesis and ketogenesis go hand in hand. When it's coffee and gluconeogenesis instead of cornflakes for breakfast the ketone bodies provide us with a useful source of energy. Thus ace-

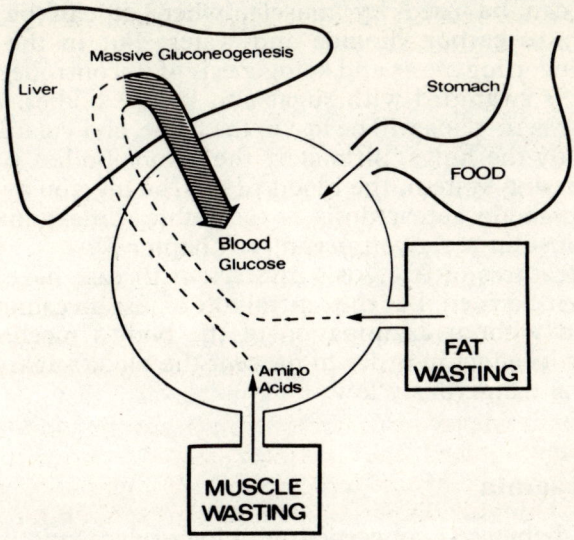

Fig. 2.8 Unrestrained gluconeogenesis of insulin lack

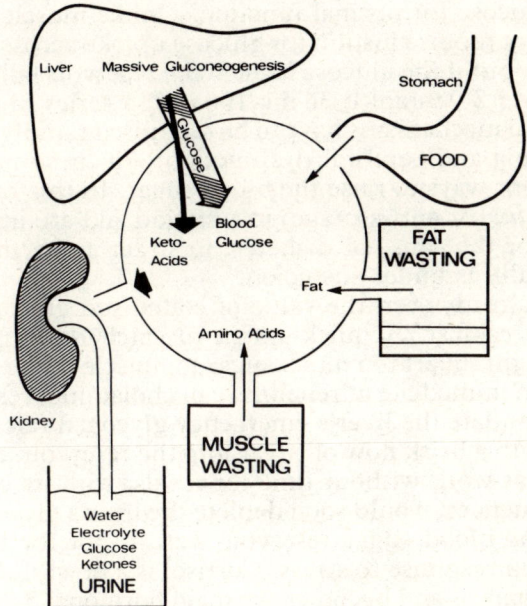

Fig. 2.9 Gluconeogenesis, ketogenesis, fluid and electrolyte loss of severe insulin lack

toacetate can be used by muscle, where it can be oxidised completely to carbon dioxide and water. But in the runaway massive gluconeogenesis and ketogenesis of uncontrolled diabetes the blood is swamped with sugar and ketone bodies. Although some of the keto-acids will be lost in the urine, and volatile acetone blown off by the lungs, ultimately the ketone bodies swamp the blood buffering system, the blood pH falls dangerously low, and death in diabetic ketoacidosis is inevitable (unless intravenous fluid and insulin are given urgently, Chapter 7).

So the features of Areteus's mysterious disease have, to some extent, been clarified. But the central role of insulin cannot be fully understood without examination of the body's mechanisms to counteract its effect in order to prevent the blood sugar reservoir from falling dangerously low.

Hypoglycaemia

Although diabetes is concerned with hyperglycaemia it must be appreciated that the reverse – hypoglycaemia – can be equally serious and possibly fatal because the brain requires a steady supply of glucose for normal function. Unlike muscle or fat, the brain does not require insulin for glucose uptake across the blood-brain barrier but if the glucose level in the reservoir falls to danger levels (around 2.0 mmol/l; 36 mg/100 ml), a series of autonomic and hormonal mechanisms have to be mobilised rapidly to prevent hypoglycaemia and cerebral dysfunction. All these mechanisms act in different ways to raise the blood sugar. In this respect they are *anti-insulin* (or anti-storage) in function and are important in the search for the cause of diabetes, in so far as anything which opposes insulin is under suspicion.

We have already seen the value of coffee and gluconeogenesis instead of breakfast. A quick sprint to catch the bus to work, however, might divert too much sugar to muscle at the expense of the brain. An immediate adrenaline (catecholamine) response will instantly stimulate the liver's emergency glycogen release (glyco-genolysis) with a brisk flow of sugar into the reservoir. A long and tedious day at work without time for meals, with its consequent stressful influences, would soon deplete the liver's glycogen stores and drain the blood sugar reservoir were it not for the plasma cortisol rise in response to stress. Cortisol is a powerful stimulant to gluconeogenesis and becomes the main hormonal drive in times of emotional stress, severe exertion or illness when the desire to eat is banished by other over-riding events. Can the brain take any direct action to prevent neuroglypenia when the blood sugar is low? How does the brain signal to muscle and fat that it is time to liberate raw materials for hepatic gluconeogenesis to provide sugar for cerebral function? Neural mechanisms are still poorly understood (although back in 1869 Paul Langerhans noticed nerve fibres close to his islets). Certainly the hypothalamus stimulates cortisol and growth hormone release in hypoglycaemia. In contrast to insulin, growth hormone is a powerful lipolytic agent stimulating the release of storage fat and fuelling gluconeogenesis. In summary, the brain can signal a catecholamine release (which switches off pancreatic insulin) and along with cortisol, growth and other hormones stimulates lipolysis and hepatic gluconeogenesis.

Whereas all these and other hormonal influences are acting in hypoglycaemia to prevent the blood sugar reservoir from falling to danger levels, they may in other circumstances be diabetogenic. Treatment with corticosteroids or with its first cousin the contraceptive pill may induce diabetes in a vulnerable individual. Acromegaly, Cushing's syndrome and a panorama of endocrine disorders involving excess hormone production may be associated with diabetes (see Chapter 19). Looked at another way, if insulin is the blood-sugar-lowering hormone, all the others tend to induce hyperglycaemia. Conversely, damage to the pituitary, as Houssay showed in the early twenties, will make pancreatic diabetes less severe, and so will pituitary surgery today. But whether these anti-insulin hormones, in the absence of endocrinopathy, are a cause of diabetes mellitus seems much less likely. Perhaps the most interesting of all these hormones, however, is glucagon, secreted so close to insulin but in the alpha rather than the beta cells of the islets and inducing hyperglycaemia rather than hypoglycaemia.

Glucagon

Shortly after the discovery of insulin it was noted that when the pancreatic extract was injected into volunteers the blood sugar first rose and then fell; the fraction causing the rise was isolated in 1924 and called glucagon. We now know that glucagon has powerful effects in stimulating hepatic glycogenolysis and gluconeogenesis with consequent hyperglycaemia. We can use this effect to advantage by injecting glucagon in emergencies to counteract severe hypoglycaemia. Used this way glucagon has many other pharmacological actions – release of pituitary hormones and catecholamines (hence its place in assessing growth hormone or as a provocative test in phaeochromocytoma). Glucagon also has powerful effects on inhibition of oesophageal and duodenal motility and depression of gastric acid and pancreatic juice output. But these are unimportant at physiological as opposed to pharmacological levels, so what is the function and purpose of glucagon?

Suppose that we eat a large steak without potatoes or other carbohydrates. After all, man was primarily designed to hunt, catching and eating fish or animals and so living on protein and fat. Only in the last thousand years of our evolution have we taken to agriculture – growing carbohydrate – as a major fuel source. When our main calories come from a steak, some of the protein-derived aminoacids will stimulate the pancreas to release insulin in response to feeding, and a simultaneous release of glucagon will divert some of the protein of the steak into gluconeogenesis. Thus a non-carbohydrate meal can, in the presence of insulin and glucagon, provide some glucose for immediate energy. So our bacon and eggs, smoked salmon or large steak – whatever way we prefer our protein and fat – are carefully garnished with insulin and glucagon to maintain the right balance of glucose homeostasis. Glucagon provided for man the hunter has become the hormone of *haute-cuisine*. The humble serf, eating bread and dripping, gets his blood sugar rise and insulin response by simple absorption of carbohydrate (lack of protein does not cause the same glucagon response). *Haute-cuisine* glucagon does it by gluconeogenesis in consort with the insulin response to protein-derived amino-acids.

Glucagon can, therefore, be seen as a hormone closely associated with insulin in maintaining a normal ebb and flow of the blood-sugar tide in response to feeding – a hormone concerned with the fine tuning of blood glucose homeostasis especially in relation to protein feeding. But is glucagon diabetogenic (a question that rich eaters and vegetarians might well ask from their different standpoints)? Yes, in the same manner as cortisol or growth hormone may be in abnormal circumstances. The extremely rare glucagonoma syndrome (Chapter 19) is, like Cushing's syndrome and acromegaly, associated with diabetes. But remember Oskar Minkowski's laboratory dog. Pancreatectomy, despite removing the source of glucagon besides that of insulin, always leads to hyperglycaemia. Thus lack of insulin is more fundamental.

Insulin glucose homeostasis

We now appreciate that an acute lack of insulin will lead to accelerated lipolysis and proteolysis – the melting down of the flesh and limbs to fan the flames of gluconeogenesis. But most diabetics have a mild disorder never needing insulin injections; this implies that they must have some insulin – at least enough to maintain cell growth, preserve protein, restrain lipolysis and prevent gluconeogenesis from getting out of hand. Which is more important, cell growth or control of the blood sugar? It is well recognised that hyperglycaemia as such causes no adverse symptoms (indeed most of us feel at our best after a meal when the blood sugar is at its high rather than low). Diabetics with high blood-sugar levels feel well unless they have glycosuria, and only when they have reached that point do they have thirst, weakness and lassitude. Thus the higher-than-normal blood sugar of mild diabetes may be the body's method of stimulating the failing beta cell to produce enough insulin to maintain cell growth (and to prevent gluconeogenesis from getting out of hand; Fig. 2.10). Lipolysis and protein-wasting only occur when the beta cell is so damaged or depleted that basal insulin levels can no longer be maintained. In examining beta cell failure in the mild diabetic, however, account must be taken of another aspect of clinical significance in the majority of late-onset diabetics: obesity.

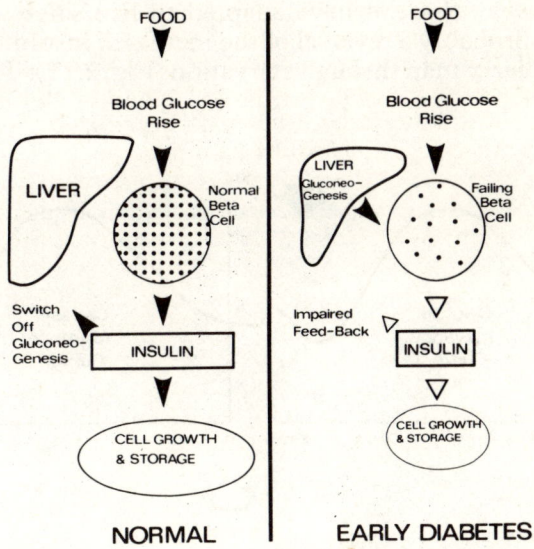

Fig. 2.10 Gluconeogenesis stimulating the failing beta cell to produce sufficient insulin for cell growth

Obesity and insulin glucose homeostasis

Is obesity a normal adaptive process, a cause or consequence of abnormal insulin-glucose homeostasis or just the result of gluttony? Mention has been made earlier of the value of fat in nutrient storage especially in the case of migratory birds. But even the migrating bird, fuelled-up for its long distance flight has to give some thought to its take-off payload. Yet obese homosapiens, with fuel tanks overflowing, rarely contemplates more than a walk to the street corner shop or driving up to the door of his favourite restaurant. Is this disease or adaptation? At least it seems that insulin-glucose homeostasis adapts to over-nutrition. In such circumstances, where feeding is pushing the glucose tolerance curve upwards, insulin counter-secretion matches the challenge so that the curve remains essentially normal (Fig. 2.11); the two sides in the tug-of-war are evenly matched. Suppose then that the over-feeding gives way to some diet reducing ritual. Do the super-charged beta cells drive the reformed glutton into hypoglycaemia as one team in the tug-of-war gives way? It seems that this is prevented by a clever adaptation to over-nutrition in which muscle and liver but not adipose tissue become resistant to insulin (Fig. 2.12). This way that we have adapted to live safely with over-nutrition is probably a reversal of the increased insulin-sensitivity designed to carry man through starvation (Fig. 2.11). The alterna-

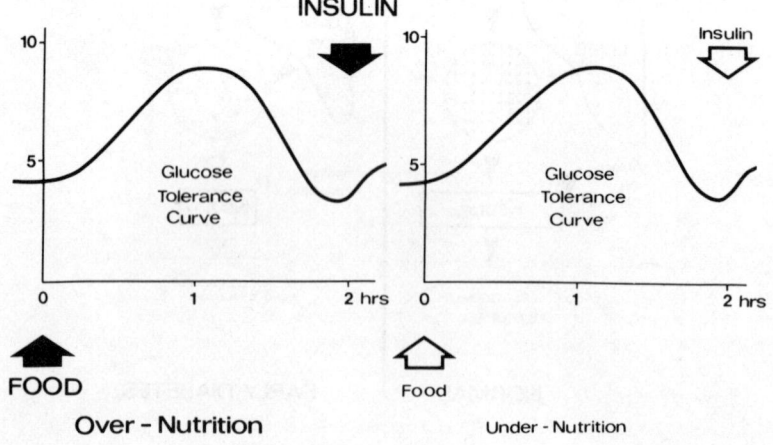

Fig. 2.11 Similar blood glucose curves in over-nutrition and under-nutrition with insulin responses appropriate to each

tive argument, so often used by the obese, of 'putting on weight easily' implies an inherited or acquired increased sensitivity to insulin in their fat depôts, that obesity arises because they are economy models with built-in fuel saving. But even if the obese have inherited or acquired fuel tanks more suited to a jumbo-jet than to a light aircraft surely it still requires gluttony or some form of inappropriate overeating to fill the tanks? Insulin is secreted in *response* to feeding. Does insulin convert dietary sugar into some form of drug of addiction, stimulating the glutton to come back for more and more? And the more that is eaten, the more the pancreas is stimulated, until in some the beta cells can no longer stand the pace and begin to fail? Is diabetes in the obese some form of just retribution for not stopping to read the fuel gauges? We still have much to learn about control of insulin-glucose homeostasis in relation to nutrition quite apart from learning to control it in diabetes.

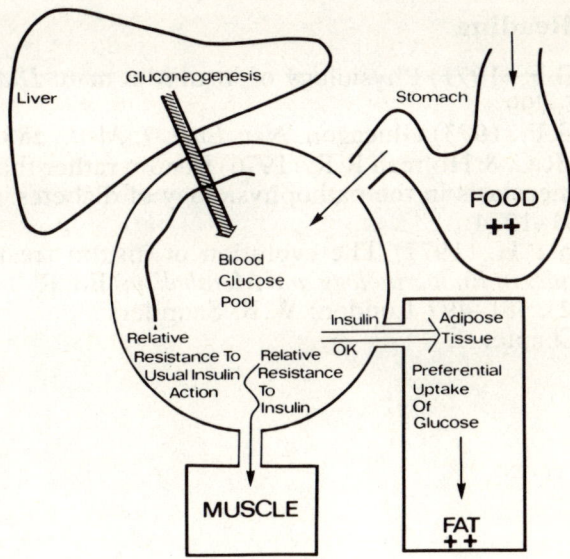

Fig. 2.12 Relative resistance to insulin's action on muscle and liver, but not adipose tissue, in obesity

The question posed at the beginning of this section on obesity remains unanswered, but we could contemplate the possibility that, in relation to insulin-glucose homeostasis, diabetes may develop in those who acquire diminished insulin sensitivity whether induced by over-nutrition or by some other factor.

In this discussion of Areteus's mysterious disease we have identified several possible diabetogenic factors, listed in Table 2.1. Perhaps before searching more closely for the fundamental cause of beta cell failure (genetic, over-nutrition, immunological, viral, hormonal or whatever) we could, with advantage, remind ourselves that diabetes is not one disease. Rather, as emphasised in Chapter 3, it is a multitude of disorders with hyperglycaemia as the common denominator.

Table 2.1   Some causes of diabetes

Lack of insulin	beta cell failure -
Excess anti-insulin hormones	catecholamines, glucagon, cortisol, growth hormone
Over-nutrition	insulin resistance

Further Reading

1 Cahill G.F. (1971) Physiology of insulin in man. *Diabetes*, **20**, 785–799
2 Cahill G.F. (1973) Glucagon. *New Engl. J. Med.*, **288**, 157–158
3 Turner R.C. & Holman R.R. (1976) Insulin rather than glucose homeostasis in the pathophysiology of diabetes. *Lancet*, **i**, 1271–1274
4 Sönksen P.H. (1977) The evolution of insulin treatment. In *Clinics in Endocrinology and Metabolism* (Ed. R. Tattersall.) **6** (2), 481–497 London: W.B. Saunders
See also Chapter 4.

CHAPTER 3

The Village Football Team

An introduction to the varied clinical patterns in diabetes mellitus

Diabetes is not a single disease. In the past the disorder has been classified into two groups which have become so entrenched in the literature and medical folklore that perhaps they are with us to stay: juvenile-onset diabetics who are insulin-dependent and ketoacidosis-prone on the one hand, and late- or maturity-onset diabetics who may often be overweight, have a milder disorder controlled by altered diet with or without hypoglycaemic tablets, on the other. Juvenile-onset diabetes (JOD) is sometimes known also as Type 1 diabetes while maturity-onset diabetes (MOD) is described as Type 2. But an increasing number of patients under 40 years of age present with a mild disorder while even more in the geriatric age group are thin, undernourished and may need insulin. At least the alternative separation into insulin-dependent or non-insulin-dependent has clinical usefulness provided it is appreciated that these should not be instant judgements nor permanent distinctions. Some patients, classed as insulin-dependent after a decade of insulin treatment, may have a further 25 years of peaceful old age without daily injections, while others thought to be mild diabetics may become insulin-dependent as a consequence of some additional stressful illness.

It is prudent to keep an open mind and appreciate that the varied clinical presentation in diabetes is such that any group of newly-diagnosed patients attending a hospital clinic would appear to be a motley assembly by comparison with a village football team. Like the village team aspiring to play football according to a set of rules so the group of patients would be diabetic according to its rules – they would all be hyperglycaemic, but there the similarity would end. To emphasise the diversity of clinical presentation, we could examine the football team; eleven different individuals with diabetes mellitus as their team colours.*

* This team of mixed sexes, varied ages and infirmities would hardly qualify to play football. The reader will appreciate that the aim is to make a point, not to score goals.

29

1 Juvenile-onset diabetes

Peter is eleven. He was always healthy until, just before his Easter vacation, he became tired, listless and was constantly running to the water tap. He still ate well, but was becoming thin and gaunt. His legs ached. The family doctor diagnosed diabetes and on finding both sugar and ketones in the urine, made an urgent appointment at the hospital clinic, where two hours after breakfast the blood glucose was elevated (20 mmol/l; 360 mg/100 ml) to three times the normal value. There was no family history of diabetes and the parents were extremely anxious until the aims of diabetic care were explained (Chapter 8). Peter was admitted to hospital for education in the principles of self-regulation with insulin (Chapter 10), was back home within a week and in the summer term at school was swimming and playing cricket better than ever. The natural history of his diabetes and its prognosis are outlined in Chapter 21.

2 Maturity-onset diabetes of youth (MODY)

Susan is 17. Glycosuria was found when she had a medical examination for entry to nursing school. Her mother and two elder sisters were diabetic but none had required insulin. Susan thought that some of her mother's relatives living in Canada were also diabetic. The two-hours-post-breakfast blood glucose was just elevated (8·0 mmol/l; 144 mg/100 ml) and a glucose tolerance test a few days later showed a frankly diabetic curve (Chapter 5, p.70). On the basis of the family history and mildness of the disorder it was thought that she had the relatively rare syndrome of mild 'maturity-onset diabetes of youth' (MODY) inherited as a dominant characteristic (see genetics, Chapter 4). It was important to her nursing career to know that Susan could be controlled by diet with the possible intermittent use of an oral hypoglycaemic agent (Chapter 11) and that serious complications (Chapter 13) were unlikely.

3 Gestational diabetes

Sally is 21. During her recent pregnancy she was found to have glycosuria and a diabetic glucose tolerance curve. She had required insulin during the last trimester of her pregnancy (Chapter 12) but after delivery the glucose tolerance test curve became normal; thus, by being diabetic only during her pregnancy Sally was a gestational diabetic. She now wants the contraceptive pill but because of her gestational diabetes her doctor has referred her to the diabetic clinic. Sally and her husband have to consider the possibility that the contraceptive pill may have an effect on her glucose tolerance similar to that of the recent pregnancy. The possibility of insulin injections would seem a high price to pay for the simplicity of the pill (Chapter 20, p.239). But the parents are reassured about the remote chances of their bouncing babe becoming diabetic (Chapter 4, p.41) and that with the recent good care in pregnancy (Chapter 12) they need not have any fears about more children.

4 The insulin-dependent professional

James is 25, and a professional footballer in a first-class team. In mid-season he developed typical diabetic symptoms (the melting down of flesh and limbs ruined his goal scoring). His doctor diagnosed diabetes on the basis of a family history of the disorder in older relatives, glycosuria, ketonuria and a two-hours-post-breakfast blood glucose (15 mmol/l; 270 mg/100 ml) elevated to twice the normal level. Valuable time was wasted while he waited for an unnecessary glucose tolerance test and to make matters worse the team doctor (an expert on minor injuries) advised that his football career was over. But James sought the advice of a wily old doctor who really knew his onions and who taught him all he needed to know about insulin, diet and frequent travel abroad in relation to insulin self-regulation (Chapters 10 & 22). James was soon back in the game and able to confirm the muscle-protein building effect of insulin. His goal scoring became more devastating than ever. And whenever he saw more than two goalposts he knew that he was verging on hypoglycaemia. With experience he found that the insulin requirements on the day of a first-class match were less than a quarter of his daily average of 100 units, confirming the effect of exercise on insulin requirements (Chapter 10, p.128). So why was he at the hospital clinic? Perhaps he'd come to teach the rest of the team about football – he certainly taught the doctors a thing or two.

5 The average 40-year-old

Mrs. Peabody is 44. Four years previously diabetes was diagnosed on the basis of typical symptoms of thirst. At that time she was slightly overweight and responded well to diet (Chapter 9) supplemented with oral hypoglycaemic agents (Chapter 11). Because she lived a considerable distance from hospital her own doctor supervised diabetic care (Chapter 8) after an initial hospital visit, but now referred her back to hospital because of recurrence of glycosuria and weight-loss despite maximal doses of oral hypoglycaemic therapy. In the clinic the two-hours-post-breakfast blood sugar was 20 mmol/l (360 mg/100 ml), there was ketonuria but the plasma ketones were normal. Insulin therapy was advised and, like Peter, Mrs. Peabody soon became an expert; thereafter she averred she'd never felt better and that she wished she'd had insulin sooner. But exogenous insulin and Mrs. Peabody's appetite consorted to encourage excess nutrient storage (Chapter 6), and at this stage her diabetes defied clear-cut definition into JOD (Type 1) or MOD (Type 2). However, there was a strong family history of thyroid disease and she was found to have organ-specific thyroid microsomal and gastric parietal cell antibodies. Moreover, she had pancreatic islet cell antibodies (ICA, Chapter 4, p.44) both in the serum obtained four years previously and at this visit. Thus she had the polyendocrine diabetes more commonly seen in females (Chapter 4, p.45).

6 Middle-aged obese diabetic

Mrs. Sweet-tooth is 50 and has become increasingly thirsty in recent months but the distress of polyuria and pruritus vulvae (Chapter 5) drive her to the doctor who finds 2% glycosuria without ketonuria. At the hospital clinic she weighs 220 lb (100 kg) as opposed to a correct weight for her age and height of 132 lb (60 kg): gross obesity by any standard. The two-hours-post-prandial blood glucose is 20 mmol/l (360 mg/100 ml) – as elevated as those previous patients requiring insulin. Mrs. Sweet-tooth must have hyper-secreted insulin over the years as she fuelled-up her fat stores to the present 220 lb payload. Yet she tells the dietician that she hardly eats a thing (now). It is estimated that the sugar in her increasing number of cups of tea and bottles of lemonade with which she assuages her constant thirst amount to 200 g (800 kcal) of concentrated carbohydrate per day. She is advised to stop the sugar in tea and lemonade; no other change is made in her management, and she is kept under regular out-patient supervision. Mrs. Sweet-tooth is co-operative, her symptoms subside rapidly and after two months the two-hours-post-breakfast blood glucose has fallen to 11·0 mmol/l (198 mg/100 ml); not ideal, but the trend is in the right direction. Unfortunately, a holiday leads to dietary relaxation and ultimately oral hypo-glycaemic agents (Chapter 11) are added.

7 Middle-aged non-obese diabetic

Jack Spratt is 55 and not overweight. Three months previously he was admitted to hospital with a myocardial infarct. Glycosuria was noted during an otherwise uneventful convalescence and a glucose tolerance test was frankly diabetic. The cardiologist thought that Jack Spratt should eat no fat (Chapters 6 and 13) for his heart's sake but wasn't quite sure how to square this with a diabetic low carbohydrate diet. Moreover, he was reluctant to prescribe oral hypoglycaemic agents because of the much publicised report (See UGDP study, Chapters 11, p.141, & 13, p. 169) of a controlled trial which was interpreted as indicating a preponderance of cardiac deaths in those taking oral hypoglycaemic agents.

At the clinic the two-hours-post-breakfast blood glucose was abnormally high (13·0 mmol/l; 234 mg/100 ml). The dietician ascertained that Jack Spratt had never eaten much fat and his carbohydrate intake was well balanced (Chapter 9). He was advised to eat as before but avoid becoming overweight, to give up the 25 cigarettes per day, and oral hypoglycaemic agents were prescribed; all was well, although his wife was quite a different problem.

8 Diabetes and hypertriglyceridaemia

Mrs. Spratt is also 55. She has always been fond of her food, especially sweet things, cream and lots of butter. When her husband became ill she worried and ate more than ever. As she became increasingly thirsty she drank more and more milk. She used her husband's urine testing set, found glycosuria and saw her doctor who referred her to hospital where she was found to exceed her correct weight by 110 lb (50 kg). The two-hours-post-breakfast blood glucose was 20 mmol/l (360 mg/100 ml), and it was noted that the serum was milky. She was admitted to the ward and the following day the students were shown the original serum sample which had been stored carefully in a cool spot overnight. They saw diffuse lactescence with a floating creamy layer suggest-ive of exogenous and endogenous hypertriglyceridaemia (Chapter

6), which was confirmed in the subsequent biochemical report. The serum sodium was only 125 mmol/l (see factitious hyponatraemia, Chapter 7, p.89, associated with hyperlipidaemia). The dietary history suggested that the chylomicrons and much of the hypertriglyceridaemia was exogenous although her high carbohydrate intake would stimulate endogenous hypertriglyceridaemia (Chapter 6). She denied taking alcohol (a common stimulus to endogenous triglyceride synthesis, Chapter 6) and although obese and diabetic she was not Cushinoid. Initially, she required insulin to overcome the resistance to insulin action caused by the lipids (Chapter 6). Within three days there was a significant biochemical improvement, insulin therapy was stopped and thereafter her management was in the hands of the dietician (Chapter 9). Ten days after admission the two-hours-post-breakfast blood glucose was 10 mmol/l (180 mg/100 ml), but her discharge from hospital was delayed by a deep venous thrombosis (a common complication of metabolic decompensation in the older patient, Chapter 7, p.101). Thereafter she was never significantly hyperglycaemic but there remained the ever present problem of a natural inclination to keep the plate clean. Mr. Spratt could never understand why he had had a myocardial infarct and his wife, with her high fat intake and obesity, had not. His doctor tried to explain that risk factors were obtained from broad epidemiological data based upon thousands of cases, but Jack Spratt was not impressed.

9 Diabetic angiopathy

Mr. Puff is a 55-year-old railway engine driver who failed a recent sight test. The ophthalmologist found the classical features of diabetic retinopathy (Chapter 15) and referred him to the diabetic clinic. The patient admitted to recent vague ill-health but denied typical diabetic symptoms, although he had noticed white spots on his trousers (Chapter 5) some time previously. The urine contained 0·25% sugar without ketones and considerable albumin. The blood pressure was 180/90 mmHg. There was slight ankle oedema, features of peripheral neuropathy (Chapter 16) and early trophic ulceration of the toes and heels (Chapter 17). The two-hours-post-breakfast blood glucose was slightly elevated (10 mmol/l; 180 mg/100 ml) and the blood urea was also elevated (10 mmol/l; 60 mg/100 ml). The diagnosis of mild diabetes with advanced complications was made. He was admitted to hospital for fuller investigation where renal biopsy confirmed that he had well-established diabetic nephropathy (Chapter 14). With simple dietary restriction of sugar the glycosuria disappeared and he was given an extra egg-white each day to compensate for the albuminuria, but it was the end of the line for Mr. Puff, who gradually succumbed to renal failure (Chapter 14).

10 Diabetes secondary to haemochromatosis

Mr. Ironside is 55 and, despite a recent holiday in the sun, consults his doctor on account of lassitude, upper abdominal discomfort and loss of weight. The doctor notes hepatomegaly without jaundice but on checking the urine for urobilinogen finds glycosuria and refers him to hospital, where he is noted to be underweight and have a two-hours-post-breakfast blood glucose of 16 mmol/l (288 mg/100 ml). The clinician also notes the firm hepatomegaly, and points out to his student apprentice that cirrhosis commonly leads to diabetes (Chapter 19) and that in recently diagnosed or poorly controlled diabetes soft rather than firm hepatomegaly occurs but regresses with improved diabetic control. Admission to hospital for investigation is advised. A liver biopsy shows typical features of haemochromatosis (Chapter 19) and on the subsequent ward round everybody discusses the 'bronzed' pigmentation of haemochromatosis now so easily seen in the light of the correct diagnosis as the holiday tan fades. Mr. Ironside starts on treatment by regular venesection for the iron overload and initially requires insulin therapy. The senior physician in the medical team invites Mr. Ironside to participate in the clinical examinations but we are not told how many candidates are failed for not observing the pigmentation.

11 Diabetes of old age

Mrs. Spritely is a 77-year-old widow now enduring her closing years in an old folks' home. She has been treated for many years for pernicious anaemia and more recently with a thiazide diuretic and potassium supplements for incipient cardiac failure (Chapter 20). The lower-limb circulation has recently been poor and when the matron called the doctor on account of an ischaemic toe he found 0.5% glycosuria and was surprised when the local laboratory 'phoned the two-hours-post-breakfast blood glucose result of 26.0 mmol/l (468 mg/100 ml). Yet the patient was not unduly thirsty. The doctor telephoned the hospital clinician for advice. Should she be admitted as an emergency? It was pointed out that the blood glucose rises with age and significantly in old age (Chapter 5) and that similarly the renal threshold to glucose rises, hence the minimal glycosuria and muted symptoms despite the hyperglycaemia. What about her weight? She's thin and just picks at her food. The suggestion is made that the aim should be simply to reduce the concentrated carbohydrate in the diet sufficiently to avoid symptoms of diabetes (polyuria so often leads to troublesome incontinence in the aged) and to deal sensibly with the other medical problems (Chapter 17). What about insulin? Often those in extreme old age are unresponsive to oral therapy but a short-acting sulphonylurea is recommended in the first instance. The call is interrupted. Two weeks' later the doctor 'phones again: the blood glucose is 15 mmol/l (270 mg/100 ml), Mrs. Spritely is eating well and the toe has improved; nevertheless Matron is edgy about having a diabetic on her hands. Regular urine testing is recommended, the dose of sulphonylurea reduced, only to be increased if there is glycosuria and a blood glucose in excess of 15 mmol/l (270 mg/100 ml) two hours after breakfast. Yes, certainly Mrs. Spritely can have some of her grand-daughter's wedding cake.

Is it possible, or sensible, to attempt to classify all diabetics? Already some reasonably definitive terms have been used:

> juvenile-onset insulin-dependent diabetes (JOD, Type 1);
> maturity onset diabetes of youth (MODY);
> gestational diabetes;
> polyendocrine diabetes;
> maturity onset (MOD, Type 2); and
> diabetes secondary to haemochromatosis (secondary diabetes).

But some patients are less easy to classify. Does Mr. Spratt have simple diabetes and vascular disease – two independent yet common disorders in the one individual – or does he have diabetes secondary to vascular disease (or perhaps *vice versa*)? And what of Mrs. Spratt, does she have a primary lipid disorder with her super-fatted circulation causing insulin resistance, or does she have a basic defect in her islet cells, or is it that she is just suffering from over-nutrition? Note also that early cases in the team were all problems of diabetes in varying severity. But in the remainder, other medical conditions or diabetic complications began to take the centre of the stage and the metabolic defect of diabetes was relegated to a virtually silent part. Perhaps the real danger in attempting to classify and pigeon-hole types of diabetics is that by attaching a label, the mind tends no longer to remain open to alternative possibilities. Diagnostic classification is a popular hobby amongst doctors, but unfortunately it has the effect of closing the medical mind to original thought. Better perhaps that we appreciate that diabetics are a motley assembly, an ever variable panorama of abnormal glucose tolerance. Nevertheless, there are many other terms, classifications and types of diabetes commonly found in the medical literature so, with the experience and insights of the football team behind us, a brief glance at the opposing 11 may be of value.

1 Pre-diabetes   This player should be dropped from the team forthwith. The term pre-diabetes was popular in the 1960s when it was believed that some people with normal glucose tolerance could, if they were primed with corticosteroids or other pressures, be squeezed into the diabetic category. It is now better appreciated that this approach has made little contribution to the understanding of insulin-glucose homeostasis.

2 Potential diabetes   This one is worth watching – a person at special risk of becoming diabetic because of a strong family or obstetric history characteristic of diabetes (Chapter 5, p.70). Prevention of diabetes is a difficult but worthy aim, advice against over-nutrition is probably the most successful approach.

3 Sub-clinical diabetes   A person with abnormal glucose tolerance but without symptoms of diabetes or complications; also known as chemical diabetes.

4 Latent diabetes   A person with normal glucose tolerance but whose glucose tolerance has in the past been abnormal.

With these groups there is a risk of misunderstanding, or the accusation of splitting hairs. After all, any latent diabetic could be looked upon as a potential diabetic. On the other hand there are many other interesting and distinctive disorders associated with diabetes mellitus which are worthy of mention.

5 Genetic syndromes   There are several rare syndromes in which diabetes is inherited in association with defects in the neuromuscular system: Friedreich's ataxia, Huntington's chorea, muscular dystrophy and dystrophia myotonica. Perhaps the most interesting is the combination of diabetes insipidus, diabetes mellitus, optic atrophy and deafness (D I D M O A D) with an onset in childhood (Chapter 4, p.43).

6 Diabetes with other metabolic disorders   Various metabolic disorders – glycogen storage disease, acute intermittent porphyria, glucose-6-phosphate dehydrogenase deficiency, galactosaemia and others (Chapter 19) may be associated with diabetes.

7 Diabetes secondary to endocrine disease   Cushing's syndrome, acromegaly, thyrotoxicosis, hyperaldosteronism, phaeochromocytoma and glucagonoma may all be found to have glucose intolerance as a feature (Chapter 19).

8 Diabetes secondary to pancreatic disease   Acute pancreatitis, chronic pancreatitis – especially those with calcification (remember Thomas Cawley's poor patient, Chapter 2) – and pancreatic carcinoma involving the body or tail have a high incidence of diabetes mellitus. Pancreatic disease is notoriously difficult to diagnose – the more easily detected diabetes is often the early clue to the underlying condition (Chapter 19, p.228).

9 Liver disease   The frequency of diabetes is increased in all forms of hepatic cirrhosis. The carbohydrate intolerance is usually due to the altered hepatic handling of glucose and lipid as well as altered potassium distribution (Chapter 19, p.229).

10 Drug-induced diabetes   Many drugs may either induce diabetes, or cause deterioration in carbohydrate tolerance in established diabetics (Chapter 20).

11 Lipoatrophic diabetes   A rare syndrome of insulin-dependent, and often relatively insulin-resistant, diabetes associated with generalised, patchy or complete lipoatrophy in which the unfortunate patient often has chronic, severe and distressing thirst and polyuria and usually succumbs to cirrhosis and liver failure (Chapter 19, p.229).

Having seen the above 11 groups, and the 11 members of the village football team, it can be better appreciated that diabetes mellitus masquerades in many guises. Some readers may be daunted by the complexity of the variables and especially by the rare disorders mentioned latterly. However, the clinician should at least be alerted to these other possibilities before too quickly classifying cases into Types 1 or 2.

Referee's comment

If the aim was to field a team of different types of diabetics, why include two insulin-dependent cases in the same team? A good question which can be better appreciated after reading the aetiology, genetics and immunology of diabetes in Chapter 4. However, on testing their HLA status, Peter was found to have typical HLA antigens while James did not. Nor did James have polyendocrine diabetes with either islet cell antibodies (ICA) or other markers of auto-immune disease. On the other hand James did have a strong family history of maturity-onset diabetes. It takes all types.

CHAPTER 4

Aetiology and Basic Aspects of Diabetes

Genetics and HLA chromosomal region; islet cell antibodies, viral infections. Insulin and other hormones. Gluconeogenesis, ketogenesis, lactic acidosis, the Cori cycle and the glucose-alanine cycle

Those who expect to be informed with certainty about the cause of diabetes mellitus will be disappointed. Not for lack of ideas, but because experts in genetics, immunology, hormonal imbalance, pancreatic peptides and a host of other topics all jostle for our attention. Thus, acceptance of a straightforward unifying concept of diabetes would be naive even though some theorists attempt to persuade us that their particular ideas explain all. The visit to the village football pitch (Chapter 3) was a reminder that diabetes is not a single entity, but instead can be seen as a panorama of disorders in which hyperglycaemia is the common denominator. Squeeze a diabetic and you will find absolute or relative deficiency of insulin. Even though many obese diabetics have high insulin levels, they have insufficient insulin to keep up with their standard of living. All diabetics are to a greater or lesser extent short of insulin, and consequently suspicion falls heavily upon the pancreatic beta cell and its ability to deliver insulin. But how much is beta cell failure *inborn* and how much is it *acquired*?

In searching out those acquired insults which assail the beta cell, whether virus infections, inappropriately large dietary intake or other environmental factors, we have to consider why these affronts should cause pancreatic failure in the few. Why do the ninety and nine without diabetes withstand these insults? It is difficult to side-step an underlying inborn *susceptibility* even in those patients where an acquired insult, which catalyses the defect towards florid diabetes, has been identified. But beware! The researcher in epidemiology, genetics, immunology or pancreatic function (and the clinician) should always be careful to winnow out those patients having diabetes secondary to other diseases – for example, acromegaly, pancreatic neoplasia or hepatic cirrhosis (Chapter 19, p.228) – or due to certain drugs (Chapter 20, p.239). Thus, in examining the arguments about the cause of diabetes,

40

three aspects should be kept in mind: what is inborn, what is acquired and what is secondary to other disease or drugs.

Genetics

The fact that diabetes clusters in some families has allowed successive generations of geneticists to postulate an ever changing panorama of theories about the inheritance of the disorder. Mendelian dominant, Mendelian recessive, variable penetrance and multifactorial inheritance have each had their brief place in the sun. However, we are now able to examine the inheritance of diabetes(or lack of it) with a new clarity, aided by the knowledge that diabetes has a variable clinical presentation and thus is unlikely to be genetically homogeneous. Moreover, the concept of possible inheritance of susceptibility to the disorder rather than of florid diabetes goes a long way to explain the inadequacy of earlier theories. Three recent approaches have been fundamental:

twin studies;
national registration of the incidence of juvenile diabetes in
    relation to age and season of onset; and
histocompatibility (human leucocyte antigen, H L A) antigens.

1   Studies of identical (monozygotic) twins[1] have shown that those who were over 45 years of age at diagnosis of diabetes were 100% concordant (both twins affected). Concordance in juvenile-onset twins, on the other hand, was low. These findings support the view that late-onset diabetes is inherited but that non-genetic factors are likely to be more important in juvenile-onset diabetes.
2   The Register of Newly-diagnosed Diabetic Children under the age of 16 years (sponsored by the British Diabetic Association)[2] showed that in 79% there was no family history of diabetes. A minimum annual incidence of around 8 per 100 000 children under 16 years was found with a bimodal age distribution having a main peak around 11 years and a smaller one at 5 years. In children of school age there was a marked seasonal variation with three times as many cases identified in the winter months (especially December to March) while the lowest incidence occurred in June and July. The clustering of notification in siblings developing diabetes almost simultaneously, together with the seasonal variation, suggests the importance of the environmental stress of winter ailments (see viral infections, page 45). The age peak at 11 years also points to the importance of the hormonal changes of puberty. These findings, where almost 80% had no family history, with a

marked seasonal variation and peak incidence at puberty, further support the view that non-genetic factors are important at the *onset* of diabetes in early life.

3   The major histocompatibility antigens (HLA) and diabetes. There is now good evidence[3] that susceptibility to juvenile-onset insulin-dependent diabetes is mainly determined by a gene (or genes) in the HLA region of chromosome 6. The HLA system is composed of three serologically defined loci (HLA A, B and C) and one lymphocytically defined locus (HLA D and HLA D related or HLADR) lying close to the HLAB locus (Fig. 4.1). The A, B and C loci control serologically detectable cell-surface glycoproteins while the D locus controls cell surface antigens detectable in mixed lymphocytic reactions. Twenty variants of the A and B alleles have been recognised.

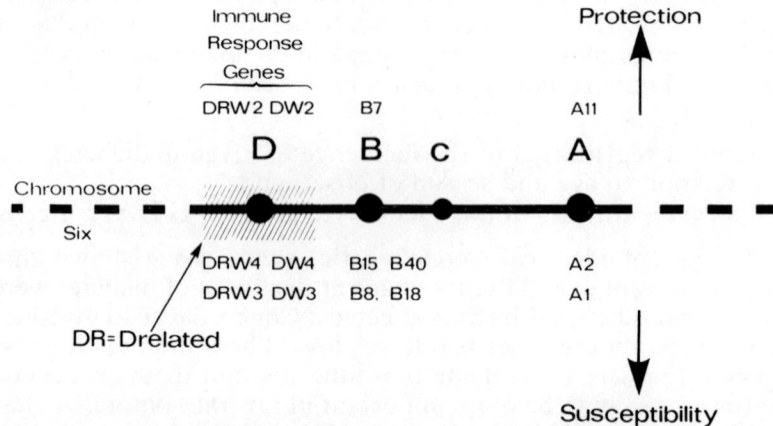

Fig. 4.1   The HLA region of chromosome six, showing the A, B, D and D-related (DR) loci. Note the proximity of the B locus to D and DR (the region of the immune response genes). Antigen types conferring susceptibility to or protection against juvenile-onset diabetes are enumerated below and above the HLA region.

All this is a spin-off from the rapid advances made in tissue typing relevant to organ transplantation. Patients having particular HLA-linked genes are, so to speak, genetically pre-charged to react with an environment cell membrane antigen such as those of viral infections or other insults. Most investigations of the relationship between the HLA system and disease have so far centred upon the three serologically defined antigens. Associations found have only involved alleles of the B locus; however, these are probably secondary to corresponding HLA D or HLA DRW associations (Fig. 4.1).

HLA typing of blood samples from diabetics and controls has shown that those with histocompatibility antigens of the type B8, B15, B18, D W3, D W4, D R W3 or D R W4 had an increased relative risk of developing juvenile-onset insulin-dependent diabetes. In those having two of these antigens the risk appears to be additive, while in those having the B7, D W2 or D R W2 antigens the risk is diminished. In other words, 'susceptibility' and 'protective' genes interact to determine the immune responsiveness to environmental agents (perhaps viral) which have a potential affinity for islet cells. There is no evidence of an association between the HLA system and maturity-onset non-insulin-dependent diabetes. Thus, the studies of the HLA system have given us scientific proof for the existence of genetic heterogeneity in diabetes mellitus.

These findings support the view that a gene in linkage disequilibrium with different HLA-B series alleles, reflecting even greater linkage disequilibrium to the HLA D and DRW associations might predispose to juvenile-onset diabetes. This could be the genetic key to susceptibility to this form of diabetes. Perhaps several diabetogenic genes on chromosome 6 are in linkage disequilibrium with different HLA alleles, each waiting to interact with its own particular environmental agent.

Confirmation of the significance of the HLA-linked gene comes from family studies showing that siblings having juvenile-onset diabetes are, with rare exceptions, identical for one, and sometimes both, antigens[4]. However, such studies have also shown that there may also be unaffected siblings having the same HLA genotypes as their diabetic sibling. Perhaps other genes outside the HLA chromosomal region are also required to contribute to susceptibility.

Besides these aspects of inheritance, there are some rare syndromes in which diabetes is genetic in origin. DIDMOAD (diabetes insipidus, diabetes mellitus, optic atrophy and deafness) is a rare syndrome usually appearing in childhood before the age of 10 years and inherited in a Mendelian recessive manner[6]. Some cases may show only a few of the features, perhaps representing incomplete clinical expression.

MODY (maturity onset diabetes of youth) is inherited as a Mendelian dominant disorder of mild nature without ketoacidosis[7] and in which long-term complications of diabetes are rare (Susan, Chapter 3, p.30). This form of diabetes may be more common than has been realised.

Diabetes may also be associated with many other hereditary syndromes. (For a general review see reference 29.)

Immunological factors

Immunologists thrive on the association of ideas. Hashimoto thyroiditis, primary hypothyroidism, pernicious anaemia and auto-immune Addison's disease occur more commonly in diabetics (and their first-degree relatives) than in non-diabetics[8]. Serological associations are also impressive. Thus thyrogastric antibodies occur most commonly in young insulin-dependent diabetics, while antibodies to gastric intrinsic factor (sometimes regarded as a 'marker' for latent pernicious anaemia) are about four times more common in diabetics. The immunologist has recently strengthened his case by focusing his attention on the beta cell of the pancreas. A chronic inflammatory lesion showing lymphocytic infiltration of the islets – 'insulitis' – has long been recognised in the pancreas of the young recently-diagnosed diabetic coming to post-mortem (now a rare event). That this may be an immune response is strengthened by experiments showing a similar lesion in animals. In addition, however, the immunologist is now able to demonstrate both humoral and cellular anti-pancreatic auto-immunity in diabetes. IgG antibodies reacting specifically with pancreatic islet cells can be detected in insulin-dependent diabetics especially during the initial period after the onset of symptoms, but less frequently thereafter. Because the titre of islet cell antibodies (ICA) in diabetics is generally much lower than that of thyroid or gastric antibodies, immunologists had to develop much more sensitive techniques of fluorescence microscopy using incident-light illumination and improved filters for their indirect immunofluorescence test[9]. The necessary fresh human pancreatic material became available as a result of tissue transplantation surgery. ICA can be shown to react with glucagon-secreting alpha (A) and somatostatin-secreting delta (D) cells of the pancreas as well as the insulin-secreting beta (B) cells.

Cell-mediated immunity in diabetes can be demonstrated by inhibition of leucocyte migration in the presence of pancreatic antigens[8]. Since this reaction is species non-specific it probably represents an auto-immune reaction to some part of the substance or hormones of the islets of Langerhans. Another technique – the lymphocyte transformation test – has also shown that lymphoid cell populations in young diabetics may recognise antigens derived from the endocrine pancreas at the time when diabetes is first diagnosed[8]. These cell-mediated responses appear to be late stages in auto-immune pancreatic damage. Thus the pancreatic self-destruction of auto-immunity seems to be not so much a primary cause of juvenile-onset diabetes as a process which one day may be preventable if we could clearly see what sets it in motion.

Alternatively, it may be a transient phenomenon of academic interest rather than a pathogenic event. Time will tell! So what triggers the immune response, and why are only 8 or 9 of every 100,000 of the population so afflicted each year? The answer seems to lie partly in the patients' environment and partly in their histocompatibility antigen status. Other patients do seem to have polyendocrine diabetes (Mrs. Peabody, Chapter 3, p.31) where there is usually strong evidence of other auto-immune disease and persistence of ICA either before or after the onset of diabetes[26]. These are, however, relatively rare cases by comparison with the majority of children in whom ICA are found usually only in the few months after diagnosis and where the HLA system, rather than auto-immune disease processes, plays a major part in determining susceptibility.

Environmental agents: viral infection

Firm evidence of virus-induced beta cell damage in diabetic patients is still lacking. But high antibody titres to Coxackie B4 virus have been found in diabetic children within a few months of the onset of diabetes. Evidence attempting to incriminate the mumps virus is also circumstantial; moreover, the mumps virus damages the acinar tissue of the pancreas and the correlation of diabetes with mumps infection is generally poor. Congenital rubella has also been implicated, especially in HLA B8-positive individuals. The strongest evidence favouring the viral trigger in those having HLA-related susceptibility is the demonstration of winter clustering of neutralising antibody titres to Coxackie virus types B1-4 in newly-diagnosed diabetic children and young adults having the HLA B15 phenotypes. Viral titres have been found to be highest in those patients who were both HLA B15 and B8 positive[5]. Perhaps further studies of the histocompatibility D antigens will eventually further clarify the susceptibility to differing viral insults.

The data so far accumulated may be interpreted as suggesting that those who inherit a particular immunogenic constitution (HLA) may be unusually susceptible to prolonged viral insulitis or may respond to the released products of such an infection with an immune response which may damage the beta cell. But if this course of events causes juvenile-onset diabetes, a totally different genetic mechanism seems to lead to late-onset diabetes where – fortunately for these patients – the pancreas remains at least reasonably intact (Fig. 4.2). Ironically, despite the rapid strides being made in explaining *how* diabetes may develop in the youngster or in the commoner maturity-onset type, we still have no *certain* way of knowing who *will* be diabetic. But the clues are there to guide the scientist, and *immunisation* may yet be a possibility for the susceptible child or young adult.

Insulin and other pancreatic hormones – glucagon, somatostatin and pancreatic peptide

In 1955, the molecular structure of insulin was demonstrated by the painstaking Nobel prizewinning work of Frederick Sanger in Cambridge, England. To-day in Cambridge, Massachusetts, and elsewhere in the United States, molecular biologists are poised to use recombinant D NA techniques to code insulin genetic precursors into the structure of the humble coliform organism, thus

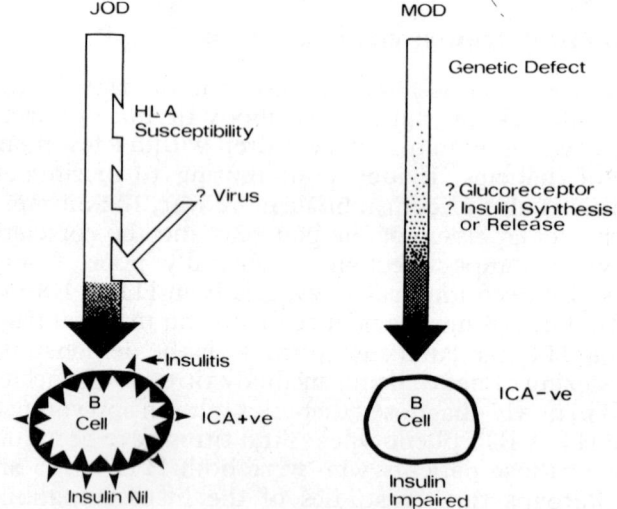

Fig. 4.2 Comparison of juvenile-onset (JOD) and maturity-onset (MOD) diabetes. Insulitis and islet cell antibody release (ICA +ve) in JOD possibly triggered by viral infection. Slowly developing beta cell defect in MOD without I CA release

elevating it to the status of a miniature pharmaceutical factory for insulin. This genetic engineering[10] depends upon new-found ability to use enzymes to break into the structure of chromosomal D NA. Also essential is a thorough understanding of how the insulin precursor *proinsulin* is derived from its pro-hormone *pre-proinsulin* and of the steps whereby it is decoded from chromosomal D NA.

How does the beta cell do it? Figure 4.3 shows a diagram of the beta cell with the nucleus containing chromosomal DNA. In the cytoplasm messenger-RNA begins to form up the pattern for the pre-proinsulin[11]. Ribosomes transfer RNA amino-acids to make the appropriate sequences of the A, B and C chains of proinsulin.

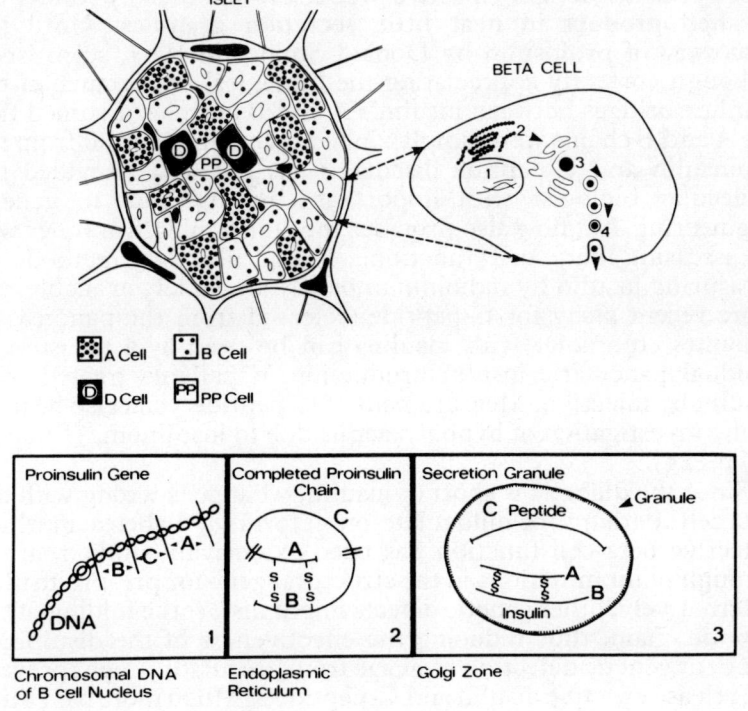

Fig. 4.3 Diagram of pancreatic islet with insulin-secreting beta cells predominating. Fewer glucagon-secreting A cells, somatostatin-producing D cells and pancreatic peptide (PP) cells. Detail of beta cell on right and stages of insulin production. **1** nucleus showing (inset) genetic decoding of *pre-proinsulin* in chromosomal DNA. **2** Formation of *proinsulin* in endoplasmic reticulum showing (inset) A and B portions having disulphide bridges. **3** Secretion granules of insulin formed in Golgi zone showing (inset) A and B chains of insulin and separated C-peptide. **4** Release of granule by emiocytosis

The chains, linked in the order A-C-B, take shape close to the microsomal membrane. The pre-hormonal sequence is cleft so that in the endoplasmic reticulum folded proinsulin with its A, B and C chains can be identified. Finally, secretion granules containing the A and B chains of insulin separated from the connecting C peptide appear in the region of the Golgi zones of the beta cell cytoplasm, ultimately to be secreted from the cell by emiocytosis (Fig. 4.3). Thus the beta cell not only unravels the appropriate genetic code to synthesise insulin, but at the same time protects itself from the powerful metabolic effects of the hormone, first by making lengthy inactive precursors and then by sealing the finished product in neat little secretion granules. Until the discovery of proinsulin by Donald Steiner in 1967, scientists – although correctly appreciating the biological importance of the sulphur bridges between insulin's A and B chains – assumed that the A and B chains were simply zipped together. Spin-off from the proinsulin and C-peptide discovery has not only provided the molecular biologist with important clues relevant to genetic engineering, but now also provides the clinician with another way of assessing beta cell function. Thus, although methods of measuring insulin by radioimmunoassay are widely available, the more recent assay for C-peptide (released from the pancreas in amounts equimolar with insulin) can be used as a measure of residual pancreatic insulin production in patients treated with insulin by injection. Measurement of C-peptide[22] can also be used in the investigation of hypoglycaemia due to insulinoma (Chapter 18, p.224).

Since the diabetic is short of insulin, what goes wrong with the beta cell? Perhaps the milder late-onset forms of diabetes, in which defective beta cell function has been extensively studied, arises through point mutations in the structural gene for pre-proinsulin. Alternatively, other genetic defects might distort the folding of the peptide chain, thus reducing the effectiveness of the disulphide bond, or genetic defects in cleavage from precursors might prevent the release of active insulin and C-peptide[11]. Much more has still to be learned about the life-span and behaviour of the beta cell. We're born with about 300 000 beta cells, which increase rapidly in the first few years of life to over a million. Although the size of the cells increases into adult life their number and function declines in old age, and this decline may be much more marked in late-onset diabetes.

Remember that the normal stimulus to insulin secretion is a rise in the blood glucose (Chapter 2, p.15). Diabetes could develop through the failure of the beta cell to sense glucose normally[12]; thus failure of the gluco-receptor would lead to decreased insulin biosynthesis and storage. The fact that the diabetic pancreas may still respond normally to such other stimuli as glucagon (Chapter 2, p.00; p.00) or sulphonylureas (Chapter 11) does suggest that there may be a defective *glucoreceptor* in the diabetic beta cell[23]. A structural glucoreceptor has not yet been identified and, moreover, studies of non-glucose stimuli are difficult to interpret because in the presence of hyperglycaemia these stimuli may only be potentiating the effect of glucose – for example by increasing the beta-cell cyclic-AMP[12].

The possibility that, in mild diabetes, hyperglycaemia may be an adaptive process which stimulates a failing beta cell to release at least enough insulin to maintain cell growth[13] and prevent the tearaway inflation of raging ketogenesis has already been mentioned (Chapter 2, p.22). However, this idea, and the concept of a failing glucoreceptor, are still at the test-bench stage. Nevertheless, we can see several ways in which the beta cell might fail the diabetic:

acute insulitis in youth following viral infection or other environmental insults;

genetic defects leading to failing insulin synthesis in the beta cell; and

failure of the glucoreceptor of the beta cell to respond normally to hyperglycaemia.

Besides insulin lack, from whatever cause, a queue of other hormones and peptides awaits our attention. Although most of them raise the blood glucose, either alone or in concert, their role in the aetiology of diabetes seems relatively minor. Foremost is the hormone of the pancreatic alpha cells – glucagon (Chapter 2, p.23).

Glucagon Approximately 15% of islet tissue is composed of alpha cells secreting glucagon from granules similar to those of insulin, but usually in different circumstances (Fig. 4.3). If insulin is the carbohydrate regulator of feeding and fuel storage, glucagon is the hormone of fasting and carbohydrate starvation[14,15]. Glucagon raises the blood glucose by stimulating hepatic glycogenolysis and gluconeogenesis (page 51). Glucagon favours amino-acid trapping by the liver to provide the carbon skeletons for glucose synthesis, at the same time stimulating adipose tissue lipolysis to provide energy for the process. Simultaneously, glucagon stimulates ketogenesis by activating the liver's carnitine acyltransferase system (Fig. 4.6) which is the essential mitochondrial gateway for ketogenic substrates. But these actions are diabetogenic only when insulin secretion is seriously impaired or when the diabetic is overwhelmed by the other hormones of stress or catabolism.

In normal blood glucose homeostasis, carbohydrate feeding stimulates insulin secretion and depresses glucagon. Protein feeding stimulates insulin to a lesser extent but also causes glucagon output. Mention has already been made (Chapter 2, p.24) of how in this way glucagon secretion saves the protein eater from insulin-induced hypoglycaemia without causing any sustained elevation of blood glucose. Even in diabetes, where insulin secretion is impaired, glucagon secretion is rarely sufficient to bring about deterioration in blood glucose regulation. Moreover, in the glucagonoma syndrome (Chapter 19, p.229) where enormously elevated plasma levels of glucagon have been recorded, diabetes is relatively mild. And pancreatectomy, simultaneously removing the source of both insulin and glucagon, always leads to diabetes mellitus, so confirming glucagon's minor role by comparison with insulin. We can live without glucagon but not without insulin.

Somatostatin   (Growth hormone-release inhibiting hormone, GH-RIH). This tetradecapeptide[16] was originally isolated from the hypothalamus and subsequently identified in the D cells of the pancreatic islets. Besides inhibiting growth hormone release, somatostatin is a potent inhibitor of both insulin and glucagon[25] secretion, but it neither causes nor aggravates diabetes; indeed, by inhibiting gastrointestinal absorption of carbohydrate it diminishes postprandial hyperglycaemia, and when given along with insulin in ketoacidosis it aids recovery by suppressing glucagon[27].

Pancreatic polypeptide   This 36-aminoacid peptide has been found in the pancreatic islets of many species, including the atrophied tissue of juvenile-onset diabetics. Although believed to be of significance in lipid metabolism and perhaps to be important in preventing obesity, currently it is an example of an identified substance waiting for its purpose to be defined.

Non-pancreatic hormones

Insulin is the hormone of *anabolism*. Catecholamines, cortisol and glucagon are the hormones of *catabolism*, and when unopposed by insulin, stimulate lipolysis and gluconeogenesis (growth hormone is a double agent, at times consorting with insulin in anabolism and at times switching to the side of lipolysis and catabolism). In normal circumstances, despite the opposing odds, insulin holds its own, so that growth, storage and development are maintained. But the stress of trauma, infection or other insults, by stimulating the catabolic hormones, can induce a diabetic state in those with a poor beta cell reserve, or a known mild diabetic may be driven rapidly toward gluconeogenesis and ketogenesis. There is general belief that the diabetes associated with either Cushinoid states or corticosteroid therapy is ketoacidosis-resistant. However, in more severe insulin deficiency, cortisol not only stimulates lipolysis but also hepatic gluconeogenesis and ketogenesis (page 00). Catecholamines mimic glucagon in their ability to contribute to lipolysis and glycogenolysis but unlike glucagon, they depress insulin secretion and may thus aggravate diabetes and, especially in severe stress states, accelerate ketogenesis.

The relationship between Cushinoid states, acromegaly, etc. and diabetes is described in Chapter 19.

So far we have examined factors which cause either a lack of insulin or antagonism to its action. Besides the antagonistic effect of hormones, other metabolites – especially free fatty acids (FFA)* released by lipolysis – may antagonise insulin (Chapter 6, p.80). Insulin resistance, on the other hand, must also be considered.

Insulin resistance and obesity

Those who are obese require increased amounts of endogenous insulin to maintain normal glucose levels. These patients develop insulin resistance through alteration in insulin receptors[24]. The initial step in insulin's cellular action – binding to specific protein receptors of the plasma membranes of target tissue – may be impeded by a decrease in insulin receptors in obesity. This appears to be a complex adaptive process to chronic hyper-insulinism in which insulin regulates its own receptors and which, moreover, may account for the fact that the obese who develop diabetes are often initially quite resistant to exogenous insulin.

Insulin lack, carbohydrate metabolism and gluconeogenesis

Glucose breakdown (*glycolysis*) is a basic energy source of varying importance in different tissues. Reconstruction of glucose (*gluco-neogenesis*) is an energy-consuming process confined to the liver and kidneys because only these organs are endowed with the

---

* The products of FFA oxidation such as citrate and acetyl CoA by inhibiting glycolysis will interfere with the cellular uptake of glucose.

enzymes capable of reversing the glycolytic pathway (Fig. 4.4).
The key to switching to gluconeogenesis is fat breakdown (*lipo-lysis*), releasing free fatty acids (FFA) which can be oxidised in the
liver and kidneys to drive the gluconeogenic process (Fig. 4.5).

Insulin lack – and those hormones antagonising insulin, especially catecholamines, glucagon and cortisol – stimulate lipolysis
(Chapter 6, p.77); the greater the insulin deficiency (or the more

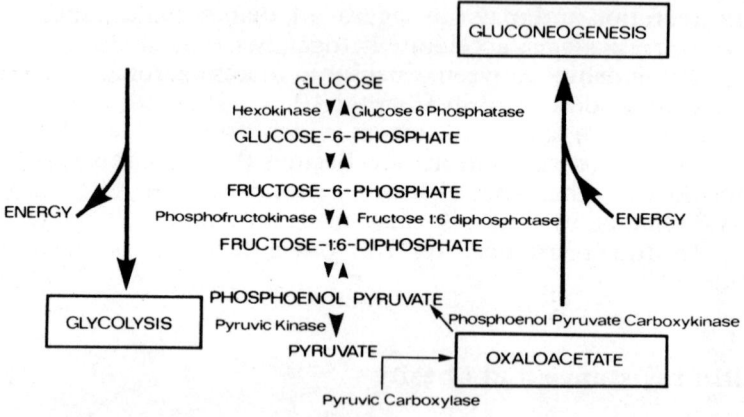

Fig. 4.4 *Glycolysis* producing energy and *gluconeogenesis* consuming energy

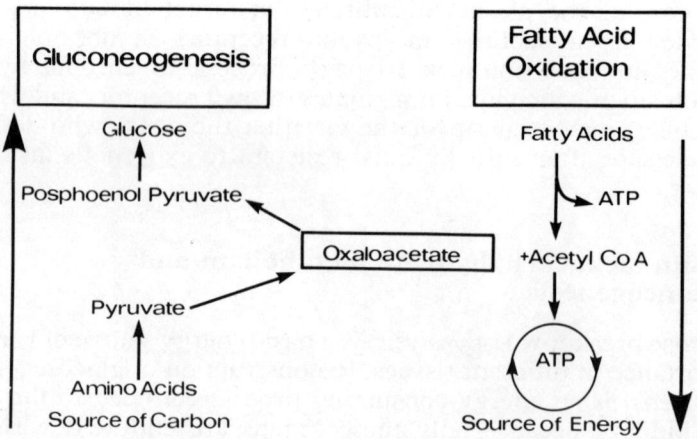

Fig. 4.5 Fatty acid oxidation producing energy for gluconeogenesis. Note that
oxaloacetate is the common link between gluconeogenesis and fatty acid oxidation

that insulin is antagonised by these other hormones) the greater the lipolysis. Moreover, insulin lack stimulates the biosynthesis of key gluconeogenic enzymes, so lipolysis and gluconeogenesis are, therefore, the heart and soul of all severe forms of defective carbohydrate metabolism in diabetes.

Fig. 4.5 shows how oxaloacetate is a common link between gluconeogenesis and fatty acid oxidation. Thus it is an obligatory intermediate in glucose synthesis, but oxaloacetate is also required for the disposal of acetyl CoA derived from FFA oxidation. As the rate of gluconeogenesis increases, all the oxaloacetic acid is eventually channelled into the gluconeogenic pathway. Acetyl CoA molecules, no longer having access to oxaloacetate, combine to form aceto-acetic acid (Fig. 4.6).

Whereas this process of carbohydrate synthesis and fat-melting can be bread and butter to those who are starving, the insulin lack

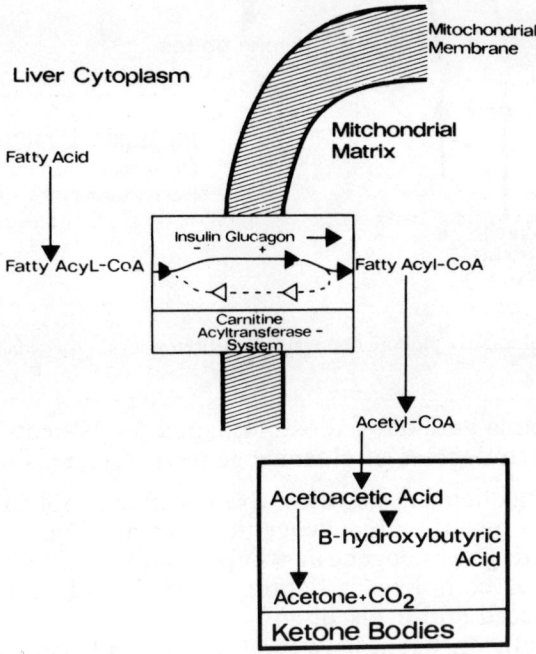

Fig. 4.6 Conversion of acetyl CoA molecules to acetoacetic acid and other ketone bodies. Oxidation of fatty acids to ketones occurs within the mitochondrial matrix of liver cells. The carnitine acyltransferase system controls *ketogenesis* because it is essential transport system carrying the substrates into the mitochondrium. Glucagon stimulates ketogenesis by activating the carnitine system

(or antagonism) of diabetes drives lipolysis and gluconeogenesis into top gear[17]. In the early stages of diabetes (or in its milder forms) the hyperglycaemia may stimulate a failing pancreas to produce enough insulin to prevent both lipolysis and gluconeogenesis from getting out of hand. At the same time acetoacetic and betahydroxybutyric acid (ketone bodies) can be utilised, as energy, especially in muscle, but when the beta cell fails completely (Fig. 4.7) glucose and ketone production cause marked

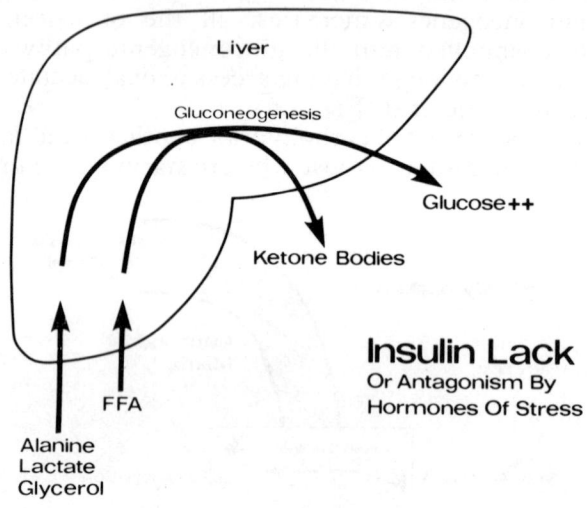

Fig. 4.7 Accelerated gluconeogenesis and ketogenesis of insulin lack or antagonism

hyperglycaemia and ketoacidosis (Chapter 7). We can, therefore, envisage three degrees of gluconeogenesis of increasing severity:

  mild gluconeogenesis where oxaloacetate is not totally channelled into the gluconeogenic pathway (Fig. 4.5);
  moderate gluconeogenesis where oxaloacetate is unavailable for the complete oxidation of FFA and acetoacetate is produced and utilised; and
  severe gluconeogenesis where glucose and acetoacetate (ketones) are produced far beyond the tissue's ability to utilise them.

The clinical consequences of this severe derangement of carbohydrate metabolism are described in Chapter 7.

Lactic acidosis

The dairymaid knows that lack of ventilation turns the milk sour. Anaerobic conditions in the milk parlour accelerate the fermentation of carbohydrate (*glycolysis*) to form lactic acid (*anaerobic glycolysis*); likewise, all body tissues tend to metabolise glucose to lactic acid in anaerobic circumstances[18, 19]. Thus lactic acid accumulates after strenuous muscular exercise both on account of relative anoxia and the inability of the circulation to keep pace with production. The liver and kidneys play a key rôle in lactate metabolism because they alone are endowed with the enzymes capable of metabolising lactate back to glucose via the gluconeogenic pathway. This energy cycle, where glucose breakdown in peripheral tissues produces lactate which can be re-converted back to glucose in the liver and kidneys, the *Cori cycle* (Fig. 4.8) is but one of the links between lactate metabolism and diabetes.

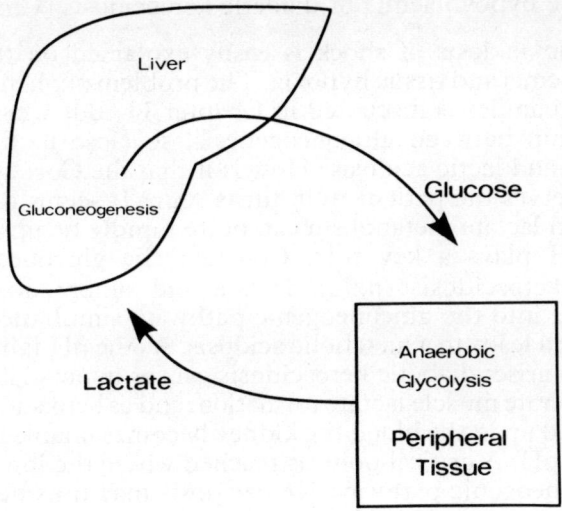

Fig. 4.8 Cori cycle: glucose produced in liver broken down to lactate (anaerobic glycolysis); lactate returned to liver to enter gluconeogenic pathway

Lactic acidosis can be defined as a state of metabolic acidosis associated with an abnormally high blood concentration of lactate. This could arise through:

abnormal over-production,
defective removal by the liver and kidneys, or
a combination of over-production and defective removal.

So from the clinical standpoint lactic acidosis might arise through the over-production resulting from poor oxygen delivery (anoxia, anaemia or shock). Liver disease (or the hepato-toxic effects of ethanol, salicylate or paracetamol poisoning) and renal disease may cause defective removal, and phenformin and other biguanides may increase production and diminish hepatic removal. It follows that several clinical problems commonly associated with diabetes might cause lactic acidosis:

1 myocardial infarction leading to shock (Chapter 13);
2 severe infection with bacteraemic shock (Chapter 20);
3 diabetes secondary to acute pancreatitis with shock (Chapter 19);
4 diabetes secondary to liver disease (Chapter 19);
5 diabetic renal disease (Chapter 14);
6 the use of phenformin and other biguanides (Chapter 11); and
7 the hypovolaemia of diabetic ketoacidosis (Chapter 7).

The lactic acidosis of shock is easily explained on the basis of hypovolaemia and tissue hypoxia. The problem of phenformin and other biguanides is discussed in Chapter 11. But what about the relationship between gluconeogenesis, so close to the heart of diabetes, and lactic acidosis? How is it that the Cori cycle, which usually serves the patient well, turns sour? It seems that a subtle balance in lactate metabolism can quite rapidly be upset and that tissue pH plays a key rôle. Consider the gluconeogenesis of diabetic ketoacidosis (p.54): lactate and other substrates can be sucked into the gluconeogenic pathway; simultaneous ketone production leads to a metabolic acidosis. As the pH falls two other problems arise: diabetic ketoacidosis causes hypovolaemia which will accelerate muscle lactate formation, and as ketoacids and lactic acids build up in the blood the kidney becomes unable to maintain the body pH. A critical point is reached where the low pH blocks the gluconeogenic pathway. Ketoacidosis may thus be overtaken by lactic acidosis; indeed, a fall in pH seems to be the key to deterioration in all forms of lactic acidosis. Thus a moderate elevation of blood lactate from whatever cause with concomitant acidosis may be swung into a critical phase by the combined effect of any renal impairment in H^+ ion excretion and the consequent fall in tissue pH switching off gluconeogenesis and lactate removal. In addition to defective removal, anything (including lactic acid) which lowers the tissue pH may turn the liver into a lactate-producing organ instead of being a consumer, which seems to be how the patient turns sour.

For some forms of lactic acidosis, especially those where peripheral production is *increased*, salvation may be at hand[20]. Dichloroacetate (DCA) stimulates the peripheral metabolism of lactate to pyruvate by activating the enzyme pyruvate dehydrogenase which will shunt more lactate into CO_2 formation. Other beneficial effects of DCA on blood lipids are difficult to explain. The chief bar to the use of DCA is the fact that lactic acidosis is often overlooked (Chapter 7).

Muscle and the glucose-alanine cycle

Muscle can be seen as a large metabolic organ comprising 45% of body weight and weighing 21 times more than the liver[21]. Muscle plays a significant part in maintaining aminoacids and glucose in the circulation because aminoacids are the only substances continuously available for hepatic gluconeogenesis. In fasting there is a net conversion of aminoacids to glucose. The gluconeogenic aminoacid *alanine* plays such a central rôle that, in addition to the glucose-lactate (Cori) cycle of active muscle a *glucose-alanine cycle* (Fig. 4.9) of resting muscle can also be visualised. Glutamate and other aminoacids are also lost from muscle during fasting.

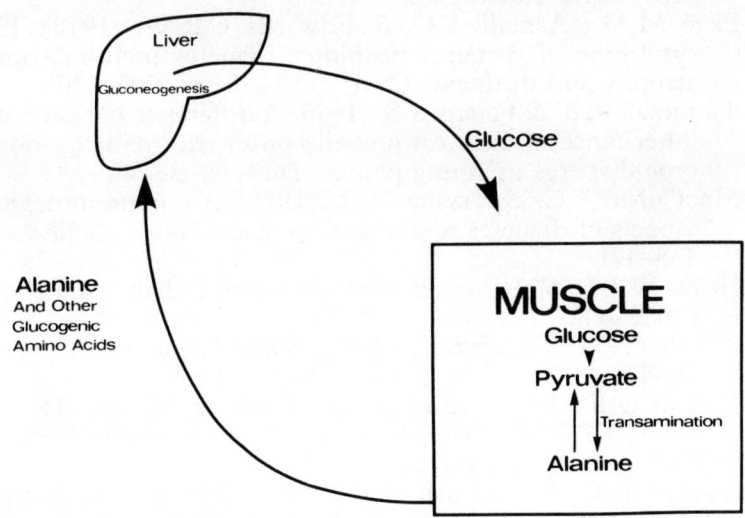

Fig. 4.9 Glucose-alanine cycle: large muscle mass releases *alanine* and other gluconeogenic amino-acids for gluconeogenesis in the liver

Glucagon (the hormone of starvation) stimulates this process. Prevention of this melting down of flesh and limbs is fundamental to the management of underweight or insulin-deficient diabetics. Insulin is therefore essential to restrain the glucose-alanine cycle ie. gluconeogenesis. But the effect of insulin upon restraining *lipolysis* is also crucial.

Insulin and fat metabolism are dealt with in Chapter 6.

Further Reading

1 Pyke D.A. (1977) The genetics of diabetes. *Clin. Endocrinol. Metabol.*, **6**, 285–303

2 Bloom A., Hayes T.M. & Gamble D.R. (1975) Register of newly diagnosed diabetic children. *Br. med. J*, **iii**, 580–583

3 Cudworth A.G. (1978) Type I Diabetes Mellitus. *Diabetologia*, **14**, 281–292

4 Nelson P.G., Pyke D.A., Cudworth A.G., Woodrow J.C. & Batchelor J.R. (1975) Histocompatibility antigens in diabetic identical twins. *Lancet*, **ii**, 193–194

5 Cudworth A.G., Gamble D.R., White G.B.B., Lendrum R., Woodrow J.C. & Bloom A. (1977) Aetiology of diabetes. A prospective study. *Lancet*, **i**, 385–388

6 Page M.M., Asmall A.C. & Edwards C.R.W. (1976) The syndrome of diabetes insipidus, diabetes mellitus, optic atrophy and deafness. *Quart. J. Med.*, **45**, 505–520

7 Tattersall R.B. & Fajans S.S. (1975) A difference between the inheritance of classical juvenile-onset and maturity-onset type diabetes in young people. *Diabetes*, **24**, 44

8 MacCuish A.C. & Irvine W.J. (1975) Autoimmunological aspects of diabetes mellitus. *Clin. Endocrinol. Metabol.*, **4**, 435–471

9 Irvine W.J. (1977) Classification of idiopathic diabetes. *Lancet*, **i**, 638–642

10 Article (1977) Tinkering with life. *Time Magazine*, 18 April, 46–49

11 Steiner D.F. (1977) Insulin today. *Diabetes*, **26**, 322–340

12 Editorial (1977) The beta cell in diabetes – more sinned against than sinning. *Lancet*, **i**, 177–178

13 Turner R.C. & Holman R.R. (1976) Insulin rather than glucose homeostasis in the pathophysiology of diabetes. *Lancet*, **i**, 1272–1274

14 Unger R.H. (1976) Diabetes and the alpha cell. *Diabetes*, **25**, 136–151

15 Felig P., Wahren J., Sherwin R. & Hendler R. (1976) Insulin, glucagon, somatostatin in normal physiology and diabetes mellitus. *Diabetes*, **25**, 1091–1099

16 Luft R. (1978) Somatostatin – both hormone and neurotransmitter. *Diabetologia*, **14**, 1–14

17 McGarry J.D. & Foster D.W. (1976) Ketogenesis and its regulation. *Am. J. Med.*, **61**, 9–12

18 Cohen R.D. & Woods H.F. (1976) *Clinical and Biochemical Aspects of Lactic Acidosis.* Oxford: Blackwell Scientific Publications

19 Alberti K.G.M.M. & Nattrass M. (1977) Lactic acidosis. *Lancet*, **ii**, 25–29

20 Relman A.S., (1978) Lactic acidosis and a possible new treatment. *New Eng. J. Med.*, **298**, 564–566

21 Daniel P.M., Pratt O.E. & Spargo E. (1977) The metabolic homeostatic rôle of muscle as a store of protein. *Lancet*, **ii**, 446–448

22 Turner R.C. & Heding L.G. (1977) Plasma proinsulin, C-peptide and insulin in diagnostic suppression tests for insulinoma. *Diabetologia*, **13**, 571–578

23 Sugden M.C. & Ashcroft S.J.H. (1977) Phosphoenolpyruvate in rat pancreatic islets: a possible intracellular trigger of insulin release. *Diabetologia*, **13**, 481–486

24 Olefsky J.M. (1976) The insulin receptor: its rôle in insulin resistance of obesity and diabetes. *Diabetes*, **25**, 1154–1164

25 Unger R.H. & Orci L. (1977) Possible rôles of the pancreatic D-cell in normal and diabetic states. *Diabetes*, **26**, 241–244

26 Bottazzo G.F., Cudworth A.G., Moul D.S., Doniach D. & Festenstein H. (1978). Evidence for a primary autoimmune type of diabetes mellitus. *Br. med. J*, **ii**, 1253–1255

27 Raskin P. & Unger R.H. (1978) Hyperglucagonaemia and its suppression. *New Engl. J. Med.*, **299**, 433–436

28 Editorial (1978) Dichloracetate. *Br. Med. J.*, **ii**, 456

29 Rotter J.I. & Rimoin (1979) Diabetes mellitus: the search for genetic markers. *Diabetes Care*, **2**, 215–226

Diagnosis, Clinical Features, Diagnostic Tests, Assessment of Severity and Prevalence of Diabetes

Diagnosis

The diagnosis of diabetes mellitus is relatively easy. In the vast majority of cases the osmotic diuresis of sugar will bring the patient to the doctor complaining typically of thirst and polyuria and other associated symptoms. Confirmation of glycosuria is quicker and simpler than almost any other diagnostic procedure. Thereafter, one sensibly-timed blood sample for glucose will clinch the diagnosis. If normal, well and good. If significantly abnormal the severity of the metabolic upset and the urgency of treatment can be assessed by reading page 71, but if the result is in the twilight zone between normal and diabetic, the glucose tolerance test remains the fundamental arbiter in cases of doubt. Many other tedious and sophisticated procedures have been devised to challenge and observe the ability of the pancreas to secrete and release insulin, but these remain the research tools of the epidemiologist and the scientist rather than aids to the clinician. What about the patient with a doubtful glucose tolerance test? Like the Olympic high-jumper, give the patient a second chance and repeat the same test. Any lingering doubt means that diabetes remains unproven; rather than therapeutic intervention maintenance of a watching brief is all that is necessary. On the other hand, if the patient is obese or eats too many sugar goodies, control of carbohydrate or other calorie intake will almost certainly move the glucose tolerance into the unequivocally normal range.

Glycosuria is commonly found at routine clinical examination for health, employment or insurance purposes in asymptomatic patients. Unless the two-hours-post-breakfast blood glucose is either well within the normal or abnormal range (page 66) a glucose tolerance test (page 67) is the best way of settling any doubts. Likewise, in the investigation of peripheral neuropathy

(Chapter 16) or other endocrine and metabolic disease (Chapter 19) where diabetes mellitus is included in the differential diagnosis, a glucose tolerance test is decisive.

Symptoms of thirst and polyuria will usually lead the doctor to test the urine for glucose. When none is found diabetes mellitus is unlikely and such alternatives as renal disease, diabetes insipidus, compulsive water drinking or some other cause for the polyuria should be considered.

Clinical features

The clinical features of diabetes mellitus can be divided broadly into three groups – those associated with

the melting down of flesh and limbs into urine,
diabetic complications, and
other disorders precipitating diabetes.

1 The melting down of the body into the urine not only causes thirst, polyuria and weight loss but also other features related to the metabolic and electrolyte upset.

Thirst   Especially for the beer drinker and the tea or coffee addict, the thirst of early diabetes can be wholesomely enjoyable and not a cause for complaint. Unfortunately, the choice of drink may aggravate the diabetic upset; often patients will turn to lemonade or other sugar containing drinks to assuage their thirst with consequent worsening of the glucose intolerance. Whatever beverage is chosen, the patient mainly replaces fluid whereas the osmotic diuresis of glucose also causes electrolyte loss (Chapter 7, p.88).

Polyuria   Although the thirst results from polyuria, most patients see it the other way round; they assume that they are passing more urine on account of drinking more. Polyuria may also create misleading complaints and inappropriate remedies: thus nocturia may send the patient to the doctor complaining of insomnia, with the prescription of a hypnotic as the remedy. In elderly males, polyuria may aggravate prostatic symptoms, so the diagnosis and treatment of diabetes will often eliminate any need for prostatic surgery. Commonly, the patient may have had a course of antibiotics in the treatment of suspected urinary infection, the correct diagnosis ultimately being made when the doctor gets round to urine testing. Or a child with sudden onset of nocturnal enuresis may be sent for applied psychology when a urine test would have been more appropriate. Diabetes is an easy diagnosis which is easily overlooked, yet the observant may occasionally make the diagnosis before urine testing by noticing white spots of sugar on the patient's shoes or trousers.

Pain   Pain will always hurry the patient to the doctor – the distress and discomfort of pruritus vulvae in the female, or, less frequently, balanitis in the male due to monilial infection aggravated by glycosuria are often presenting complaints (Chapter 20, p.242). Middle-aged obese woman may develop extensive inflammation, spreading sometimes to cause pruritus ani besides excoriation of the perineum. Painful peripheral neuropathy or diabetic amyotrophy (Chapter 16, p.205) may also be distressing presenting complaints.

Weight loss   Whether obese, thin or of normal weight at the outset, all but those with a very mild disturbance of glucose tolerance will tend to lose weight coincident with the onset of diabetic symptoms. Always be alert to other underlying disease (see below); when weight loss persists despite control of the metabolic disorder, such other underlying conditions as tuberculosis, thyrotoxicosis or neoplasia should be considered.

Hepatomegaly   Liver enlargement is a common accompaniment of newly-diagnosed or untreated diabetes. The liver is soft on palpation (so soft it may be overlooked), no biochemical disturbance of liver function is evident but biopsy would demonstrate fatty infiltration of the sinusoidal structure. The enlargement and histological abnormality should revert to normal with control of the diabetes. Firm hepatomegaly suggests haemochromotosis, cirrhosis or hepatic secondaries due to pancreatic neoplasia, all of which may be associated with diabetes (Chapter 19).

Tiredness and leg cramps   These are common complaints which improve with control of the severe osmotic diuresis and electrolyte loss.

Visual changes   Dehydration tends to cause short sight and blurred vision. In the elderly with gradual onset of symptoms, hypermetropia (a common defect in ageing) will perhaps improve, so that treatment of diabetes may lead to deterioration in vision (Chapter 15).

2 Diabetic complications as presenting features   Especially in older patients, a complication of diabetes rather than the thirst or polyuria of the metabolic upset may sometimes be the presenting feature. Remember Mr. Puff (Chapter 3) the railway engine driver with failing vision? His diabetes was diagnosed by the opthalmologist who shunted him off to the diabetic clinic. Likewise, every doctor worth his salt knows to test the urine for sugar when called to see lower limb gangrene. Often in such cases the metabolic upset may be relatively muted. Moreover, patients are naturally much more concerned about their vision or gangrenous toes than to give much thought to thirst or polyuria. The various lesions are described in greater detail in later sections as follows: diabetic nephropathy, Chapter 14; retinopathy and visual disturbances, Chapter 15; diabetic neuropathy, Chapter 16; the diabetic foot, Chapter 17.

3 Other disorders precipitating diabetes   Any illness, from a simple viral infection to a malignant tumour, can precipitate diabetes. No matter what the complaint, it is a wise precaution to test a urine sample for sugar. Sometimes the patient is driven towards glucose intolerance, not so much by the stress of the illness, but by the doctor's remedy. The effects of drugs and other illness upon diabetes are discussed in Chapter 20, p.238.

Diagnostic tests

    1 Glycosuria
    2 Blood glucose
    3 Glucose tolerance tests
    5 Other tests

1 Glycosuria   Testing the urine for sugar is fundamental to the clinical detection of diabetes. It has shortcomings as a definitive diagnostic procedure, but should not be overlooked on this account. Remember that the concentration of sugar in the urine does not depend only on the height of the blood glucose. The 'renal threshold' to glucose is affected by the glomerular filtration rate (GFR) and the renal tubular reabsorptive capacity for glucose. Youngsters generally have a lower renal threshold to glucose so that asymptomatic glycosuria is more likely to be due to a tubular 'leak' than to diabetes (and the young rarely present with mild asymptomatic diabetes; when they do, the problem is less urgent anyway). At the other extreme, the elderly are more likely to have a higher renal threshold (poorer GFR), so that glycosuria in the older patient usually means hyperglycaemia. Figure 5.1 illustrates these points.

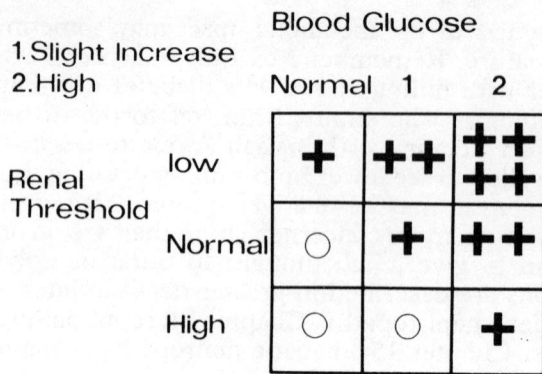

Fig. 5.1 Glycosuria: the effect of a low, normal or high renal threshold upon glycosuria in patient with normal, elevated (1) or grossly elevated (2) blood glucose

The best urine sample for screening is one obtained after a meal. The most sensitive and glucose-specific methods of testing are those using glucose oxidase – Clinistix, Tes-Tape, Glucotest and Diastix (Table 5.1). Quantitative measurement of urinary glucose can be made with reasonable accuracy using Tes-Tape, Diastix or the copper reduction method such as the Clinitest tablets (Table 5.1). This is a useful way of confirming whether glycosuria found by one of the specific tests is slight or significant. Thus there is a colour range as follows:

NEGATIVE	$\frac{1}{4}$	$\frac{1}{2}$	$\frac{3}{4}$	1	2	over 2 per cent.

Table 5.1   Urine tests for glucose and keytones

CONFIRMATION OF GLYCOSURIA Use tests which are:

1 GLUCOSE-SPECIFIC – glucose-oxidase method
2 BUFFERED – to avoid false negative results in presence of ketones or other acids
3 SENSITIVE – detect $0.1\% = 100\,mg/100\,ml = 5.5\,mmol/l$

A

Clinistix (Ames Co)	Dip and read in 10 seconds	QUICK
Glucotest (Boehringer Mannheim	Dip and read in 1 minute	and RELIABLE

ASSESSMENT OF PERCENTAGE GLYCOSURIA For use after
CONFIRMATION, or to assess control in known diabetic.

B

Tes-tape (Lilly)	Glucose-specific but not buffered: false negative or low reading if ketones or other acids present	$0 \cdot 1 - 2 \%$ scale
Diastix (Ames Co)		$0 \cdot 1 - 2 \%$ scale
Ketodiastix (Ames Co)		As above plus ketones scale

C

Clinitest (Ames Co) Test tube and dropper	$0 \cdot 25 - 2 \%$ scale 5 drops urine plus 10 of water: add reagent tablet	NOT GLUCOSE SPECIFIC False positive with other reducing substances in urine: salicylates, antibiotics, lactose (high in pregnancy)

Note: tests in Group A +ve and Clinitest −ve = less than $0 \cdot 25 \%$ glycosuria
tests in Group A −ve and Clinitest +ve = other reducing substance
present

If glycosuria confirmed − SUSPECT DIABETES:
if significant (1% or more) CHECK URINARY KETONES

TESTING FOR KETONES

Ketones are rapidly excreted by the kidney and may appear in the urine
without a significant increase in plasma ketones in *starvation, vomiting* or
fever. Ketonuria without *glycosuria* is due to these causes rather than diabetes.
Tests based on nitroprusside reaction in which *acetoacetic acid* and *acetone*
form a violet colour complex.

D

Ketostix (Ames Co)	Dip and read at 15 seconds	All sensitive to ketonuria above the physiological range
Ketur-test (Boehringer Mannheim)	Dip and read at 60 seconds	All detect ACETOACETIC ACID on weak to strong scale.
Acetest (Ames Co)	Moisten tablet with drop of urine. Read at 30 seconds	WEAK = $1 \cdot 0$ mmol/l (10 mg/100 ml) MODERATE = $5 \cdot 0$ mmol/l (50 mg/100 ml) STRONG = $10 \cdot 0$ mmol/l (100 mg/100 ml)

GLYCOSURIA · KETONURIA *more severe insulin lack than glycosuria without
ketonuria*
GLYCOSURIA · STRONG URINARY KETONES · CHECK PLASMA KETONES
(Chapter 7, p.87)

Check the manufacturer's literature for the precise details of all the tests and
their interpretation.

The Clinitest can give false results in the patient taking aspirin, antibiotics or having lactosuria, but for practical purposes those with 1% glycosuria or more are usually hyperglycaemic.

For those confused by the above provisos, follow these simple rules:

1 anybody found to have glycosuria is under suspicion of having diabetes mellitus and should have an appropriate blood test; and

2 a negative result in a post-breakfast urine test makes diabetes unlikely unless the patient has an elevated blood urea (poor GFR and raised renal threshold to glucose).

2 Blood glucose Hyperglycaemia remains the fundamental basis of the clinical diagnosis of diabetes. Our only problem is the definition of what is normal and what is hyperglycaemia. For want of anything better we have to follow arbitrary rules – tempered with caution. Instead of a fixed cut-off dividing normality from diabetes, it is wiser to think in terms of normal, doubtful and diabetic. Moreover, there is an upward trend with age so that analogy with blood pressure is particularly apt. Because older patients can be allowed a higher normal blood glucose and blood pressure, results in the doubtful range are much more likely to be of significance in the young, and relatively unimportant in those aged over 65 years (Table 5.2).

Table 5.2   GTT diagnosis of diabetes related to age: venous blood*

	Fasting		Peak		2 Hours	
Age in years	mmol/l	mg/100 ml	mmol/l	mg/100 ml	mmol/l	mg/100 ml
Less than 20	5·0	90	9	162	7	126
20–39	5·5	100	10	180	8	144
40–59	6·0	108	11	200	9	162
60+	6·5	117	12	216	10	180

Values in excess of those quoted for particular ages should be regarded as diabetic.

* For *venous plasma* add 1·0 mmol/l (18 mg/100 ml) to the above. For *capillary blood* add 1·0 mmol/l (18 mg/100 ml) to the *peak* and *2-hour* values (See Fig. 5.3). Blood or plasma estimated by specific enzymatic method. Test conducted according to criteria in Table 5.3.

When should the blood glucose sample be obtained? fasting, at random, or two hours after a normal meal? Look at the blood glucose curve in Fig. 5.2. The most practical and scientifically acceptable time to obtain a single sample is two hours after a meal. A fasting sample is not only less practical to obtain but will

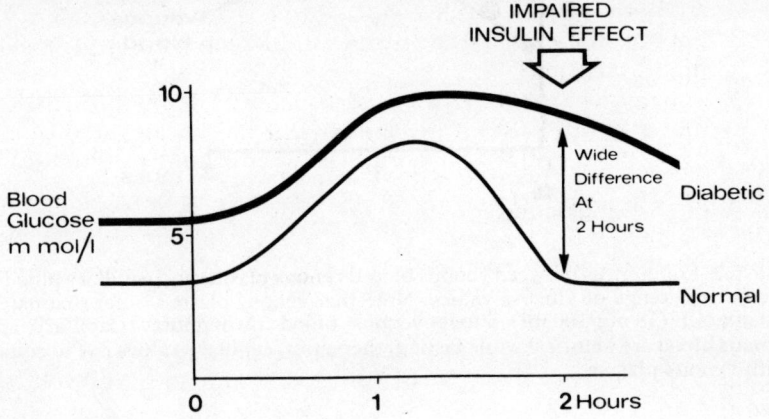

Fig. 5.2 Normal blood sugar curve compared with mild glucose intolerance showing greatest deviation at two hours

chapter (page 71). Doubtful results are the main indication for miss an abnormal rise following the glucose challenge of the meal; without careful timing the peak might be missed. The result at two hours best reflects the overall response to the meal (glucose challenge) in terms of pancreatic-islet-release of insulin, tissue sensitivity to insulin and homeostatic control of blood glucose (Chapter 4). A result unequivocally in the abnormal range (Table 5.2), means diabetes mellitus and further estimation of blood glucose or tests of glucose tolerance are unnecessary for diagnostic purposes. The remainder of the assessment of the severity of diabetes depends upon those other factors outlined later in this chapter (page 71). Doubtful results are the main indication for formal glucose tolerance testing. The effects of age, or different sampling sites (venous or capillary) and of methods of estimation of blood or plasma glucose are shown in Figure 5.3 and Table 5.2.

3 Glucose tolerance test (GTT) If the two-hours-post-breakfast blood glucose is the best way of diagnosing diabetes the oral GTT is the ideal method of confirming normality. The cardinal error in using the GTT is to conduct it under the artificial

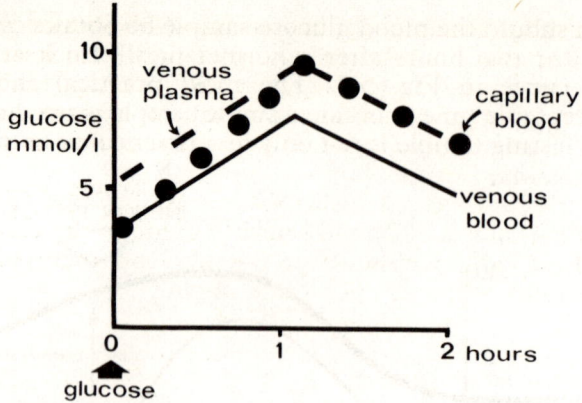

Fig. 5.3 Differences between venous blood, venous plasma and capillary blood in the normal range of glucose values. Note that venous plasma is approximately 1·0 mmol/l (18 mg/100 ml) above venous blood throughout. Capillary and venous blood are identical while fasting; thereafter, capillary values rise to equate with venous plasma

and abnormal conditions of a hospital ward, perhaps while the patient is still recovering from recent surgery or a major illness, and then to interpret some dubiously borderline value as evidence of diabetes. Instead, the test should be carried out using reasonably standardised methods and the results interpreted with caution, bearing in mind the patient's age, nutritional status and emotional composure.

Although an intravenous GTT may have some merit in early pregnancy (when oral glucose may be nauseating), the procedure has no diagnostic value which cannot be matched by oral testing. For the oral GTT 50, 75 and 100 g loads have all been compared. Although there are slight differences, the higher loads are no more discriminatory and are more likely to be nauseating. The 50 g load is the usual British standard and can be given as 235 ml of Lucozade or Glucola. Since there is a circadian variation in glucose tolerance with deterioration as the day advances, the test should be conducted in the morning after a 12-hour fast, but the patient should have had a normal diet at least for the preceding three days because starvation can adversely affect glucose tolerance. Likewise, bed rest has an adverse effect, so the patient should have been reasonably ambulant, and those drugs which interfere with glucose tolerance – especially combined oral contraceptives, other oestrogens, diuretics and corticosteroids (Chapter 20, p.239) – should either be avoided or taken into account in the interpretation of the results. Trauma – or any stress – will impair the GTT so that if the patient is admitted to a metabolic unit for a barrage of blood-letting sessions, perhaps for the investigation of diabetes secondary to other endocrine or metabolic disease (Chapter 19), the GTT should be completed before the patient is subjected to more exacting procedures.

The criteria of the British Diabetic Association (Fitzgerald & Keen, 1964) give a clear and sensible guide to the conduct of the oral GTT (Table 5.3); however, the subject is undergoing revision (see reference 4 for an up-to-date review).

Table 5.3   Oral glucose tolerance test   Procedure recommended by the *British Diabetic Association* (Fitzgerald & Keen 1964)

Conditions	Unrestricted diet and physical activity for at least 3 days, 12 hours of fasting and 30 minutes sitting quietly before the test. Subject to remain seated and non-smoking during the test.
Method	After withdrawing the fasting blood sample, 50 g glucose in 200–500 ml of flavoured water (235 ml Lucozade will do) to be drunk in 5 minutes. Zero time to be taken as the beginning of the drink and samples to be withdrawn at 30-minutes intervals for 2 hours.
Standard of abnormality	Capillary blood glucose level of 6.7 mmol/l (120 mg/100 ml) or more at 2 hours and of 10 mmol/l (180 mg/100 ml) or over at some other time in the test (see Table 5.2 for age-related data). The blood glucose measurements should be made by either the glucose oxidase method or the ferricyanide method after dialysis using the Autoanalyser.

The effects of other disorders upon the nature of the blood glucose curve are shown in Fig. 5.4. Rapid gastro-intestinal absorption of the glucose load (typically in patients with ulcer dyspepsia) may cause such a sharp rise in blood glucose that the peak may be missed unless blood samples are obtained at 15-minute intervals in the first hour of the test. Liver disease is discussed in Chapter 19. Special variants of the GTT used in the assessment of *hypoglycaemia* are discussed in Chapter 18.

4 Other tests in the diagnosis of diabetes   When the standard oral GTT is on the borderline of normality, could not some other test add diagnostic precision? What about augmenting the

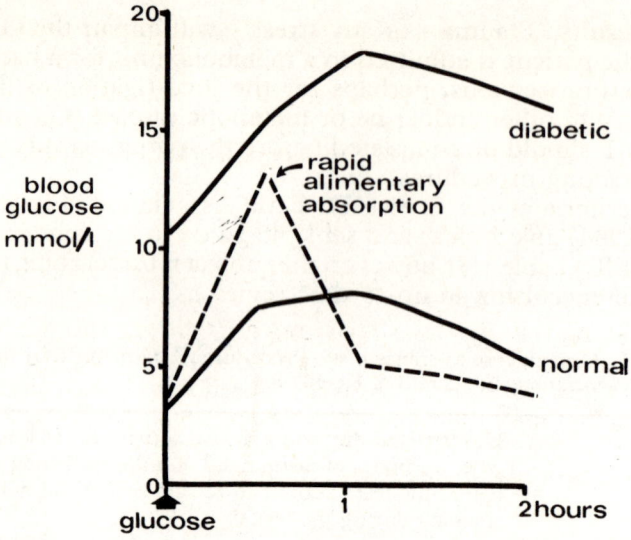

Fig. 5.4 Effect of rapid alimentary absorption on GTT curve. Note the early peak at 30 minutes; thereafter, the results fall below the normal range. The diabetic curve was a waste of time. A random blood glucose in such a case would have been diagnostic

test by giving the patient the additional stress of oral corticosteroids? Unfortunately, such tests attempt to squeeze too much out of the patient and the GTT procedure. We're all a bit 'diabetic' if we're pushed hard enough, but the main fault in the use of corticosteroids is the wide variability in response, making standardisation impossible for individual diagnostic purposes. Other procedures, such as

> the intravenous tolbutamide test,
> the intravenous glucagon test,
> oral leucine test,
> insulin radioimmunoassay, and
> C-peptide assay

are all concerned with the diagnosis of hypoglycaemia and insulinoma (Chapter 18) rather than diabetes.

Remember that if any patient is suspected of being diabetic (perhaps because of a family history or other predisposing factors, Chapter 4) and glucose tolerance is well within the normal range, this is no guarantee of future immunity to diabetes mellitus. This is our major diagnostic dilemma. Predictive tests are needed in order to identify susceptibility to diabetes. Examination of the HLA chromosomal region (Chapter 4, p.42) and tests for islet-cell antibodies (Chapter 4, p.44) are the first steps in the identification of those at risk of diabetes. Progress in this direction will be essential to the prevention of diabetes in the susceptible.

Assessment of severity of diabetes

So your patient has significant glycosuria. You are well on the way to having diagnosed diabetes mellitus but you don't know what to do next. One solution is to dash off a letter to the nearest hospital diabetic clinic indicating that the patient's urine is 'loaded' with sugar. This is an emotive phrase, charged with hidden innuendo, implying that the situation is explosive (but you don't know how to defuse it) and expert advice is urgently required.

Where do we go from there? Will a blood glucose estimation both confirm the diagnosis and give an estimate of severity? Yes and no. Suppose that the two-hours-post-prandial blood glucose value is 15 mmol/l (270 mg/100 ml) – well into the diagnostic range. If your patient is a youngster he might, within a few days, be in severe diabetic ketoacidosis requiring emergency management whereas an elderly patient with the same blood glucose value may be virtually asymptomatic and ultimately responsive to nothing more than dietary adjustment. Admittedly those patients with greater elevation of the blood glucose – over 25 mmol/l (450 mg/100 ml) for example – usually have a more urgent problem, but nevertheless the decision about management and assessment of severity is based on other clinical features rather than on the degree of hyperglycaemia.

Table 5.4 shows the main features to be taken into account. Notice that the patients requiring treatment most urgently are those with ketoacidosis, dehydration or features of hypovolaemia (Chapter 7). At the other extreme are those with relatively asymptomatic glycosuria. Remember also that youngsters tend to have a lower renal threshold to glucose than the aged. The massive renal loss of glucose may prevent the blood glucose from rising as high as in others, but the price is more serious dehydration and electrolyte loss. On the other hand patients who increase their fluid intake in the form of glucose drinks in response to the thirst and polyuria of mild diabetes may artificially elevate the blood glucose perhaps to what seems at first sight a rather high value, yet simple advice about switching to non-carbohydrate beverages (water will do) may lead to a significant improvement both in symptoms and blood glucose.

Table 5.4 Assessment of severity of diabetes and urgency of treatment: some broad guidelines

Urgency	Hours	Days	Weeks	Months	Years
Clinical features	Ketoacidosis Hypovolaemia Dehydration Vomiting	Severe thirst Marked polyuria Marked weight loss: eating or drinking adequately	Overweight Slight thirst or polyuria Eating too well	Asymptomatic	Previous borderline GTT Gestational diabetic Strong family history of diabetes
Urine	Glycosuria Ketonuria	Glycosuria Mild ketonuria	Glycosuria No ketonuria	Intermittent glycosuria No ketonuria	No glycosuria
Blood	Hyperglycaemia Ketonaemia	Hyperglycaemia No ketonaemia	Hyperglycaemia	Marginal or slight hyperglycaemia	Euglycaemic

But how do we assess those who are neither acute medical emergencies on the one hand nor mild, relatively asymptomatic, patients on the other? How do we pick out those who will need nothing more than dietary advice (Chapter 9), those who will need insulin (Chapter 10) and those in the middle ground needing oral hypoglycaemic agents (Chapter 11)?

Four main factors can be helpful:

    ketonuria,
    the age of the patient,
    the severity and duration of symptoms, and
    the weight of the patient.

Having found glycosuria, always check for ketonuria (Table 5.1). Its absence means that ketogenesis is not accelerated and that insulin lack is less acute. On the other hand, ketonuria is always an indication for careful assessment even though it is not an invariable danger signal. For example, starvation may be associated with brisk renal excretion of ketones without a significant increase in plasma ketones. The patient in real danger and in need of immediate hospital treatment will have both ketonuria and *positive plasma ketones* (Tables 5.1 & 5.4).

The younger the patient, especially if under 25, the more likely is the need for insulin therapy. Of course there are exceptions, but these are judged on the basis of other features. Rapid onset of severe symptoms of less than four weeks duration usually warrants consideration for insulin, whereas patients with symptoms of many months' standing and without significant deterioration are much less urgently in need of correction of the metabolic upset. Perhaps the best guide, besides ketonuria, is the weight of the patient: those who are significantly overweight (20% or more above their ideal weight, see Appendix 1) are unlikely to require insulin. The more hyperglycaemic they are, the more they should have their excess calorie intake curtailed. On the other hand, patients who are underweight at the time of diagnosis, especially those having lost weight coincident with the onset of diabetic symptoms, may need treatment with insulin even though they are middle-aged or elderly. And even if relatively mild diabetic symptoms and freedom from ketoacidosis make the initial use of an oral hypoglycaemic agent feasible, one cannot confidently predict that such treatment will succeed in the underweight.

Most doctor's letters referring patients to hospital diabetic clinics give all the clues that we need, the age of the patient, duration and severity of symptoms, glycosuria, ketonuria and mention the presence or absence of obesity: we can decide about management almost before the patient walks in the door. The blood glucose hardly matters – it only begins to have importance as the response to treatment is assessed. Getting the blood glucose back to normal, and especially keeping it there, is a problem that taxes our ingenuity far more than the diagnosis of diabetes.

Prevalence of diabetes

Widely differing estimates of prevalence are quoted by various sources, mainly because of lack of any universally acceptable definition of what is diabetes and what is not. The experts know that blood glucose increases with age, yet many of the population surveys which quote high prevalence rates for diabetes seem to ignore this aspect. Diabetes detection drives, whether conducted for epidemiological research purposes or as part of health care programmes, usually bring to light many previously undiagnosed cases, but the vast majority of these are elderly asymptomatic patients. In other words there are very few amongst the general public who are suffering for want of insulin injections. Such patients will present with florid symptoms. On the other hand, the mildly asymptomatic or borderline abnormal patient will almost certainly show improvement in glucose tolerance by moderating his intake of carbohydrate calories.

Table 5.2 shows a suggested range of blood glucose values in different age groups. Until there is universal agreement about what is to be regarded as diabetes the range quoted is only a general guideline.

Prevalence by age   The vast majority of diabetics are in the older age groups. With an overall prevalence of about 1% in the population, amongst children of school age there are only 1–2 per 1,000 (Chapter 12) but about 1 in 50 of those aged over 50 years are known to be diabetic. Looked at another way the *incidence* of new cases related to the age bands shown in Table 5.2 is as follows:

Age in years	Percentage of total
Less than 20	5
20–39	10
40–59	40
60 +	45

Most disagreement between different surveys relates to the older age groups because of the previously mentioned lack of consensus about what is diabetes and what is not. There is more agreement in most studies about the low prevalence of juvenile-onset diabetes. Because of the relationship to histocompatibility 'susceptibility' antigens (HLA) (Chapter 4, p. 42) in juvenile-onset diabetes, differing prevalence rates in some populations may be related to differing frequencies of HLA patterns. Thus in Japan, where HLA B8 is virtually absent and HLA B15 is more common, juvenile-onset diabetes is extremely rare[3]. But even if more widespread studies of HLA bring a new clarity to the epidemiology of juvenile-onset diabetes we shall still be left with the problem of where normality ends and diabetes begins in the rest of the population. If this problem worries you, test an evening urine sample for glucose: if negative you're almost certainly (so far) one of the ninety and nine without diabetes.

Further Reading

1 Kutter D. (1977) *Rapid Clinical Diagnostic Tests.* Munich: Urban & Schwarzenberg
2 Jarrett R.J. (1976) Epidemiology of diabetes. *Br. J. hosp. Med.,* **16**, 200–204
3 Cudworth A.G. (1978) Type 1 diabetes mellitus. *Diabetologia,* **14**, 281–292
4 Keen H., Jarrett R.J. & Alberti K.G.M.M. (1979) Diabetes mellitus: a new look at diagnostic criteria. *Diabetologia,* **16**, 283–285

CHAPTER 6

Lipid Metabolism and Diabetes

Fat is an immensely useful commodity. It provides an efficient source of energy, it insulates the body and – properly distributed – it can help in winning beauty contests. But too much can be embarrassingly counter-productive. Those who build up vast reserves of this high-energy fuel increasingly impede the efficient function of their cardiac output through fat deposition amongst the fibres of heart muscle besides diminishing the general mobility of the body. We were certainly designed to use fat for energy storage, but its efficiency implies that we should do so sparingly. Consider migrating birds where mobility is the essence of survival. Fat is their main fuel, yet they never carry such great quantities that take-off would be prevented.

Many diabetics have too much fat fuel on board. Not surprisingly, there is a close metabolic relationship between obese diabetics and obese non-diabetics. The latter have several 'diabetic' abnormalities in their metabolism of insulin and carbohydrate. For instance, obese patients are characterised by having hyperinsulinism with normal or decreased glucose tolerance – in other words they have a degree of insulin resistance. Likewise, hyperinsulinism and hyperglycaemia go hand in hand in early maturity-onset diabetes besides arising frequently in patients treated with insulin. Excessive insulin favours fat storage. This does not necessarily mean that insulin controls obesity. After all, insulin is secreted physiologically in response to feeding, but those who are obese have something wrong with their appetites and their ability to read their fuel gauges sensibly. If diabetics are treated inappropriately with insulin obesity will be aggravated; thus we can identify several circumstances in which there may be insulin excess and fat storage:

    eating to excess in the non-diabetic,
    excessive insulin therapy in the diabetic, and
    stimulation of excessive insulin secretion by the inappropriate
        use of sulphonylurea drugs (Chapter 11, p.142) in mildly
        obese diabetics.

However, there will often be a lack of insulin in diabetes. The essence of insulin lack is mobilisation of storage fat into the blood – the melting down of flesh and limbs – and diabetes is an ideal model system in which to study fat storage, fat release and fat transport in the blood. It also serves to remind us that the liver is essential in nutrient regulation.

Fat metabolism in the liver: the parting of the ways

The liver alone has the ability to direct fatty acids into one or other of two fundamentally different pathways:

> triglyceride synthesis for transport to the periphery – fuel storage; or
> oxidation to ketone bodies as instant fuel for muscle or brain – fuel burning.

How does the liver decide between triglyceride synthesis for fuel storage or fatty acid oxidation to ketone bodies? The answer lies in hormone balance. Insulin has to make its way in the metabolic jungle as the main hormone lowering the blood glucose and favouring fat storage. Catecholamines, glucagon and cortisol – the hormones of stress – at times aided and abetted by growth hormone, T S H and A C T H are the hormones of fat release. Thus in the balance between storage and release, insulin takes on the field virtually single-handed. When healthy man over-eats, insulin secretion is stimulated and the liver guides excess calories into triglyceride synthesis. When insulin is lacking, however, as in severe diabetes – and especially when overwhelmed by the hormones of stress – ketogenesis will be the major metabolic pathway.

The parting of the ways in liver – triglyceride synthesis or oxidation of fatty acids (FFA) to ketones – is fundamental to understanding what happens in mild or more severe diabetes. The mild diabetic will have sufficient insulin in the portal circulation to allow triglyceride synthesis; moreover, this pathway tends to be stimulated by excess intake of carbohydrate (as in Mrs. Sweet-tooth's case, Chapter 3), or by alcohol consumption. In severe insulin deficiency on the other hand, FFA arriving from the periphery will be partially oxidised to swamp the circulation with ketone bodies. These pathways which FFA follow, depending upon the insulin status of the liver are contrasted in Fig. 6.1.

Understanding fuel storage and release also depends on examination of two other fundamental aspects:

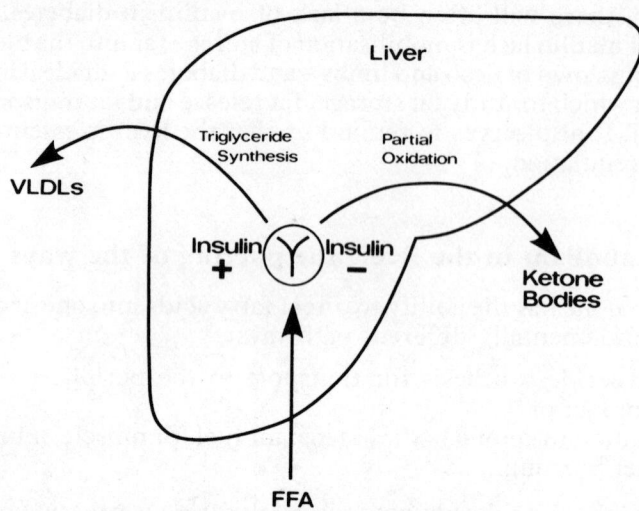

Fig. 6.1 The parting of the ways. Free fatty acid (FFA) metabolism to triglyceride and VLDLs in insulin excess or partial oxidation to ketone bodies in insulin lack. Insulin lack (or antagonism by glucagon) will stimulate the coupled carnitine acyltransferase system which transfers metabolites into the mitochondrial matrix for partial oxidation to ketones (see Fig. 4.6, Chapter 4)

lipid transport in the blood, and
fat metabolism in adipose tissue.

These are worthy of study, not only because they are the foundation of nutrient distribution, but particularly because they are essential to the explanation of the varying degrees of severity of diabetes and of the development of ketoacidosis. Moreover, as the reader will become aware in later chapters, abnormal lipid metabolism forges a common bond between diabetes and its henchman – degenerative vascular disease, especially atheroma.

Lipid transport in the blood   The suitability of fat for energy storage relates to its insolubility in water and because of this insolubility the body requires a special transport and delivery system for fat, fatty acids and their associates – the various *lipoproteins*. Just as modern man must know his way about town, discriminating between taxi-cabs, omnibuses and vans, so those who seek to know their way about lipid metabolism must be able to distinguish the nature and purpose of each of the following (Fig. 6.2):

chylomicra;
very-low-density lipoproteins (VLDL);
low-density lipoproteins (LDL);
high-density lipoproteins (HDL);
fatty acids (FFA); and
ketone bodies.

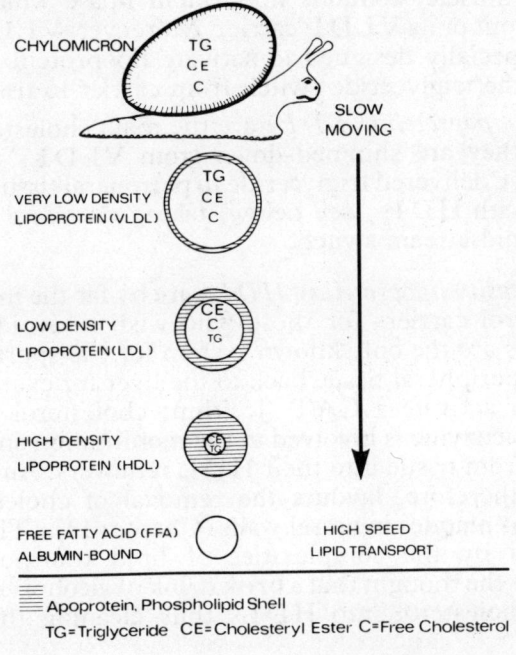

Fig. 6.2 The plasma lipoproteins. The relative densities and composition of the various lipoproteins and albumin-bound free fatty acid

Expert lipid-spotters can also recognise IDLs (intermediate density lipoproteins) and know where to look out for off-loading enzymes like lipoprotein lipase, or those which switch cholesterol from one truck to another in mid-plasma traffic stream.

Chylomicra The chylomicron is a large snail-pace lipid transporter concerned with dietary fat. Triglyceride and cholesterol absorbed from the diet in the small intestine are rolled into chylomicra travelling via the thoracic duct to the blood stream. Triglycerides are off-loaded into adipose tissue and muscle while the cholesterol-containing remnants are taken up by the liver so that 12–14 hours after fat ingestion, chylomicra virtually disappear from plasma.

Very-low-density lipoproteins (VLDL)   These mainly carry triglycerides. They may be formed either in the small intestine to pick up dietary triglyceride or in the liver to collect endogenously synthesised triglyceride. The capillary endothelium of adipose tissue (and muscle) contains lipoprotein lipase which transfers triglyceride out of its VLDL carrier. Moreover, VLDL apolipoprotein is specially designed to activate lipoprotein lipase, thus facilitating the triglyceride switch from carrier to tissue depot.

Low-density lipoproteins (LDL) are the main cholesterol carrier: in a sense they are slimmed-down from VLDLs. Thus after VLDLs have delivered triglyceride to peripheral tissue they come in contact with HDLs (see below) taking on board cholesterol esters in a mid-stream switch.

Tiny high-density lipoproteins (HDL) are by far the most important cholesterol carriers for those who wish to avoid atheroma. Thus HDLs are the only known system for transporting cholesterol out of peripheral tissue back to the liver for excretion in the bile. HDLs activate LCAT (lecithin: cholesterol acyl transferase). This enzyme is involved in the mobilisation and uptake of cholesterol from tissue into their HDL removers. An abundance of HDLs, therefore, favours the removal of cholesterol from atheromatous plaques in vessel walls (Chapter 13). (Those feeling rather jaded by the complexities of lipid transport may be heartened by the thought that a brisk drink of alcohol enhances the uptake of cholesterol into HDLs thus cleaning the coronary arteries.)

Free fatty acid (FFA) transport   This is a high speed transport system in which FFA released from adipose tissue is bound to albumin to form the simplest and fastest moving of the plasma lipids. Although the plasma concentration of FFA may be only 0·5 mmol/1 (14 mg/100 ml), 5–10 g per hour can be shuttled from fat stores to the liver or muscle for fuel. Neutral fat is a combination of glycerol and fatty acids. So when FFA is released from adipose tissue glycerol is simultaneously released into the blood stream. Because glycerol cannot be re-utilised in adipose tissue, blood glycerol concentration reflects the rate of lipolysis.

Ketone bodies are a water soluble form of fat fuel produced by the liver when FFAs are directed into the oxidative pathways of ketogenesis. Normally oxidised in muscle for energy, the accumulation of ketone bodies in the plasma is good evidence of accelerated lipolysis (Chapters 2, p.20; 4, p.52; 7, p.85).

Fat metabolism in adipose tissue   Preoccupied with watching saturated fat in the diet or having his blood lipids measured, modern man often ignores his fat stores. Whether the glutton's excess calories are of fat, sugar or protein matters little, for metabolic pathways will steer extra fuel towards storage in adipose tissue. Insulin, secreted in response to feeding, will stimulate storage in several ways.

1 In the liver glucose can be converted through the glycolytic pathway to *pyruvate* or *glycerol*.
2 In the presence of insulin *pyruvate* is metabolised to acetyl-CoA. These two carbon fragments are built up into long chain fatty acids because the key enzyme acetyl-CoA carboxylase is stimulated by insulin.
3 Glucose-derived *glycerol* (or glycerol released by lipolysis) can then condense with the fatty acids to form neutral fat (triglyceride).
4 Thus triglyceride-rich V L D Ls formed in the liver will arrive at adipose tissue where, in the presence of insulin, lipoprotein lipase will allow fatty acids to be discharged from their V L D L transporters.
5 Simultaneously, insulin increases the uptake of glucose into the adipose cell to form *glycerol* which can condense with the V L D L-derived fatty acids, again to form neutral fat.
6 There is some evidence that in the presence of high insulin levels of overnutrition steps (1) and (2) may also occur in adipose tissue.

In situations of insulin deficiency, or if the anti-insulin counter-regulatory hormones, catecholamines, cortisol, glucagon, and growth hormone, are increased *lipolysis* will be stimulated and the fat cell switches from storage to release. Free fatty acids and glycerol are then melted into the circulation, providing the liver with the essential fuels of fasting or starvation.

Variations on the theme of storage and release

Complex situations of imbalance between the liver and the peripheral metabolism can arise in diabetes. In mild diabetes, or in those partially or inadequately treated with insulin, there may be sufficient insulin in the portal circulation to allow the liver to favour triglyceride synthesis, yet out in the periphery insulin may be scarce so that fat release (*lipolysis*) is enhanced. This imbalance between the centre and periphery – well known to the student of bureaucratic government – can foul the channels of communication in the diabetic, allowing an ever changing panorama of lipids in the blood transport system. Thus V L D Ls are frequently increased in mild diabetes due to a combination of hepatic synthesis and lack of sufficient insulin in the periphery to allow lipoprotein lipase to handle them. Peripheral insulin lack simultaneously favours lipolysis with F F A and glycerol pouring out of adipose tissue. Hence, estimation of blood lipids in diabetics may reveal various abnormalities affected by fluctuations in diabetic control, diet or degree of insulin deficiency.

Blood lipids in diabetes

Although classification of the various blood-lipid abnormalities is now widely accepted, the system cannot always be applied sensibly to diabetics. Non-diabetic abnormalities tend to be relatively steady states, whereas the diabetic may cascade through several lipid abnormalities with fluctuations in diabetic control – especially those who are ketoacidosis-prone. If the reader finds lipid abnormalities difficult to understand at the best of times, diabetes certainly adds spice to the problem.

In diabetes the following abnormalities may be found:

1 *In ketoacidosis*   Due to severe insulin lack lipoprotein lipase is inhibited and thus lipid cannot be cleared from the circulation. Even though the patient may not have eaten for two days, the plasma is turbid with significantly increased triglyceride levels.

2 *Poor control*   V L D L triglyceride is frequently elevated due to the imbalance between hepatic production and peripheral clearing. Excessive dietary intake, especially of carbohydrate and alcohol will stimulate endogenous V L D L production from the liver.

3 *Diabetic renal disease* (Chapter 14)   Hypercholesterolaemia will accompany the hypoproteinaemia of diabetic protein-losing nephropathy.

4 Besides the above secondary forms of hyperlidipaemia, the patient may have one of the primary hyperlipidaemias with glucose intolerance as an associated feature. Xanthelasma, and eruptive or tuberous xanthomata (Chapter 20) should

alert the observer to a primary lipid disorder. These lipid abnormalities include:

Type IIa: LDL↑, plasma cholesterol↑

Type IIb: LDL↑, plasma cholesterol↑
VLDL↑, plasma triglyceride↑

Type III: abnormal LDL, plasma cholesterol↑ and triglyceride↑

Type IV: VLDL↑, plasma triglyceride↑

The well-controlled diabetic, without renal or other complications should have normal fasting blood lipid values. The possible relationship between cholesterol, triglycerides, HDLs or VLDLs and atheroma in diabetes is discussed in Chapter 13.

Management

Management of lipid abnormalities in diabetic patients involves the following elements:

1 bring diabetes under control (Chapters 10, 11);
2 control diet in the overweight (Chapter 9);
3 assess and limit alcohol consumption; and
4 medication should be reserved for diet-resistant disorders or those who will not follow dietary advice; hypercholesterolaemia responds to clofibrate (Atromid-S); hypertriglyceridaemia responds in some cases, alternatively nicotinic acid or the bile-acid sequestrant cholestyramine (Questran) may be tried.

In all cases, however, reading the fuel guage and acting accordingly is the basis of management.

Further Reading

1 Newsholme E.A. & Start C. (1973) *Regulation in Metabolism.* London: John Wiley
2 Lewis B. (1976) *The Hyperlipidaemias, Clinical and Laboratory Practice.* Oxford: Blackwell Scientific Publications.
3 Alberti K.G.M.M. & Hockaday T.D.R. (1975) The biochemistry of the complications of diabetes mellitus. In *Complications of Diabetes* (Ed. H. Keen & J. Jarrett) London: Edward Arnold, 221–264

Diabetic Coma, Ketoacidosis and other forms of Severe Metabolic Decompensation, including Lactic Acidosis and Hyperosmolar States

Before the insulin era, diabetic coma was a death sentence. Now commuted to a life dependent upon insulin injections, diabetic coma is still one of the most challenging and at times alarming emergencies in medical management, but one which can dramatically demonstrate the value of judicious fluid and electrolyte replacement therapy when successfully conducted. Unfortunately, the expression diabetic coma has become inappropriate to our better understanding of the complexities of the metabolic derangements and at times the phrase is misused or is frankly misleading. Originally depicting the final stage in untreated diabetes resulting from insulin lack in the pre-insulin era, diabetic coma described patients who were hyperglycaemic, wasted and severely dehydrated: with the hand of death upon them, these luckless diabetics slowly lapsed into coma. But faced today with a diabetic in coma it is important at the outset to attempt to distinguish between the following main causes:

> hyperglycaemia,
> hypoglycaemia,
> coma due to other factors – for example uraemia, stroke, meningitis, drugs or lactic acidosis

Some doctors still have difficulty in distinguishing between the *gradual* process of hyperglycaemia and the *sudden* loss of consciousness of hypoglycaemic coma arising from insulin excess (Chapter 18). Hypoglycaemia can overtake a diabetic in a few minutes while hyperglycaemia builds up slowly over several hours (or days). Fear of confusing these alternatives still leads some doctors to steer clear of insulin-treated diabetes. For those in a diagnostic dilemma it is just as important, however, to consider other possibilities. Diabetics have no immunity to other disease, thus other causes of coma – uraemia, meningitis or drugs, for example – must be considered. And there is another problem: we are now able to distinguish clinically and biochemically between patients having the hyperglycaemia of tear-away gluconeogenesis with its associated ketoacidosis (Chapters 2 & 4) and a much slower process, more often seen in the elderly, where impaired renal function and severe dehydration rather than gluconeogenesis lead to profound hyperglycaemia. Moreover, where acidosis is the major problem, lactic or renal acidosis must be distinguished from typical ketoacidosis.

One way out of the difficulty is to drop the term coma and concentrate on various forms or degrees of metabolic decompensation. Looked at this way the following basic elements mix to greater or lesser extent:

hyperglycaemia,
dehydration, electrolyte upset and impaired renal function,
and
metabolic acidosis.

Whether the patient is alert, drowsy or comatose will depend, not only on the metabolic upset and its effect on the vital functions (pulse rate, blood pressure and respiration), but also on the underlying condition precipitating the disturbance.

Typical diabetic ketoacidosis

First of all, let us examine typical diabetic ketoacidosis as seen in the young untreated patient where there is no other disease affecting renal, cardiac or hepatic function. Remember the salient features of gluconeogenesis and ketoacidosis – the melting down of flesh and limbs – resulting from insulin lack as outlined in Chapter 2 and detailed in Chapter 4.

Insulin lack   Absolute deficiency of insulin leads to rapidly-accelerating fat breakdown in adipose tissue stores (*lipolysis*) releasing large quantities of free fatty acids (FFA) into the circulation (Chapter 6; Fig. 7.1). Simultaneously, protein wasting leaches amino acids into the circulation providing the liver with the carbon skeletons for gluconeogenesis. Fuelled by hepatic oxidation of FFA, gluconeogenesis swamps the circulation with glucose and simultaneously ketogenesis generates ketone bodies

(3-hydroxybutyrate, acetoaceotate and acetone) (Fig. 7.2). The organic acids 3-hydroxybutyric and acetoacetic acid are fully dissociated at physiological pH causing metabolic acidosis.

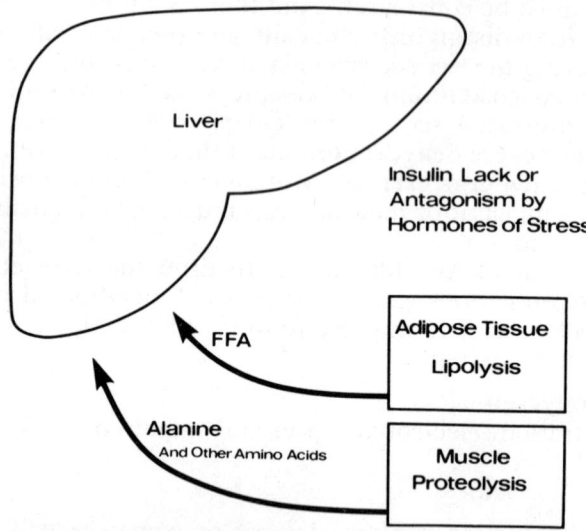

Fig. 7.1 Lipolysis producing free fatty acids (FFA) and proteolysis releasing alanine and other amino-acids in insulin lack

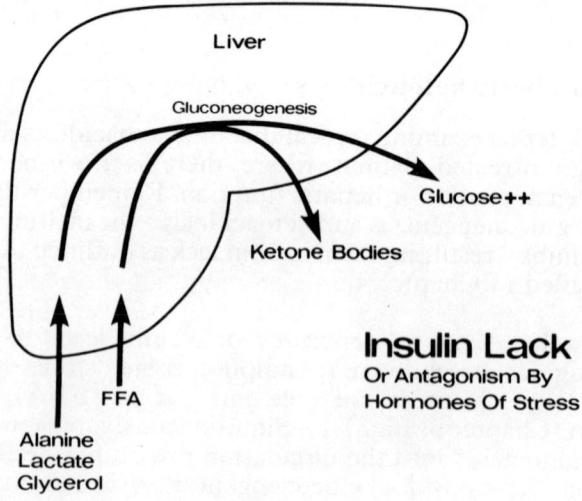

Fig. 7.2 Gluconeogenesis and ketogenesis go hand in hand

Besides driving the patient into lipolysis and gluconeogenesis the underlying insulin lack prevents utilisation of glucose by the peripheral tissues causing overflow into the urine.

Osmotic diuresis   This is inevitably induced by the sharp rise in the blood glucose. The massive osmotic diuresis of glucose involves distal renal tubular loss of water and sodium leading to a fall in the extracellular fluid volume. The associated reduced plasma volume (hypovolaemia) leads to haemo-concentration, tachycardia, hypotension and impairment of renal function; the last decreases the renal ability to excrete H^+ ions, aggravating the metabolic acidosis which further stimulates hyperventilation and potassium loss from inside cells. The acidosis adversely affects cardiac function and causes peripheral vasodilation. Despite hyperventilation, oxygen exchange in the lungs becomes impaired as a result of the ventilation-perfusion imbalance of hypovolaemia. At this stage urgent resuscitation is essential.

Diagnosis

Diabetes is often much easier to diagnose in theory than in practice. Without a nose for sweet apples (or nail varnish remover) detecting the acetone in the patient's exhaled breath or the obvious clues of sugar and ketones in the urine, the doctor called to a sickbed may not suspect diabetes or immediately notice the degree of dehydration (the peripheral vasodilation of acidaemia can be misleading). The drowsiness, anorexia, or vomiting are common to so many other ailments both minor or serious, and tachycardia, hypotension and hypovolaemia might reasonably be attributed to the associated infection which often triggers diabetes. Of course, it is much easier in the known diabetic, or if a relative cues the doctor with a remark related to the classic symptoms: 'he's been drinking so much these past few days . . .' Urine containing sugar and ketones in large amounts as well as a small quantity of protein is usually easily obtained. If not, a Ketostix (Chapter 5) showing a strongly positive reaction when dipped in a sample of the patient's plasma is perhaps the best confirmation of diabetic ketoacidosis. Indeed, on admission to hospital the diagnosis is incomplete without this evidence (those without facilities for separating plasma can allow a sample of blood to clot and dip the Ketostix in the supernatent serum). From then on, with the aid of a bio-chemistry laboratory and intravenous fluid therapy, it's plain sailing . . .

Biochemistry

The value of biochemistry is now acknowledged, yet too often the hospital doctor is so bemused by watching the serum potassium or plasma pH that he ignores valuable information relevant to management in the deviations of other significant electrolyte data. Figure 7.3 shows the expected changes in typical diabetic

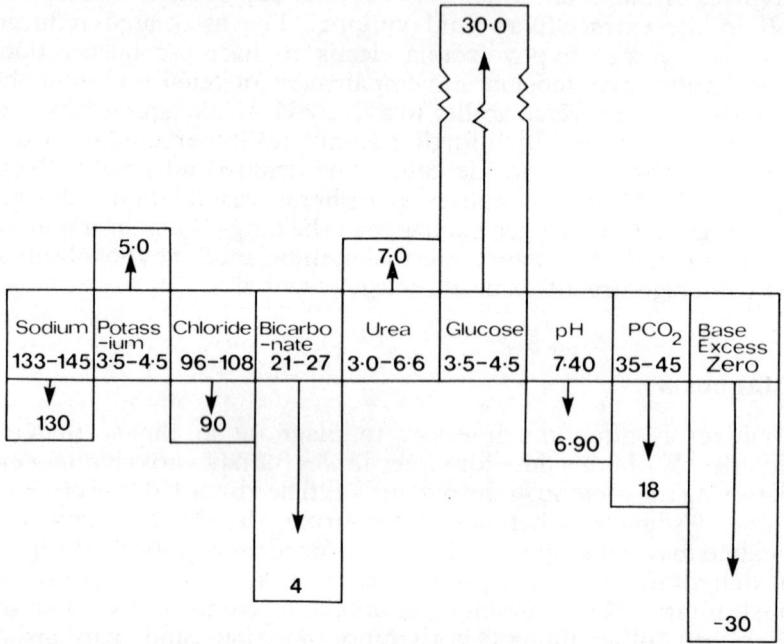

Fig. 7.3 Biochemical changes in diabetic ketoacidosis. Normal values and typical deviations upwards or downwards in arrowed boxes (mmol/l except pCO_2 in mm of mercury)

ketoacidosis. But things in medicine are rarely typical, so studying the reasons for each deviation is valuable. A better understanding of possible variations on the theme of acidosis is essential for improved patient management.

Blood glucose   The marked rise in blood glucose is due to the combined effect of increased production (gluconeogenesis) and impaired tissue utilisation. The rise soon exceeds the reabsorptive capacity of the renal tubules (the renal threshold) and glycosuria results.

Youngsters usually have a relatively low renal threshold (Chapter 5) to glucose so that their urinary loss is greater than in older patients who tend to have poorer renal function. Because of the enhanced osmotic diuresis of youth, the loss of water, sodium, potassium and chloride can be massive. Typically, the blood glucose is in the region of 25–30 mmol/l (450–540 mg/100 ml). If the value is higher expect a greater impairment in renal function (see blood urea).

Sodium Plasma sodium concentration measured in mmol/litre depends upon the relative amounts of sodium and water in the extracellular fluid (ECF). Thus a low sodium value may be due either to water excess or to salt depletion. Likewise, a high value may result from dehydration or salt excess. ECF volume depends upon the content of sodium which is the principal cation in the ECF. In ketoacidosis water and salt are lost in the osmotic diuresis and perhaps also in vomitus. Both the urine and vomitus are *hypotonic* with regard to sodium, thus water loss outstrips that of salt and the tendency is towards *hypernatraemia* (additional water loss by evaporation in the compensating hyperventilation of acidosis will increase the water loss). Thus in the early stages of hyperglycaemia and osmotic fluid loss both the falling EFC volume and hypernatraemia will stimulate *thirst*. Unless cast away in an open boat, the patient responds by drinking water rather than brine and hence converts a tendency to *hypernatraemia* into *hyponatraemia*. Thus the more the patient is able to drink the lower the plasma sodium. In contrast, where there is clouding of consciousness the patient fails to drink adequately, creating a tendency to hypernatraemia (see also hyperosmolar effect of hyperglycaemia, page 100).

Factitious hyponatraemia In some patients (Mrs. Spratt, Chapter 3) the plasma is milky in appearance due to excess of triglycerides. Hyponatraemia (low sodium when expressed in mmol/litre of *plasma*) is often found in these cases as the water content of the plasma in which the sodium salts are dissolved is reduced by displacement by fat. However, osmolality (corrected for glucose or urea) which is expressed in mosmol/kg water will be normal.

Blood urea The blood urea tends to rise slightly due to increased protein breakdown and then later increasing sodium depletion causes a further rise as the glomerular filtration rate diminishes. Because this is an essentially pre-renal uraemia, the urea rises out of step with the creatinine. A blood urea of 6·0–8·0 mmol/l (36–48 mg/100 ml) is typical in adolescence. Higher values usually mean a greater degree of renal impairment and especially in older patients when over 20 mmol/l (120 mg/100 ml) imply that there is pre-renal uraemia superimposed upon renal uraemia. Healthy kidneys make the doctor's work relatively easy – the higher the urea the greater the biochemical and medical skills required in management.

Potassium   Here there is a paradox! Note that the serum value is usually elevated yet there is an overall body deficit. This is because several factors accelerate the passage of potassium from the intra- to the extra-cellular fluid:

acidosis,
anoxia,
increased protein breakdown, and
interrupted carbohydrate metabolism.

The potassium which has passed from the cells to the extra-cellular fluid is then lost in the urine due to

osmotic diuresis,
stress of infection or ketoacidosis, and
covering some of the acetoacetate anion.

Vomiting will aggravate the body loss. Remember that successful treatment of the acidosis will shift potassium back into cells. The more successful the treatment the greater the need to start intravenous potassium replacement early.

pH   The metabolic acidosis is mainly due to the ketone production and partly due to lactate formation (see lactic acidosis, Chapter 4). Any renal tubular defect (especially pyelonephritis) may impair the ability to excrete H^+ ions (Chapter 14). Always check the plasma ketones with Ketostix. Metabolic acidosis without excess plasma ketones implies either lactic acidosis or a renal defect in H^+ ion excretion.

PCO_2 and PO_2   Hyperventilation blows off CO_2 (and water) from the lungs causing the PCO_2 to drop to around 20 mmHg or less. Once the patient is in a terminal phase of hypovolaemia, oxygen exchange becomes impaired (the shock-lung syndrome) inducing a fall in the PO_2 and justifying the use of oxygen therapy.

Base excess   Characteristically the base excess will fall to around – 30 mmol/l in severe ketoacidosis. Patients in a lesser degree of ketonaemia – such as minor diabetic upsets or starvation – often may be rescued without intravenous fluid therapy if the base excess is not worse than -12, provided that their fluid and electrolyte status is otherwise satisfactory.

The plasma bicarbonate and the *anion gap*[2]   A metabolic acidosis is accompanied by low bicarbonate levels. In some cases consideration of the *anion gap* may be of diagnostic help. Normally the difference between the sum of the plasma anions (chloride and bicarbonate) and cations (sodium and potassium) gives a calculated anion gap of 10–20 mmol/l. The unmeasured anions in the gap are mainly sulphate, phosphate and proteins (Fig. 7.4).

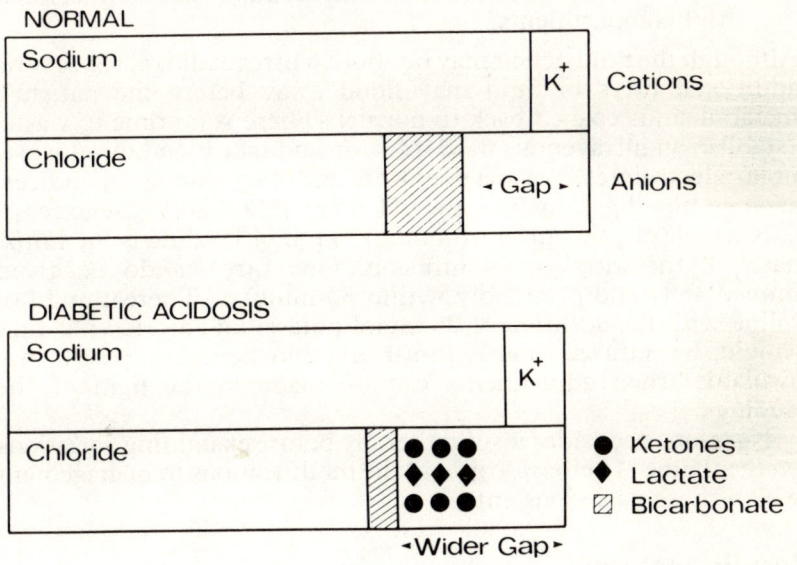

Fig. 7.4 The anion gap. Normally the difference between the sum of the plasma cations (sodium and potassium) and anions (chloride and bicarbonate) gives a calculated gap of 10–20 mmol/l. In diabetic acidosis there is a wider gap due to ketones or lactate

Ketoacidosis, lactic acidosis or the accumulation of sulphate and phosphate that accompanies azotaemic renal failure are three forms of acidosis which widen the anion gap. On the other hand bicarbonate loss in renal tubular acidosis results in an acidosis with a normal anion gap.

Management of diabetic ketoacidosis

Effective treatment depends upon:

intravenous fluid therapy and
insulin.

Intravenous fluid therapy is the patient's lifeline. Three
components are fundamental to the correction of ketoacidosis:

Sodium to restore the plasma volume without overloading the
interstitial fluid volume,
water to correct the plasma osmolality and maintain urine
flow, and
Potassium to correct the body deficit and to maintain the
proper balance between the intracellular and extracellular
fluid compartments.

Although the fluid deficit may be about 6 litres at diagnosis, several
additional litres of fluid may flood away before the patient's
metabolism is coaxed back to normal. There is no time to waste:
establish an intravenous fluid infusion and take blood for glucose,
urea, electrolytes, plasma Ketostix and haematological indices;
arrange blood gas analysis for pH, PO_2, PCO_2 and base excess.

Normal (physiological isotonic, 154 mmol/l) saline is the initial
basis of the intravenous infusion. One litre should be given
immediately and preferably within 30 minutes. Thereafter 1 l of
saline with the addition of 20 mmol potassium chloride per litre
should be infused hourly until the biochemistry results are
available when adjustments can be made in the light of the
findings.

Next let us consider insulin therapy before examining variations
on the theme of ketoacidosis and the modifications in management
which these variations entail.

Insulin therapy

Ideas about insulin dosage and delivery have turned somersaults in
recent years. Previously, most experts thought in terms of large
doses, often advising 100 units of insulin at a time or even more if
the patient failed to respond adequately: now small is beautiful.
Recently, many patients in ketoacidosis have been rescued successfully and even more efficiently on much smaller doses of
insulin, averaging around 5–10 units per hour. This does not mean
that insulin therapy should be turned into a competition aimed at
giving the smallest dose possible. Instead this new approach allows
us to take stock and make two observations:

1 Intravenous fluid therapy is the foundation of management. Attempts to establish normal metabolism with insulin cannot succeed, regardless of dosage, without first restoring blood volume, plasma osmolality and normal renal function by appropriate intravenous fluid therapy.

2 In the first few vital hours of treatment, the precise dose of insulin is relatively unimportant provided that a reasonable amount is delivered by a reliable route. Large, small or intermediate doses are effective.

In normal, less urgent circumstances, insulin is usually given subcutaneously (Chapter 10). However, in ketoacidosis or other forms of severe electrolyte disturbance, absorption of insulin from injection sites would be too slow and erratic even using soluble or one of the highly purified neutral short-acting insulins (Chapter 10). Two alternatives are successful:

intramuscular injections repeated at hourly intervals, or
continuous intravenous infusion.

Intramuscular injections are simple, safe and effective if, after an initial dose of 20 units, 5–10 units are injected hourly (proportionately less in children: 0·1 unit per kg) until the blood glucose has fallen to below 15 mmol/l (270 mg/100 ml).

Intravenous insulin is rapid and reliable, but because the half-life is about four minutes, continuous infusion is required to maintain an adequate serum concentration of around 50–100 micro units/ml. If insulin is added directly to the intravenous fluid infusion some will be lost by adhesion to the glass or plastic of the giving set. This difficulty can be overcome by a variety of manipulations each having advocates and critics, advantages and disadvantages:

1 giving larger doses of insulin (20 units per 500 ml added to each bottle freshly at the time of use);
2 using an infusion pump (24 units in 20 ml saline made up freshly every four hours) infused at a rate of 5 units per hour;
3 adding albumin or polygeline to the insulin solution to avoid absorption on to glassware and plastic; and
4 some of the patient's own blood can be added or drawn back into the giving set if no albumin or polygeline is available.

The demonstration that a satisfactory and reliable fall in the hyperglycaemia of ketoacidosis can be achieved with small amounts of insulin has been dramatically instructive in causing us to re-think the previously accepted blunderbuss approach. But the use of an infusion pump, additives, or small amounts of the patient's own blood makes treatment more complicated. Thus either the hourly intramuscular regime or the continuous infusion of larger doses of insulin have much to commend them.

There is much more to the treatment of ketoacidosis or other forms of severe metabolic decompensation, however, than infusion of intravenous saline, insulin and potassium. Let us consider other aspects by looking at some practical problems.

Some examples of acute metabolic problems

1 Tom Brown's schooldays as an insulin-dependent diabetic were uneventful (medically) until his final term. Now admitted to hospital in typical diabetic ketoacidosis: drowsy, dehydrated, polyuric, occasionally retching and apparently in abdominal pain; gluconeogenesis and ketogenesis in full flight with hypovolaemia, hyperventilation and metabolic acidosis; pulse rate 125/min, BP 90/60 mmHg; urine containing more than 2% glucose and strongly positive for ketones. On removing blood for biochemical estimation, blood gas analysis and haematological indices, the junior hospital doctor confirms the provisional diagnosis by checking for plasma ketones. He starts treatment with intravenous physiological saline and in searching for a cause of the ketoacidosis notes the tense abdomen. Quick thinking: vomiting, abdominal pain, tense abdomen and a white cell count of 15,000 cells per cubic mm – appendicitis. But the consultant surgeon points out that the white cell count is usually raised in ketoacidosis and that the tense abdomen is common in children or adolescents in ketoacidosis. He also points out that if ketoacidosis is secondary to infection the temperature may not be elevated because the acidosis causes vasodilation. Indeed, the patient may be hypothermic. Thus in ketoacidosis absence of pyrexia does not exclude, and neutrophilia does not indicate, infection. The biochemical data are as follows:

Plasma sodium	130 mmol/l or meq/l
Plasma potassium	5 mmol/l or meq/l
Plasma chloride	90 mmol/l or meq/l
Plasma bicarbonate	4 mmol/l or meq/l
Plasma urea	7 mmol/l or 42 mg/100 ml
Plasma glucose	30 mmol/l or 540 mg/100 ml
Blood pH	6·90
Blood PCO_2	18 mmHg
Blood base excess	− 30 mmol/l

The typical data in a ketoacidotic adolescent (see Fig. 7.3) show that the urea is only slightly elevated and as a consequence of the greater osmotic loss, the blood glucose does not rise as much as in those with a poor GFR.

The junior doctor arranges an intravenous régime of insulin therapy and having given a litre of saline quickly, also adds potassium. He recalls that frequent biochemical estimations are advised, but the surgeon has further advice – 'go back and look at the patient'. If the vital functions (pulse rate, BP) have improved, biochemistry will only confirm the clinically obvious. Exit the surgeon in high esteem. Within 2 hours and after 2 litres of intravenous fluid therapy, Tom looks better, and his tense abdomen is settling, but the young doctor is uneasy about the amount of intravenous potassium and consults a more experienced colleague. No problem: a youngster with healthy kidneys, a good urine flow and clinical evidence of improvement is unlikely to be overdosed. And if the blood glucose falls into the hypoglycaemic range? Go back and look at the patient – if the improvement has been marked the tense abdomen with thoughts of appendicectomy can be banished and he will be hungry. Start to feed him: remember that he has just been rescued from an acute catabolic phase and dietetic restriction of carbohydrate is temporarily unnecessary.

But the junior doctor has a good question: if it wasn't appendicitis, why did Tom develop ketoacidosis? He gets his answer in a chance remark made by a visiting school-friend 'Pity he wasn't allowed to go to the school dance because of his diabetes'. The adolescent had rebelled, skipped taking his insulin with the result that unrestrained lipolysis and gluconeogenesis led to ketoacidosis. How is it proved when the patient will never admit anything? The doctor puts his suspicions to the senior clinician on the ward round. 'Yes, ketoacidosis is often a social problem, yet the duty doctor is so excited about dealing with a medical emergency by intravenous manipulation that too often manipulation by the patient is overlooked'. Although ketoacidosis is a medical emergency, its roots often lie in social problems especially in adolescence (Chapter 22).

2 Remember Mrs. Peabody (Chapter 3), aged 44, taking insulin and now admitted in acidosis following a recent urinary infection despite treatment with an antibiotic for the preceding 5 days. Once again the white cell count is elevated, but this time there is infection and no emotional problem. The patient is profoundly dehydrated with marked loss of tissue turgor.

The initial biochemical findings are as follows:

Plasma sodium	134 mmol/l or meq/l
Plasma potassium	5·5 mmol/l or meq/l
Plasma chloride	105 mmol/l or meq/l
Plasma bicarbonate	4 mmol/l or meq/l
Plasma urea	15 mmol/l or 90 mg/100 ml
Plasma glucose	40 mmol/l or 729 mg/100 ml
Blood pH	6·90
Blood PCO_2	20 mmHg.
Blood base excess	−30 mmol/l

The urine contains pus cells, more than 2% sugar and ketones. The junior doctor (now with his recent experience) goes back to look at Mrs. Peabody after the intravenous saline has been infusing for more than three hours. She still looks ghastly and the repeated biochemistry bears this out: pH 7·06, base excess −25 mmol/l. Moreover, the biochemist warns that the plasma ketones are only moderately elevated. What has gone wrong? The junior doctor seeks the help of his senior clinician, outlining the patient's history by telephone: '. . . has required insulin since a urinary infection 4 years previously and has had a recurrence of infection. . . .' He is advised that the underlying problem is acute on chronic pyelonephritis with glomerular dysfunction (note the high urea) and uncontrolled diabetes where the acidosis mainly represents impaired renal tubular function with inability to excrete H^+ ions – a common problem in older diabetics (Chapter 14). The junior doctor is re-assured that the biochemical disturbance should improve with intravenous fluids and is advised to add sodium bicarbonate until the pH is above 7·10 (100 mmol infused over one hour should suffice, although 200 mmol or more may be needed).

Mrs. Peabody responds well and as the urine flow recovers and renal function improves, the vital functions return to normal. During her convalescence an intravenous pyelogram shows bilateral focal pyelonephritis and tests of renal function show that the ability to acidify and concentrate the urine is impaired. When there are underlying renal problems the patient is much more vulnerable to the water and electrolyte upsets of uncontrolled diabetes.

3 Poor Jack Spratt (Chapter 3) is re-admitted to hospital after another myocardial infarct, and simultaneously the hormones of stress (catecholamines, glucagon, and cortisol) strain his already beleaguered beta cells. Nevertheless, the doctors in the intensive care unit are not worried about his diabetes; the fasting blood

glucose is 9·0 mmol/l (162 mg/100 ml) and there is only 0·5% glycosuria without ketonuria. He is treated with a slow infusion of 5% dextrose (1 litre per 24 hours) and subcutaneous insulin in place of his usual oral sulphonylurea therapy.

But the staff become concerned about Jack's falling blood pressure and unstable cardiac rhythm. During the night his general condition deteriorates and he becomes unconscious. The duty doctor re-checks the biochemistry:

Plasma sodium	138 mmol/l or meq/l
Plasma potassium	4·0 mmol/l or meq/l
Plasma chloride	95 mmol/l or meq/l
Plasma bicarbonate	3 mmol/l or meq/l
Plasma urea	9·0 mmol/l or 72 mg/100 ml
Plasma glucose	12·0 mmol/l or 216 mg/100 ml

The low bicarbonate (page 91) suggests acidosis, yet there are no abnormal plasma ketones and although the urea is slightly elevated this is unlikely to be renal acidosis. But it is likely to be the *lactic acidosis* or poor tissue perfusion (Chapter 4). Blood gas analysis is as follows:

Blood pH	7·00
Blood PO_2	40 mmHg
Blood PCO_2	25 mmHg
Blood base excess	− 26 mmol/l

Without waiting for estimation of lactate or the lactate/pyruvate ratio, 200 mmol sodium bicarbonate is given intravenously followed by 5% dextrose with insulin. The low PO_2 is due partly to the poor myocardial function and partly to the shock-lung syndrome. With oxygen therapy, the blood pressure rises and the monitor of central venous pressure shows improvement. Urinary output increases. The following morning the blood gas analysis is nearly normal but there has been a marked swing to hyperglycaemia (blood glucose 25 mmol/l, 450 mg/100 ml). Diabetics in lactic acidosis can be hypoglycaemic, euglycaemic or hyperglycaemic. However, this upswing in blood glucose is often seen as acidosis is corrected and the liver recovers its ability to metabolise lactate through the gluconeogenic pathway. Such diabetics, although possibly relatively euglycaemic at the outset, usually need energetic insulin therapy – not to block gluconeogenesis, which in the context of lactic acidosis is beneficially removing lactate, but rather so that glucose can be utilised in peripheral tissue and metabolised to acetyl CoA and citrate, instead of lactate, as tissue perfusion is simultaneously improved.

Jack Spratt made a good recovery. Interestingly, raised serum transaminase values, previously attributed to myocardial infarction were found to be associated with liver dysfunction traced to a previous problem with alcohol excess. This almost certainly had a bearing on the development of lactic acidosis which is usually multifactorial in its development. Note that Jack Spratt had not been treated with phenformin (Chapter 11). But suppose the previous patient, obese Mrs. Peabody, had been. Remember that her diabetes was originally controlled with oral therapy (Chapter 3) before insulin was started. In her case the underlying renal disease would make her vulnerable to acidosis so that the use of phenformin (which tends to block the hepatic uptake of lactate into the gluconeogenic pathway) would lead to the accumulation of lactic acid, perhaps with any extra exertion. Moreover, the impaired renal function would diminish lactate excretion and also cause retention of phenformin, thus aggravating a vicious circle.

Routine use of sodium bicarbonate   Some clinicians have recommended routine intravenous sodium bicarbonate therapy in diabetic metabolic decompensation but this is unwise. All severe cases of ketoacidosis will have an element of lactic acidosis especially when hypovolaemic (lactic acidosis, Chapter 4) thus when the pH is less than 7·10 or the base excess more abnormal than −20 mmol/l, 50 or 100 mmol of bicarbonate can be helpful. Similarly, it should be given immediately in severe renal or lactic acidosis and in the latter case 500–2000 mmol may be necessary. But its inappropriate use may have adverse effects on the central nervous system by causing a paradoxical fall in the pH of the CSF. If sodium bicarbonate is considered necessary two other measures must be contemplated: oxygen therapy and potassium replacement. Sodium bicarbonate may impair tissue oxidation by altering the shape of the oxyhaemoglobin dissociation curve, and lactic acidosis is so often associated with hypoxia that oxygen therapy is sensible. Improvement in pH with sodium bicarbonate will cause potassium to shift back into cells and intravenous potassium should therefore be given except in the acidosis of renal failure with hyperkalaemia. But the routine use of sodium bicarbonate in all cases leads the doctor into the trap of giving it in error to the hyperosmolar patient (see below) where the serum sodium is already elevated and the plasma pH virtually normal. Reserve sodium bicarbonate for severe acidosis, whether due to keto-, renal or lactic acids. (DCA is an alternative in lactic acidosis, Chapter 4.)

4 Our last example of acute metabolic decompensation is an old man of 70, sent to hospital as an emergency with broncho-pneumonia. On admission it is noted that he is hypothermic, dehydrated and has 2% glycosuria with some acetonuria.

The initial biochemistry is as follows:

Plasma sodium	148 mmol/l or meq/l
Plasma potassium	4·0 mmol/l or meq/l
Plasma bicarbonate	105 mmol/l or meq/l
Plasma chloride	21 mmol/l or meq/l
Plasma urea	24 mmol/l or 145 mg/100 ml
Plasma glucose	45·2 mmol/l or 820 mg/100 ml
Blood pH	7·34
PCO_2	40 mmHg
Blood base excess	− 4 mmol/l

Thus, despite the ketonuria, the striking features are the lack of acidosis and that the plasma urea and glucose are markedly elevated. Note also that, unlike typical ketoacidosis, the serum sodium is elevated so that careless treatment with normal saline might aggravate the biochemical upset. This is a typical case of hyperosmolar diabetes which can best be understood by examining plasma osmolality.

Plasma osmolality   The number of osmotically-active particles in plasma water, or *osmolality*, expressed as mosmol/kg plasma water, can be calculated with reasonable accuracy in healthy subjects by doubling the plasma sodium (mmol/l). For several reasons, including the fact that not all salts are fully dissociated (the osmotic coefficient), potassium and *normal values* for urea and glucose can be ignored. For example, in a normal subject with a sodium of 140 mmol/l, the plasma osmolality can be calculated as $140 \times 2 = 280$ mosmol/kg plasma water, give or take the odd osmole (this calculation is misleading if alcoholic intoxication is present because alcohol contributes significantly to plasma osmolality). Osmolality will be moderately increased if there is elevation of urea or glucose. But when both urea and glucose are markedly elevated, osmolality will be dramatically abnormal. Remember that the sodium is raised in such cases for good measure. Thus, for our patient having a sodium of 148 mmol/l, a urea of 24 mmol/l and a glucose of 45 mmol/l, the osmolality can be calculated:

$$(148 \times 2) + 24 + 45 = 365 \text{ mosmol/kg plasma water}$$

Hyperosmolar effect of hyperglycaemia How does the hyper-osmolar state arise? The answer lies in the effect of hyperglycaemia on body fluid composition. Hyperglycaemia causes a water shift from the intracellular compartment to the ECF leading to intracellular dehydration and extracellular hyponatraemia (plasma sodium usually falls by 1·6 mmol/l (meq/l) for each 5·0 mmol/l (90 mg/100 ml) rise in glucose). But remember that hyperglycaemia causes an osmotic diuresis of hypotonic sodium-containing fluid in the urine, leading to a fall in ECF volume and a tendency to *hypernatraemia*. Often in the elderly this is aggravated by a *failure to drink* in response to the fluid loss and especially in a protracted illness (bronchopneumonia or stroke, for example) the slow but insidious fluid upset can lead to profound intracellular dehydration and a critical fall in the ECF volume. Thus the initial management involves *restoration of ECF volume* using saline or plasma. Thereafter the overriding water loss and hyperglycaemia are best corrected with half-strength saline and insulin, switching to 5% dextrose once the blood glucose is below 15 mmol/l (270 mg/100 ml). The hyperosmolar state is therefore a con-sequence of several days of hypotonic fluid loss during which time the patient has failed to drink adequately. Sometimes in the early stages, however, the hyperglycaemia is aggravated by drinking lemonade or glucose-containing drinks.

General measures and modifications in treatment

In the light of the above examples, it follows that management will depend on

1 the underlying cause of the upset,
2 the severity of the osmotic disturbance, and
3 the nature and cause of any metabolic acidosis, ie. whether predominantly keto-, renal or lactic acidosis.

Thus treatment must be modified to take account of such underlying causes as infection, pyelonephritis or cardiogenic shock. Patients with a predominantly hyperosmolar disturbance should be switched from isotonic to half-strength (0·5 N) saline as soon as the ECF volume has been restored, but when acidosis predominates bicarbonate supplements are important initially, especially in lactic acidosis. Indeed, present evidence suggests that if recognised and treated promptly with bicarbonate (which is widely available) there is no advantage in using DCA (Chapter 4).

How fast should the metabolic upset be corrected? With one

exception a severe hyperosmolar state or metabolic acidosis should be corrected *as fast as possible*. And the exception? A patient who has been hypertonic for several days will have developed a compensating mechanism in the brain by secreting *idiogenic osmoles*[8] causing the brain to expand towards its normal volume. Correction of hypertonicity by rapid replacement of fluid deficits may result in brain swelling. This possibility need only be considered if the hypertonic state has existed for more than four days and is therefore unlikely. Nevertheless, if suspected, initial treatment to restore ECF volume should be prompt, and then replacement should be slowed.

Additional aspects of management depend upon the presence or absence of the following:

Coma The unconscious or semi-conscious patient should have *gastric aspiration* to avoid the inhalation of vomitus from the large amounts of fluid which sometimes accumulate in the stomach. *Catheterisation* of the bladder is sensible either if there is incontinence due to osmotic diuresis or if there is no flow of urine in the first three hours.

Shock Especially for the elderly or following myocardial infarction, a *central venous pressure* line allows prompt yet safe restoration of ECF volume. *Oxygen* should be given in the shock-lung syndrome (page 90) which induces a fall in PO_2. ECG monitoring is also valuable in the shocked, elderly or unconscious patient.

Infection Blood, urine and a throat swab should be sent for culture and antibiotics appropriate to the clinical nature of the infection should be given.

Hypercoaguable state Particularly in the elderly or those with severe hyperosmolar states, blood viscosity and platelet adhesiveness are increased, justifying consideration of the addition of *heparin* to the intravenous régime.

Diffuse intravascular coagulation (DIC) Ketoacidosis or underlying small-blood-vessel disease (Chapter 13) may predispose to DIC. A watch should be maintained for features of bleeding, thrombosis or haemolysis, especially in the deeply unconscious or elderly. When DIC has reduced fibrinogen and platelets below haemostatic levels, *heparin* should be given for 24–48 hours provided that underlying liver disease is excluded, but prevention of DIC by prompt treatment of the acidosis is better.

Treatment is summarised in Table 7.1.

Table 7.1 Management summary

A. ASSESSMENT AND INITIAL TREATMENT

Take account of age, history and clinical findings; examine urine; assess volume depletion by pulse, BP and tissue turgor.

Take blood for biochemistry – urea, electrolytes, bicarbonate and glucose; haematology – Hb WCC.

Measure plasma ketones (KETOSTIX) and blood gases.

If plasma KETOSTIX −ve look for causes of LACTIC ACIDOSIS, HYPEROSMOLAR STATE or other causes of COMA.

INITIAL TREATMENT

Normal Saline: 1 litre in 30 minutes and hourly till biochemistry available.
Insulin: 5 units per hour by infusion pump OR 20 units IM and 5 units IM hourly thereafter. (Soluble, actrapid or neutral insulin – see Chapter 10).
Potassium: Add 20 mmol/l to the second litre of saline in patient with +ve plasma KETOSTIX and passing urine.

Aspirate stomach if unconscious; treat infection with antibiotic; CVP line in elderly or shocked; catheterise if no urine.

B BIOCHEMICAL ASSESSMENT

The correct diagnosis is made and treatment modified at this stage. Discriminate between predominant KETOACIDOSIS, LACTIC ACIDOSIS, HYPEROSMOLAR STATE or OTHER CAUSE.

Sodium: The higher the value the greater the WATER depletion. Consider $\frac{1}{2}$ strength saline as soon as ECF volume restored if initial sodium high.
Urea: The greater the value in excess of 8 mmol/l the poorer the renal function.
Bicarbonate: Low in KETO and LACTIC acidosis.
Glucose: Highest in hyperosmolar state, lowest in lactic acidosis.
pH: If below 7·10 give 50 mmol bicarbonate and repeat blood gases in 30 minutes; repeat treatment till pH above 7·10: 500–2000 mmol may be needed in LACTIC ACIDOSIS; as pH rises, potassium falls.
Potassium: If initially low (less than 3·0 mmol/l) increase concentration to 40 mmol/l for 1 litre only and revert to 20 mmol/l till repeat value known.

C CONTINUING CLINICAL REVIEW

Re-assess clinical improvement, ECF volume and urine output hourly. Repeat biochemistry at 2, 5 and 8 hours.

Slow IV saline after 2 litres infused, aim to give total of 3 litres in first 6 hours.

Increase insulin to double initial rate if blood glucose not falling at rate of 5 mmol/hour.

Switch to 5% dextrose when blood glucose less than 15 mmol/l, and slow infusion to 1 litre per 6 hours, continuing potassium 20 mmol/l.

Consider low dose heparin in elderly or hyperosmolar state.

Always be prepared to revise management in light of fresh clinical evidence.

D DIABETIC ROUTINE PLANS

Promptly-treated patients should have ACIDOSIS corrected (pH > 7·25) in 3–6 hours.

Hyperosmolar patients need approximately 6 litres of fluid in first 12 hours; rising sodium is indication for $\frac{1}{2}$ strength saline.

I V fluids must be continued in drowsy or unconscious patient, but if alert, significantly improved or hungry, plan for routine care. Aim to give routine insulin regime on morning after admission.

In new diabetic see Chapter 10.

Mild diabetic on oral agents – give S C insulin until full clinical recovery. Look for social problems in adolescent with recurrent episodes of ketoacidosis.

Feed generously during convalescence.

Plan to assess renal function and monitor for pyelonephritis in those whose urea does not return to normal in 48 hours.

Conclusion

Remembering the features discussed in this chapter, 'diabetic coma' should alert the clinician to various possible patterns of presentation each with its particular influence on management. Perhaps the term *coma* might gain a new image by retaining it as an aid-memoire or form of shorthand for the following important aspects which should be considered in each case:

Causation; Osmolality; Metabolic Acidosis

Armed with a good understanding of the varied clinical, metabolic and biochemical interrelationships, an intravenous line and a little insulin, lives can be saved.

Further Reading

1 Gennari F.J. & Kassirer J.P. (1974) Osmotic diuresis. *New Engl. J. Med.*, **291**, 714–720

2 Editorial (1977) The anion gap. *Lancet*, **i**, 785–786

3 Editorial (1977) Insulin regimens for diabetic ketoacidosis. *Br. Med. J.*, **i**, 405–406

4 Sönksen P.H., Srivastava M.C., Tomkins C.U. & Nabarro J.D.N. (1972) Growth hormone and cortisol responses to insulin infusion in patients with diabetes mellitus. *Lancet*, **ii**, 155–157

5 Page M. McB., Alberti K.G.M.M., Greenwood R., Gumaa K.A., Hockaday T.D.R., Lowy C., Nabarro J.D.N., Pyke D.A., Sönksen P.H., Watkins P.J. & West T.E.T. (1974)

Treatment of diabetic coma with continuous low-dose infusion of insulin. *Br. med. J.*, **ii**, 687–690

6 Semple P.F., White C. & Manderson W.G. (1974) Continuous intravenous infusion of small doses of insulin in treatment of diabetic ketoacidosis. *Br. med. J.*, **ii**, 694–698

7 Alberti K.G.M.M. & Hockaday T.D.R. (1977) Diabetic ketoacidosis. *Clin. Endocrinol. Metabol.*, **6**, 421–456

8 Feig P.U. & McCurdy D.K. (1977) The hypertonic state. *New Engl. J. Med.*, **297**, 1444–1453

9 Champion H.R., Caplan Y.H., Baker S.P., Long W.B., Benner C., Cowley R.A., Fisher R. & Gill, W. (1975) Alcohol intoxication and serum osmolality. *Lancet*, **i**, 1402–1404

CHAPTER 8

Aims in Diabetic Care

R.D. Lawrence pioneered the most positive and successful, yet often neglected, way of encouraging the diabetic in the right direction. This famous London physician, who was one of those diabetics saved from an untimely death in the early twenties by the discovery of insulin, taught that patients should be trained to look after their own disorder. His book *The Diabetic Life* brought hope and encouragement to countless thousands in his lifetime.

Today, in an enlightened world where health care is better organised Lawrence's philosophy should be more easily promoted. The essential elements are:

education about diabetes, and
aiming to lead a normal life.

Unfortunately, many diabetics are still denied job opportunities or discouraged from some outdoor or recreational activities because of the metabolic disorder. Often the decision, based on medical advice, may be correct in so far as the diabetic has never had adequate education in the principles of self-regulation (Chapters 10, 22), yet without education it is almost impossible for the insulin-dependent patient to lead a normal life. Becoming a diabetic should not involve entering a monastic order of self-denial, but leading a normal life does imply some reasonable organisation of behaviour, regular habits, avoidance of excesses and applied common sense.

It is like learning the skills of driving a motor car and understanding how to maintain it thereafter. Handing out a book of instructions is of little value. Instead, the novice starting an engine or injecting insulin needs practice and supervision. Once the basic principles are established the driver and patient must continue the practical training beyond the garage forecourt or away from the cloistered hospital bed. The way that a modern suspension irons out the stresses and strains of braking, accelerating or cornering matter little to the learner driver; likewise, the complexities and intricacies of hormonal control of insulin-glucose homeostasis are equally unimportant to the patient. But training and practice in judging distance or speed in relation to road conditions are important to the driver and very similar to controlling the blood sugar relative to the influences of exercise, nutrition and stress. Does this mean that the patient, like the experienced driver, becomes totally independent of the instructor and service-station? On the contrary, most sensible drivers realise the value of the regular service check-up. There will always be some who will be negligent, forgetting the routine maintenance until ultimately there is some serious breakdown – when back they come, often with some dangerous yet avoidable medical or other emergency.

Can diabetic patients be taught to look after their own disorder? Anybody who can read or write, or who is capable of driving a car, can learn all the essentials of diabetes. Most would be quick to agree that there are some bad, not to mention downright dangerous, drivers on the road and there are badly-controlled diabetics around too. But there are many badly-controlled diabetics afoot for the very reasons that they are bad drivers: either poor instruction at the outset or the acquisition of careless habits with the passage of time.

When a candidate seeks driving tuition, provided that he is reasonably fit and has normal eyesight the remainder of the exercise is a challenge to the instructor; likewise, the new diabetic is a challenge to the doctor. Those diabetics who cannot be taught independence are a reflection on their instructors or on our ability to organise effective diabetic health care. Medical science has so far failed to solve the problem of preventing diabetes or of producing a cure without using regular insulin injections in the more severe cases. But at least insulin is widely available; we are failing our patients and certainly falling well short of the pioneering spirit of Banting and Best or of Lawrence if we cannot educate our patients to lead a normal life.

Diabetic control

How strictly should diabetes be controlled? Perhaps this is the most fundamental, yet difficult, question in relation to diabetic care today. Clearly the patient will be glad to reach a degree of control sufficient to relieve the symptoms of thirst and polyuria, sufficient also to maintain normal body growth and well-being. But must insulin-glucose homeostasis be so finely tuned that the blood glucose never rises above 8 or 9 mmol/l (144 to 162 mg/100 ml) as in the normal non-diabetic, and is such perfection compatible with a reasonable way of life for the diabetic? Read your motor car handbook: check the oil level, tyre pressures, brake fluid and battery every few hundred miles; never accelerate until the engine has reached its normal operating temperature and so on. Why bother? you say. Despite the high capital and running costs the shiny motor car is due for the junk yard within the next ten years, and there is always a new model waiting in the showroom; patients are different. Unfortunately, as will become apparent (Chapter 13 onwards), all too often the diabetic also accelerates to the junk yard, tragically corroded by atheroma or seized up by one or other of the specific diabetic complications. The fundamental question is whether these problems are a consequence of poor maintenance or are the result of planned obsolescence. Some experts believe that those who develop diabetes inevitably also acquire, perhaps genetically, the corroding complications. Aiming for strict control is a waste of time and effort, they say; why check the dip-stick? they ask. There has always been a strong body of opinion taking the alternative view, believing that the various complications of diabetes are a result of poor control. Without scientific evidence this has been an act of faith sometimes followed with demagogic zeal – witness the number of medical texts insisting on 'strict', 'rigid' or 'tight' control of diabetes. A third faction would have rightly decried this debate as useless on the grounds that valid data correlating control and complications in diabetic patients were lacking. However, in recent years numerous studies on animals, including dogs, rats, mice, monkeys, Chinese hamsters and others have shown that severe and chronic hyperglycaemia leads to more severe diabetic complications in various tissues. Apart from the fact that rats and mice are not men and that diabetic animals are rather different from diabetic humans, most experimental work has, nevertheless, shown that severe and chronic hyperglycaemia is harmful. Moreover, a recent study of diabetic small-blood-vessel disease in the kidney (Chapter 14) has shown a direct correlation between the degree of hyperglycaemia and the severity of the renal lesion. We remain uncertain, however, about the need or otherwise for perfect control throughout the 24 hours of every day. Experimental data have been based on levels of poor control which would be intolerable to most patients for extended periods.

Looked at another way there is now good evidence that constantly 'doing the ton' is dangerous. On the other hand, we lack evidence to the effect that never exceeding the speed limit is a guarantee against accidents. Perhaps patients can be allowed some leeway from time to time. There is another problem: remember that metabolically-normal non-diabetics get heart attacks. Here we plunge into another murky area: how can we be sure who is metabolically normal and who is not? So far as diabetes is concerned should blood glucose be the measure of control? Quite reasonably some would add that body growth, blood lipids and many other metabolic parameters (haemoglobin A_1, for example, Chapter 22, p.249) should also be normal. On all sides we are assailed with doubts and difficulties. More fundamental aspects of the effect of diabetic control or tissue damage are examined in greater detail in Chapters 13 and 14, and discussed in Chapter 23.

Perhaps we should return to the aim and ideals of R.D. Lawrence. Patients can only begin to be well controlled (and lead a normal life) if education is thorough, competent and above all *practical*. Those who have a good grasp of steering their diabetes through the twists and bends of varying activity are best suited to coping with the stresses and strains of life. Simultaneously, such diabetics are more able to maintain good control (as currently measured). Thus, education about regularly checking the dip-stick is of practical value, and regular servicing where the expert searches for the early warning signs of corrosion or wear and tear is more valuable to the patient's well-being and peace of mind than the alternative of neglect. We cannot coerce our patients beyond what is either sensible or practical, nor can we expect them to make sacrifices in order to achieve better control unless we explain the reasons and the risks (Chapter 22) related to poor control.

Organisation of diabetic care

As medicine, and its para-medical services, become more and more specialised, the problems of working together in the patient's interest become increasingly difficult. Known as clinical integration in the medical jargon, care of the diabetic patient is a good test of its efficiency. Two doctors are at the centre of things – the family practitioner and the hospital specialist in diabetes.

Most often the family doctor will make the diagnosis and be the first to explain the meaning of diabetes to the patient and his family. Maintenance of health care and dealing with intercurrent illness will be a continuing responsibility. The hospital specialist usually confirms the diagnosis, establishes management policy and provides routine follow-up.

But patients tend to place their confidence in one doctor rather than another. Those having a good rapport with their own doctor, or especially those given a brusque or unsatisfactory interview at a hospital clinic may prefer to rely upon the family physician. Where the family doctor wants as little as possible to do with diabetes, patients will tend to become more dependent on the hospital clinic. Those patients in the happy situation where a good dialogue exists between their family doctor and the hospital clinician will probably get the best care.

Wherever the emphasis lies, neither doctor can fulfill the aims of R.D. Lawrence or hope to delay or minimise the serious complications of diabetes without a variety of supporting services, both medical and para-medical. Thus dieticians, chiropodists, chemical pathologists and health visitors, as well as ophthalmologists and obstetricians having a special interest in diabetic problems, are essential to comprehensive diabetic management. Health care requirements will depend much on the individual patient's diabetes. Newly diagnosed adolescent diabetics setting out on the highroad of life or those frequently having to modify their insulin régime according to varying work and recreational patterns require the most education and guidance. The insulin dependent, and especially the pregnant diabetic (Chapter 12), require the advice of those most experienced in diabetic care. On the other hand, those who develop diabetes in the context of obesity and overnutrition mainly require dietetic advice. For the patient with diabetes of onset coincident with coronary thrombosis or having the disorder secondary to other disease the underlying medical condition may take precedence over conventional diabetic care. In the case of those in the closing years of life, failing faculties and many non-diabetic impediments tend to place an increasing burden on various para-medical services. Whatever the nature of the diabetes, or age of the patient, the diabetic has no immunity to other disease. Often medical, surgical, gynaecological, psychiatric and other problems cannot be managed adequately without co-operation between the particular specialist and those providing diabetic supervision. Good diabetic care is clinical integration at its best.

Figure 8.1 illustrates the various medical and para-medical services most often involved in diabetic care. Their individual contributions will become apparent in later chapters, but some aspects are worth considering at this stage. Take dietetics for example. Any doctor has access to diet sheets (there are even some in the Appendices) and patients can also find slimming diets – usually in tantalisingly close proximity to recipes for fattening cakes and other goodies – in almost any women's magazine. To be effective, however, a patient's diet has to be tailored to taste quite apart from financial, racial or religious considerations. It is in dealing with those various aspects that dieticians come into their

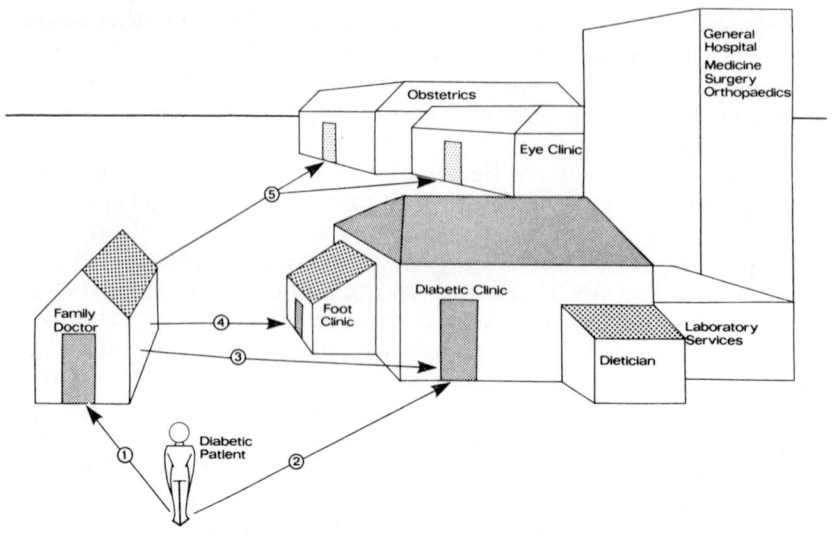

Fig. 8.1 The patient, the family doctor and the diabetic clinic. The patient may attend the family doctor 1 or the diabetic clinic 2 or be referred to the clinic 3. Alternatively the doctor may refer the patient to specialist services 4 or 5

own. They are best able to modify feeding patterns sensibly without totally or unnecessarily disrupting a family's eating habits, and they are best able to suggest alternatives to meet individual taste or feeding foibles. Equally, supervision of insulin-injecting technique and the practical application of diabetic self-regulation is seen at its best in the hands of nursing staff with a special interest in diabetic care. They not only have the rewarding task of guiding the nervous child (or even more nervous adult) over the first hurdles of self-injection, but also are able to identify faults in injecting technique or syringe care in the established diabetic.

Expert foot care (Chapter 17) given by chiropodists has so far been more effective in reducing the incidence of diabetic gangrene than any other measures directed towards preventing diabetic complications. Today, opthalmologists are able to arrest many of the more serious features of diabetic retinopathy (Chapter 15) which previously made diabetes a major medical cause of blindness.

In summary, education of the patient and co-ordination of health care services, both medical and para-medical, provide the best foundation for the creation of improved diabetic care. Whereas the aim is to prevent or delay serious diabetic complications, unfortunately many diabetics are not referred to the expert until some disaster has happened. These usually prove to be the patients with most problems and in greatest need of well-organised diabetic health care (Chapter 21).

Further Reading

1 Knibbs S. & Jackson J.G.L. (1975) Social and emotional complications of diabetes. In *Complications of Diabetes* (Ed. H. Keen & R.J. Jarrett) London: Edward Arnold, 265–285

2 Hill R.D. (1976) Running a diabetic clinic. *Br. J. hosp. Med.*, 16, 218–226

3 Ruben L.A. (1976) Diabetes and the general practitioner. *Br. J. hosp. Med.*, 16, 241–250

4 Judd S.L., O'Leary E.O.., Read P. & Fox C. (1976) The changing role of nurses in the management of diabetes. *Br. J. hosp. Med.*, 16, 251–255

5 Cahill G.F., Etzwiler D.D. & Freinkel N. (1976) Control and diabetes. *New Engl. J. Med.*, 294, 1005–1005

6 Siperstein M.D., Foster D.W., Knowles H.C., Levine R., Madison L.L. & Rott J. (1977) Control of blood glucose and diabetic vascular disease. *New Engl. J. Med.*, 296, 1060–1062

7 Ingelfinger F.J. (1977) Debates in diabetes. *New Engl. J. Med.*, 296, 1228–1230

CHAPTER 9

Diet and Diabetes

Diet and insulin-glucose homeostasis

Eating food is fun. Most diets are not so much fun. Are doctors who prescribe diets for diabetics spoil-sports, or is there a better reason? Mrs. Sweet-tooth's problem (Chapter 3) was clear enough: she had had too much fun for too long. For her, or in the case of anyone else who develops diabetes in the context of excess fuel consumption and storage, restriction of carbohydrate intake quickly relieves the symptoms of uncontrolled diabetes besides inducing weight reduction. Thus in the overfuelled, diet can be shown to be effective, and in a bygone era, before insulin became available, severe diabetes could be relieved, at least partially or temporarily, by carbohydrate-free diets. But what is the basis of the argument for restricting carbohydrate in dealing with the young insulin-dependent diabetic of today? Presumably the growing diabetic who is as energetic as his non-diabetic brother should need similar amounts of kilocalories or megajoules. Fig. 9.1 shows the energy requirements across the years for the moderately active male or female. Notice the sharp rise in adolescence, a plateau in middle life and a decline in old age. There has been a

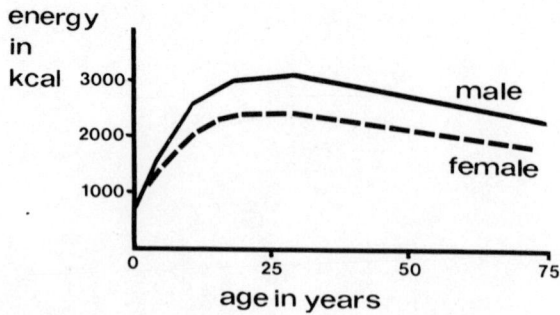

Fig. 9.1 Energy requirements in kilocalories at different ages for the moderately active male or female. Note the steep rise in adolescence, a peak in the prime of life and a decline thereafter. From puberty the female requirements are less throughout except during pregnancy

long-established habit of giving the insulin-dependent diabetic rather less carbohydrate than his non-diabetic brother, and this manipulation has usually involved a compensating increase in protein and especially in fat (raising doubts and fears about atheroma). Worse still, some diabetic adolescents have been given low-carbohydrate diets, without any compensating increase in other fuel sources. And some, across those years between 12 and 18 when there is a sharp rise in energy requirements, are never advised about diet increases. Little wonder if the adolescent diabetic rebels against what is in effect a starvation régime by taking the law into his own hands. At least by eating more than the prescribed diet he might save himself from the stunted growth which often blemished childhood diabetes in less enlightened times. The average 16-year-old will require around 3,000 kilo-calories (12·5 megajoules) containing 350 grams of carbohydrate per day. Yet most diabetics are restricted to around 200–250 grams of carbohydrate daily. Less toast and no marmalade for breakfast. Why? The argument has concerned the ebb and flow of blood sugar in relation to feeding. The insulin-dependent diabetic (Chapter 10) will take his injection shortly before breakfast, whereas his non-diabetic brother will secrete insulin in response to breakfast. Unfortunately for the diabetic, despite the insulin injection, the post-breakfast blood glucose rise may be excessive. Much depends on what happens after breakfast: if our friends rush out of the house and hurry to school or work the burst of exercise will then divert the toast and marmalade into muscle for energy. This is the crux of the problem for the diabetic because the size of the breakfast and its disposal will depend closely on personal transport. Toast and marmalade is ideal for those who walk or cycle to work; however, if the diabetic fails to exercise after breakfast he will not only be hyperglycaemic but the marmalade will be lost in the urine as glycosuria. On the other hand, the non-diabetic who does not exercise will store the marmalade as fat. The diabetic is not alone in having problems of fuel dispersal, just different, the important difference being that he lacks the options open to his non-diabetic brother. Once insulin is injected the diabetic must have breakfast; whether he has glycosuria after breakfast will depend on how much he eats and how he exercises. But if too much to eat induces glycosuria, too little may cause hypoglycaemia. The diabetic cannot rush off to school or work without breakfast, he cannot skip his mid-morning snack or be late for lunch. His non-diabetic brother can have as large (or small) a breakfast as he wishes – excesses stored as fat can be used as energy later without having to bother about snacks or lateness for meals.

Thus dieting for the insulin-dependent means taking aboard fuel regularly in relation to insulin and energy requirements. Eating can still be fun, but unlike the non-diabetic gourmet, the diabetic cannot eat just for fun. And as he matures and becomes less active – effortlessly operating power-assisted steering or sliding in and out of escalators – energy requirements decline so that the feeding fun must be curtailed if excessive weight-gain is to be avoided. Toast and marmalade for stair climbers not for escalator riders!

Diet and vascular disease

Eating food is such fun that as we mature and become less active, feeding increasingly becomes a pleasant habit in which the last thing we want is to stop to read the fuel gauges. We deceive ourselves. Enough is not enough. Sometimes, however, the medical profession counter-attacks with another deceit by leading an anxious public to believe that certain foods are harmful, often without the authority of scientific evidence to support the interference. Take, for example, diet in relation to degenerative vascular disease, a subject not to be passed over lightly in the diabetic (Chapter 13). There is the simplistic view about cholesterol, for instance. Because cholesterol is found in atheromatous vessel walls and egg yolks, some doctors believe that eggs should be banned for the heart's sake. This approach not only ignores the complexities of cholesterol synthesis, storage and transport (Chapter 6), but also some clever advertising on behalf of the hen – 'go to work on an egg'. Notice the subtle catch in the wording – for those almost extinct members of the species who actually work, an egg might be a good thing. This emphasis on energy consumption rather than storage is supported by the wave of enthusiasm for having abundant HDLs (Chapter 6) in the circulation in order to keep the coronary arteries clean (Chapter 13). How can I get more HDLs, doctor? Exercise is the answer. Thus the hen's advertising agents have probably got their slogan absolutely right.

For the heart's sake we are advised to avoid saturated fat. But some, like the Masai and other pastoral tribes in East Africa, have a diet rich in saturated fat yet they avoid atheroma. You will never see an overweight member of the Masai in his own environment but probably more importantly the Masai have developed an unique transport system (for want of anything better) which they use constantly. The system is based on two special appendages (legs). Perhaps for those far removed from pastoral Africa we might risk the comment: bacon and eggs for stair climbers but not for escalator riders. Certainly there's a lot of energy in fat. Wherein lies the fault? Is it in taking on board too much fat, or in not using the energy? Urban man seems to have begotten double trouble by eating high-energy fat fuel and diminishing exercise and energy consumption. For those who believe strongly that fats are harmful there will be ready sympathy for the poor diabetic who for many years was encouraged (or ordered) by his medical adviser to take a low-carbohydrate high-fat diet.

What about carbohydrate and vascular disease? Some believe that the great increase in degenerative vascular disease in western civilisation relates to an increasing consumption of carbohydrate – especially of sucrose. Interestingly, the Japanese enjoy a low level of atheroma by comparison with western civilisation, yet their diet contains a much higher amount of carbohydrate energy. But the Japanese do have that irritating habit of being so industrious and hard working (it's those H D Ls again).

There is a vast and not easily digestible literature on diet and degenerative vascular disease; these glimpses of the egg-yolk story, the Masai and the Japanese are but tiny morsels. Perhaps we should leave the gourmet to take his chance and admit to the more introspective that there really is insufficient evidence to justify modification of the balance of the diet in the hope of preventing vascular disease. On the other hand, if excess weight or obesity is the problem, reducing the energy intake (and there's a lot of energy in fat) or increasing the energy output will lead to a fall in weight.

Remember that *alcohol* is often an important source of excess fuel especially in overweight middle-aged diabetics. The energy value of alcohol in kilocalories per gram (kcal/g) can be compared with other sources as follows:

carbohydrate	4 kcal/g
fat	9 kcal/g
protein	4 kcal/g
alcohol	7 kcal/g

(if that doesn't mean anything to you, there are 100 kcal in every 50 ml of whisky or gin that you sip).

Dietary goals and the diabetic

Cardiologists advise against eating fat, diabetologists frown on carbohydrate, while ecologists want us to be sparing with the world's protein resources. How can we construct diets which satisfy so many conflicting interests and at the same time satisfy our patients? In 1977, the US Senate Select Committee on Nutrition and Human Needs, concerned about public health and heart disease risk, laid down the following six dietary goals:

1 to increase carbohydrate intake to between 55% and 60% of energy (kilocalories) intake;
2 to reduce fat consumption to 30% of energy intake;
3 to reduce saturated fat to 10%, balanced with 10% poly-unsaturated and 10% monounsattrated fat;
4 to reduce cholesterol intake to about 300 mg daily (one egg contains about 250 mg of cholesterol);
5 to reduce refined sugar intake to 15%, increasing the intake of less refined carbohydrate; and
6 to reduce salt intake – closely related to hypertension – from 12 g daily to around 3 g.

How can we square these health goals with the faulty insulin-glucose homeostasis of diabetes? The health goals suggest that 55–60% of energy should be carbohydrate in origin but traditional diabetic diets have tended towards 40% carbohydrate. The problem for the diabetic has always been the post-prandial blood glucose rise associated with carbohydrate; however, this difficulty can be overcome effectively by avoiding refined sugar and those processed carbohydrate foods lacking in fibre. This aspect of the nature of carbohydrate is fundamental and worthy of closer examination.

Fibre to the rescue

As the 20th century draws to a close the belated discovery that we were designed to chew our food slowly and thoroughly, and that *fibre* is good for the alimentary system from the teeth to the bowels, is largely due to the writings of Surgeon Captain T.L. Cleave. In his book *The Saccharine Disease* he has implicated lack of fibre in many of the other ills of fat, toothless, constipated modern man. We now realise, moreover, that fibre is of particular relevance to insulin-glucose homeostasis in diabetes. Carbohydrate from foodstuffs rich in fibre is more slowly absorbed from the alimentary tract, and apart from reducing the post-prandial glycaemic peak, the value to the diabetic lies in the fact that the blood glucose curve matches much better the more sustained time-action of exogenous insulin (Chapter 10). Patients taking carbohydrate in the form of high-fibre food-stuffs need smaller doses of insulin, smaller doses of oral hypoglycaemic agents (Chapter 11), and some may be more easily controlled by diet alone. Not surprisingly, everybody (including the diabetic patient) wants to know about fibre.

Essentially, fibre is the supporting framework of the plant cell which has a fine structure akin to that of glass-fibre-reinforced plastic – in other words, a strong fibrous network embedded in a resilient matrix. Chemically, fibre is a mixture of polymers. Cellulose, for example, is a straight chain of glucose molecules, similar to starch (amylose), except that by having different linkages it is resistant to digestive amylases. Hemicelluloses are polysaccharides like cellulose but the chains are branched and the sugar units are hexoses rather than glucose which have linkages resistant to digestive enzymes. Some hemicelluloses, such as *pectin*, have the property of forming gels with water. *Lignins* are substituted hydrocarbon polymers which encrust the fibrous matrix as it ages, adding to its rigidity. *Guar* and other gums are not cell-wall substances but unusual storage polysaccharides. Physiologically, fibre resists hydrolysis by enzymes of the human stomach, pancreas and intestine and, by passing into the colon relatively intact, becomes the undigested residue of plant or carbohydrate foods. Fibre has no nutritional value and is sometimes known as empty calories. Cooking does not reduce the amount of indigestible residue, but it does alter the physical properties of fibre with consequent effects upon the appearance and texture of food. The only foodstuffs of plant origin which do not contain fibre are honey and refined sugar (brown sugar, syrup and molasses).

Fibre is not inert, but has a significant ability to bind water. Although it is often described as 'roughage', once fibre has been chewed it is no longer rough and due to its water-binding properties it provides the colon with 'smoothage'. Fibre is a weak cation exchanger and some have said that by binding to calcium, zinc and metallic ions, fibre might deplete the body of essential elements; however, this claim seems exaggerated.

Food processing involves fibre depletion in the refining technology. Processing is inevitable in urban civilisation, especially to keep food fresh, and unfortunately agricultural products are systematically deprived of fibre on their journey from the field to the grocery store. Supermarkets (and corner-shops) sell bread unsurpassed in the fineness and whiteness of the flour. As modern mass-production roller-milling grinds all the fibre out of the wheat, the diabetic has to go to the 'health-food' shop to get good wholesome old-fashioned stone-milled bread. If the diabetic can be encouraged to have carbohydrate in the form of wholemeal bread or biscuits, porridge oats, beans (guar gum comes from the cluster bean) and the various other vegetables and fruit high in fibre, then his total intake may reasonably be around 50% of energy. Health foods are in. Sweets, candies and other sugar goodies are out. Chew an apple instead. Perhaps the 'rigid diet' principle of most medical texts on diabetes should be reinterpreted to mean rigid in fibre content.

In the normal-weight diabetic, if approximately 50% of energy is obtained from unrefined carbohydrate and 10–15% from protein, the remaining 35–40% may be fat in origin. Energy requirements can vary as much as 100% from one individual to another. Thus, total amounts of carbohydrate and fat especially should relate to the patient's usual intake and whether they are over- or underweight. Increased intake should always be allowed to match increased exercise (Chapter 10).

Aims in diabetic diets

Immediate, ie. at diagnosis

1 to improve insulin-glucose homeostasis
2 to restore patients towards their correct weight

Long-term

1 to maintain insulin-glucose homeostasis
2 to maintain normal weight and growth
3 to avoid excesses or deficiencies of proven harm, ie. to correct serious imbalance in the intake of protein and fat, to include adequate iron, essential minerals and vitamins.

Immediate improvement in insulin-glucose homeostasis will result from reducing the intake of refined sugar. Often the patient will have *increased* the sugar consumption in sweetened drinks taken in response to the thirst of uncontrolled diabetes. If the patient is underweight the diet should be generous in total amounts of unrefined carbohydrate, protein and fat; if overweight, total calories should be reduced. If sugar intake has been high, cutting it out will probably have a significant effect. But other high calorie fuels – especially cream, butter and alcohol – should also be reduced. For the overweight housewife (Mrs. Sweet-tooth or Mrs. Spratt, Chapter 3) cutting out sugar and reducing butter and cream – without any other change in their feeding habits – would fulfil the immediate and long-term dietary aims (See Simple Diet, Appendix 2).

However, the *insulin-dependent* diabetic (Chapter 10) requires to have the carbohydrate spread throughout the day; for example, 25% of carbohydrate with each of the 3 main meals and the remaining 25% as snacks between meals. The simplest way of regulating the carbohydrate content is based on the 10 g *exchange system* (see Appendix 3). Thus, if the diet appropriate to age, weight and energy requirements (See Table 9.1) = 240 g carbohydrate,

Table 9.1   Energy and carbohydrate intake per day
Recommended energy requirements at different ages where approximately 50% is of carbohydrate. Daily intake of carbohydrate in grams and as EXCHANGES, where 1 EXCHANGE = 10 g of carbohydrate (see Appendices 3 & 4).

A = Sedentary   B = Moderately active   C = Very active

MALES

Age in years		Energy in		Carbohydrate in	
		kcal	Mj	grams	Exchanges
9 to 12		2500	10·5	300	30
12 to 15		2800	11·7	340	34
15 to 18		3000	12·6	350	35
18 to 35	A	2700	11·3	330	33
	B	3000	12·6	350	35
	C	3600	15·1	420	42
35 to 65	A	2600	10·9	320	32
	B	2900	12·2	340	34
	C	3600	15·1	420	42
65 to 75		2400	10·0	280	28

FEMALES

9 to 18		2300	9·6	270	27
18 to 55	A	2000	8·4	240	24
	B	2300	9·6	270	27
	Pregnancy	2500	10·5	300	30
55 to 75		2000	8.4	240	24

Note: These are broad guidelines for patients who are NOT overweight. Those exceeding their correct weight for age and height by up to 20% require ⅔ of the above; those exceeding 20% require ½ of the above.

60 g or 6 exchanges could be taken with each of the three main meals and the remaining 6 exchanges divided between mid-morning and evening snacks, but these should not be regarded as hard and fast rules. In the fine-tuning of blood glucose (Chapter 10), therefore, modifications in meal size or distribution can often be made in the light of urine or blood glucose values and exercise variables.

These are general guidelines. Remember that individual diets must take account of the feeding habits of the whole family and that personal circumstances, social class, culture and religion are as important to patients and their eating behaviour as ideas about carbohydrate, protein and fat are to the medical profession. Skilled dietitians, accustomed to diabetics and doctors, are best able to reconcile both standpoints.

Further Reading

1 Paul A.A. & Southgate D.A.T. (1978) *McCance & Widdowson's The Composition of Foods.* London: H M S O
2 Editorial (1977) Dietary goals. *Lancet*, **i**, 887–888
3 Editorial (1976) Diet and the diabetic. *Br. med. J.*, **ii**, 780
4 Mann G.U. (1977) Diet-heart: end of an era. *New Engl. J. Med.*, 297, 644–650
5 Editorial (1977) Sensible eating. *Br. med. J.*, **ii**, 80–81
6 Editorial (1977) Food and fibre. *Br. med. J.*, **ii**, 418
7 Jenkins D.J.A., Wolever T.M.S., Hockaday T.D.R., Leeds A.R., Howarth R., Bacon S., Apling E.C. & Dilawari J. (1977) Treatment of diabetes with guar gum. *Lancet*, **ii**, 779–780
8 Heaton K.W. (1977) Perspective on the therapeutic use of bran. In *Clinical Medicine and Therapeutics* (Ed. P. Richards & H. Mather). Oxford: Blackwell Scientific Publications, 251–257
9 Gouldner T.J. & Alberti K.G.M.M. (1978) Dietary fibre and diabetes. *Diabetologia*, **15**, 285–287
10 Keen H. & Thomas B. (1978) Diabetes mellitus. In *Nutrition in the Clinical Management of Disease* (Ed. J.W.T. Dickerson & H.A. Lee). London: Edward Arnold, 118–143

CHAPTER 10

Insulin Therapy

Insulin therapy is feared by some patients and doctors in much the same way as men of ancient times feared God. Then the power of the deity was not in question – nor to-day is the potency of insulin. Therein lies the doctor's dilemma: fear that by giving the wrong dose of insulin there may be dangerous under- or overdosage. Nor is there any immediate *aide-memoire* or instant formula by which the dose can be calculated. There is no real comfort in knowing that the vast majority of insulin-dependent diabetics need between one and four units of insulin per hour or 10 to 20 units for each main meal, and the bewildering choice of insulin preparations on the market compounds the doctor's fears.

Quite naturally – like taking the plunge in anything new – the patient may be nervous of injecting insulin until the simplicity of the technique is realised. Nevertheless, the patient-consumer may reasonably ask why insulin must be injected so laboriously when the pharmaceutical industry thrives on packaging medicines into attractive capsules or foil wrappings. The explanation that our relatively crude digestive systems are unable to discriminate between T-bone steaks or soya bean substitutes, and would treat oral insulin with similar indifference, breaking it down into simpler amino-acids so that on absorption insulin would no longer be insulin, helps the patient to understand the need for injections. Re-assured that injections are necessary, relieved that the technique is simple and above all invigorated by the metabolic benefit of insulin, diabetic patients usually quickly grasp, with enthusiasm, the principles of insulin dose adjustment. Of course, the diabetic who wishes to lead a normal life has an added incentive to learn, nevertheless it should not be beyond the wit of those with a medical training to understand insulin usage.

Insulin therapy embraces all the skill, judgement and hazards of the golf course. The array of insulins available is like the vast selection of clubs bristling from the golf fanatic's bag. Just as these can be divided into irons for the short to medium shots and woods for the long shots, so insulin preparations can be divided into short-acting or long-acting. But neither golf nor insulin therapy is an exact science. The distance that a ball travels with a particular club, or the duration of action of an insulin preparation, depends on how it is used. Thus a short-stroke iron may be muscled into a medium shot; similarly a large dose of short-acting insulin tends to have a longer duration of action than a small dose. Some advise the novice to get to know a few clubs really well – much the same advice is often given about types of insulin. Yet the golfer needs a variety of clubs to cope with all the features and hazards of the average course and doctors running diabetic clinics – despite having a particular preference for certain insulins – will come across clinical situations where most insulins find a use at some time or other.

Looking at insulin secretion in response to feeding, Figure 10.1

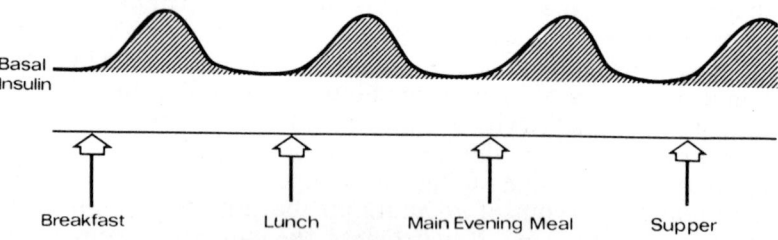

Fig. 10.1 Normal insulin secretion with each meal (not to scale)

reminds us that physiological requirements match the four main meals each day. But the patient expects the doctor to design something simpler than such frequent injections. Just as the golfer dreams of a hole-in-one so the patient hopes for once-daily insulin. How is the patient's desire for nothing more than a daily injection reconciled with physiological needs? Often it is not, yet no diabetic need have insulin more often than twice daily. Let us develop this theme by first examining some simple, but often far from ideal, methods in order better to appreciate more complex four-insulin twice-daily injection routines. Suppose that the patient has an injection of a short-acting insulin before breakfast; this will build up to a peak effect in the forenoon, giving sufficient insulin to cope with both breakfast and lunch (Fig. 10.2). One problem is the strong insulin action with the risk of hypoglycaemia before lunch, prevented by an adequate mid-morning carbohydrate snack. If the patient has a second similar but perhaps smaller injection before the main evening meal this will also cope with the bed-time snack and wear off gradually during the night (Fig. 10.2).

Alternatively, the patient could have an appropriate long-acting insulin along with the morning short-acting injection which could eliminate the need to inject again before the evening meal (Fig. 10.3) – a hole-in-one every day!

These manipulations still fail to reproduce the pattern of insulin secretion enjoyed by the non-diabetic, but a clever combination of twice-daily injections of a short- and medium-acting insulin-mix can get close to that ideal. Remember that the duration of action of any insulin will depend in part on the size of the dose; the larger the

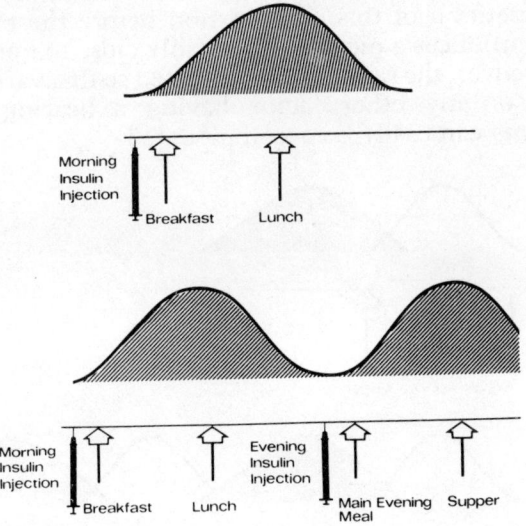

Fig. 10.2 *Upper part:* time-action of short-acting insulin injected before breakfast. *Lower part:* time-action of twice daily short-acting insulin. Not to scale

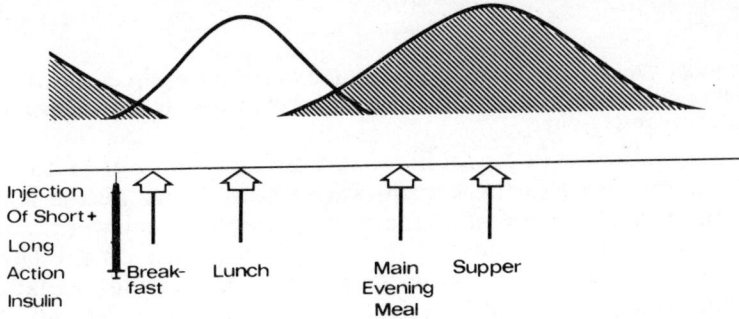

Fig. 10.3 Combined injection of short (clear) and long-acting)hatched) insulin injected before breakfast

dose the longer the action. The situation demonstrated in Fig. 10.2, in which two doses of short-acting insulin are given each day implies that each dose will be relatively large (half the daily requirement). Suppose that the patient has a small dose of short-acting insulin plus a small dose of a medium-acting insulin before breakfast instead of the short-acting insulin alone. In other words each insulin will be about a quarter of the daily needs instead of half. Smaller doses – shorter action. Thus the effect is as in Fig. 10.4. A repetition of this combination before the main evening meal then produces a picture remarkably close to normality (Fig. 10.4). Moreover, the ratios can be adjusted so that variations in the meal size or any other factor having a bearing on insulin requirements can easily be accommodated.

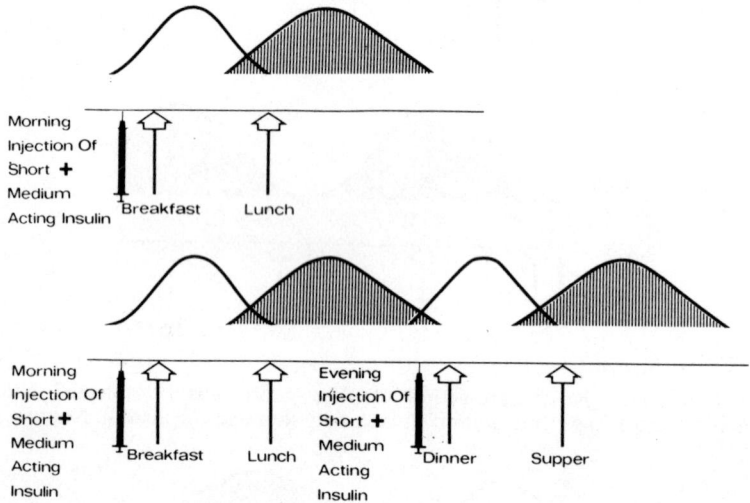

Fig. 10.4 *Upper part:* time action of *small* doses of short plus medium-acting insulin given before breakfast. *Lower part:* effect of twice daily doses of short plus medium-acting insulin

Now we come to the key question: how do we decide about insulin dose? Unfortunately for many patients the answer lies in a crude technique of trial and error, with emphasis on the latter. Insulin requirements show a marked individual variation; nevertheless, with an intelligent combination of foresight and the ability to profit by experience, good diabetic control – the object of the exercise – can be achieved. Consider the example of Peter (Chapter 3, p.30), the newly-diagnosed insulin-requiring adolescent and eager to learn. Adolescence is one of the most difficult periods in terms of maintaining good control. Peter must be taught a régime combining good control with flexibility so that he can lead as normal a life as possible. The insulin-mix illustrated in Fig. 10.4 would be appropriate. Suppose that his main meals are breakfast (8 am), lunch (1 pm) and dinner (6 pm) with a smaller supper before bed (10 pm). Let us call the short acting insulin A and the medium acting B. Thus in the morning he takes insulins A_1 B_1 and before dinner A_2 B_2. A reasonable start would be to give 10 units of each insulin A_1 B_1 and 8 units of insulins A_2 B_2; thereafter, each insulin can be adjusted upwards or downwards by 2 units until good control is achieved. But how? Peter learns that each insulin covers a particular meal and stretch of his day. Thus;

Insulin A_1 covers breakfast and the forenoon,
Insulin B_1 covers lunch and the afternoon,
Insulin A_2 dinner and the evening, and
Insulin B_2 covers supper and overnight.

The aim is to bring the pre-meal blood glucose close to the normal range. There are two phases in the process:

1 *Rough adjustment: Urine* tests
2 *Fine tuning: Blood* glucose monitoring

First let us examine the use of urine tests which are a simple and effective way of re-establishing the diabetic in the paths of metabolic righteousness. Once the patient is back to normal weight and has passed through the early running-in phase of diabetes, consideration of switching to home monitoring of blood glucose by reflectance meter is then appropriate.

Control by urine tests

Fig. 10.5 shows the insulin injections, their actions in relation to meals and the urine tests for each insulin. So that the urine sample matches the time accurately, Peter is taught to empty the bladder about half an hour beforehand and then pass a fresh sample to test before each main meal. Remember the Clinitest scale (Chapter 5, p.64).

$$0 \quad \tfrac{1}{4} \quad \tfrac{1}{2} \quad \tfrac{3}{4} \quad 1 \quad 2 \text{ per cent.}$$

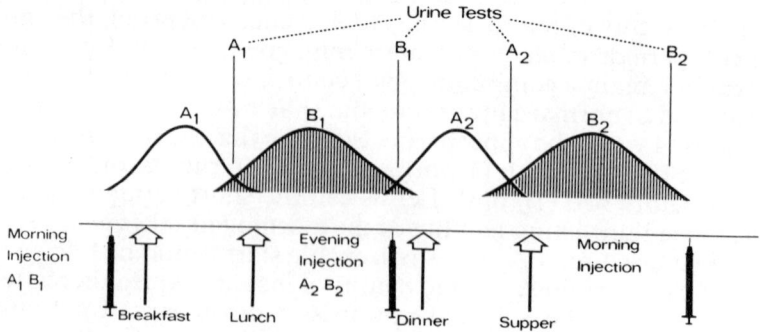

Fig. 10.5 Urine tests in relation to Fig. 10.4. Twice-daily short-acting insulin (A_1 and A_2), medium-acting insulins (B_1 and B_2)

Peter learns that if the test shows 2% he increases the appropriate insulin by 2 units, reduces by 2 units if 0 and leaves the dose unchanged if $\frac{1}{4}$, $\frac{1}{2}$, $\frac{3}{4}$ or 1%. Look at insulin A_1 and the before lunch test as an example:

Insulin A_1 (units)		Before lunch test	Action next day
Day 1	10	$\frac{1}{4}$	No change
Day 2	10	2	Increase
Day 3	12	$\frac{3}{4}$	No change
Day 4	12	$\frac{1}{4}$	No change
Day 5	12	0	Reduce
Day 6	10	0	Reduce
Day 7	8	$\frac{1}{4}$	No change

Remember, Peter is constantly acting on experience, in other words the insulin is adjusted each day according to the previous day's results. Fig. 10.6 gives an example of a composite picture of the adjustments of insulins A_1 B_1 A_2 B_2 in Peter's case. Notice that in 7 days, 28 observations have been made leading to several sensible dose adjustments without recourse to frequent blood tests. By matching occasional blood tests to the urine chart, the validity of the urine tests can be confirmed.

Because Peter was not in severe ketoacidosis at the outset there was no need to rush his metabolism back to normal by treating him as an emergency. Even if the initial doses of insulin prove to be inadequate, their effect should not be judged on urine tests (or blood glucose) alone. Improvement in the symptoms of thirst or polyuria is good evidence that the melting down of flesh and limbs

DATE	A₁	Before Lunch Test	B₁	Before Dinner Test	A₂	Before Supper Test	B₂	Before Breakfast Test
Day1	10	$\frac{1}{4}$	10	$\frac{1}{4}$	8	$\frac{1}{4}$	8	$\frac{3}{4}$
" 2	10	②	10	$\frac{1}{2}$	8	⓪	8	⓪
" 3	12	$\frac{3}{4}$	10	$\frac{1}{3}$	6	$\frac{1}{4}$	6	②
" 4	12	$\frac{1}{4}$	10	$\frac{3}{4}$	6	$\frac{1}{4}$	8	$\frac{1}{2}$
" 5	12	⓪	10	$\frac{1}{3}$	6	$\frac{1}{2}$	8	$\frac{1}{3}$
" 6	10	⓪	10	$\frac{1}{2}$	6	$\frac{1}{2}$	8	⓪
" 7	8	$\frac{1}{4}$	10	$\frac{1}{3}$	6	$\frac{1}{3}$	6	$\frac{1}{3}$

Fig. 10.6 Patients's chart of urine test results using insulins A₁, A₂, B₁ and B₂, as in Fig. 10.5. Results recorded on scale 0, $\frac{1}{4}$, $\frac{1}{2}$, $\frac{3}{4}$, 1 or 2 per cent. Dose increased by 2 units next day when test shows 2 per cent, similarly reduced when negative (0)

has been put in reverse. And if the dose is too great? Stop and think. Peter is thin and underweight: if his blood glucose is low he is probably getting inadequate carbohydrate. If hypoglycaemic: feed him.

Peter has much more to learn about insulin dose adjustment. The problem can be divided broadly into two contrasting parts:

factors causing hyperglycaemia, ie. glycosuria, and
factors causing hypoglycaemic reactions.

Look at Table 10.1 carefully. All the influences which might cause hyperglycaemia on the one hand or hypoglycaemia on the other are

Table 10.1   Causes of glycosuria (hyperglycaemia) and of hypoglycaemia

Causes of glycosuria	Causes of hypoglycaemia
Extra carbohydrate to eat	Late for meals
Lack of insulin	Extra insulin
Lack of exercise	Extra exercise
Any illness, accident or stress	Recovery from any illness, etc

summarised under these headings. Peter has recently experienced severe hyperglycaemia and appreciates only too vividly how it feels to lack insulin. While under hospital supervision it is worthwhile letting him experience the symptoms of hypoglycaemia (Chapter 18) by giving an artificially high dose of insulin A_1. Peter has to understand to expect an upset in diabetic control in the event of an intercurrent illness, minor accident or the stress of examinations. If the insulin dose has been increased to cope with an intercurrent illness, he must appreciate that there is the risk of hypoglycaemia on recovery.

The effect of exercise, however, can often be most profound. James, the professional footballer, is the expert . . .

Exercise and insulin requirements Playing first-class football as an insulin-dependent diabetic requires first class diabetic control and understanding of the principles of self-regulation. During the summer break from football, while still more active than the rest of us, James takes insulins A_1 B_1 and A_2 B_2 in the following doses: A_1 28 units; B_1 28 units; A_2 24 units and B_2 24 units – just over 100 units daily. But as soon as he starts training for the football season there is a profound change. Morning and afternoon training sessions involve cutting insulin A_1 and B_1 and 28 to only 10 units each. Yet when James gets back to the changing room the blood glucose may be only 3·0mmol/l (54mg/100ml) despite cutting the morning insulin by almost two-thirds. James still eats normally while training, but once he is playing in earnest he has nothing more than a light breakfast and lunch on the day of a first class fixture. Then he takes only 10 units of insulin A_1 and none of B_1. Kick-off is 3 pm, he is in goal-scoring form which is ball control and diabetic control at their best yet the insulin dose is profoundly different from that of a more gentle routine. An extra large meal after the game is covered by an increase in insulin A_2.

Peter is thrilled to have advice from a professional footballer, who has given him his autograph which he will keep as a constant reminder of the effect of exercise upon insulin requirements.

For those contemplating more gentle pursuits, such as fishing their favourite stretch of river or a bird-watching expedition, the relaxation (absence of stress, Table 10.1) will diminish the need for insulin. More important, however, is the possibility of being so engrossed that lateness for meals can happen all too easily. The extra exercise of hurrying off to find food in such circumstances is the certain way to induce hypoglycaemia – take your sandwiches with you and make the most of a day of freedom. Ski-ing? Half the doses of insulin effective during daytime and eat extra to provide fuel for the increased energy consumption. Indeed, that is the message for all outdoor or other pursuits involving exercise: more fuel and less insulin. And carry a little sugar at all times.

To confirm that Peter has a confident grasp of the principles of self-regulation it is best to give him a notebook in which he can copy the time-actions of his insulins (Fig. 10.5) and the appropriate urine tests, make his own chart for results and insulin doses as in Fig. 10.6, and record the details of Table 10.1. As soon as his injection technique (page 139) is satisfactory, his diet is organised and reasonable diabetic control is established, Peter can be discharged from immediate hospital supervision. As confidence is established urine testing can be reduced from daily to alternate days.

Fine-tuning: blood glucose monitoring

By comparison with urine testing, blood glucose monitoring is a much more advanced method of diabetic control.

For the patient there is the problem of even more needles, but most find this a small sacrifice well worth facing in order to know their own blood glucose from time to time. One drop of blood obtained by finger prick (there are several easy-to-use painless aids) can be applied to either Dextrostix (Ames Company) or Reflotest (Boehringer Mannheim) reagent strips for exactly 60 seconds before washing or wiping off.

Four instruments are currently available for reading the reagent strips, each capable of giving an instant blood glucose reading to within 1·0mmol/l (18mg/100ml) of the true value:

Eyetone reflectance meter (Ames Company)
Reflomat reflectance meter (Boehringer Mannheim)
Glucochek pocket meter (Medistron Ltd)
Hypo-count meter (Hypoguard Ltd)

The Eyetone and Reflomat are rather bulky mains-operated instruments which require warming up and calibration each time they are used. The more recently introduced Glucochek and Hypo-count are battery-operated, permanently-calibrated digital read-out instruments having the added advantage of built-in 60-second timers. The Glucochek has brought self monitoring down to the pocket calculator size which makes it easier for the patient to assess the blood glucose at work or leisure. Those without meters can get close to the blood glucose value by using the ingenious BM-Test-Glycemie 20-800 (Boehringer Mannheim) reagent strips.[9]

In aiming to establish good control, remember the blood glucose variables (arrows indicate raising or lowering of blood glucose):

DIET ↑
INSULIN ↓
EXERCISE ↓
STRESS ↑

1 *Diet* has an intermittent effect like the normal glucose tolerance curve, with a peak at 1 hour and a return towards the baseline at 2 hours.

2 *Insulin* will have a variable duration of effect dependent upon type and dose.

3 *Exercise* has an intermittent effect related to its duration or severity, physical fitness and capacity of the individual. In practice, unaccustomed exercise has the most profound effect.

4 *Stress* may be acute (heated argument with employer), chronic (depression or other serious illness) or acute followed by sustained stress for a few days (influenza-like illness).

In practice – assuming absence of stress – the insulin is geared to the main meals (diet) while exercise is an additional variable. Suppose that the four-meal, four-insulin, two-injection régime (Fig. 10.4) is again followed. The first aim is to bring the pre-meal blood glucose close to the normal range (4–6mmol/l or 72–108mg/100ml). Although the insulins overlap variably in action, in practice a pre-meal value can be assigned to each insulin, thus:

Insulin A_1 covers breakfast and controls the pre-lunch value
Insulin B_1 covers lunch and controls the pre-dinner value
Insulin A_2 covers dinner and controls the pre-supper value
Insulin B_2 covers supper and controls the pre-breakfast value

Suppose that in a particular instance the dose of insulin A_1 is 10 units and that three consecutive pre-lunch readings are 7·0, 10·0 and 8·0mmol/l (126, 180 and 144mg/100ml) – clearly too high. The patient is advised to increase the insulin by 1 unit if above the normal range and reduce it by 2 units if below, and the results might be as follows:

Insulin A₁ (units)		Before-lunch test	Action next day
Day 1	10	7·0mmol/l 126mg/100ml	increase 1 unit
Day 2	11	7·5mmol/l 135mg/100ml	increase 1 unit
Day 3	12	5·5mmol/l 99mg/100ml	no change
Day 4	12	3·5mmol/l 63mg/100ml	reduce 2 units
Day 5	10	5·5mmol/l 99mg/100ml	no change

It cannot be emphasised too strongly that these instructions relate to active out-patients. Attempts to obtain similar values in the hospital environment may induce profound hypoglycaemia as soon as the patients venture out of the building. Thus the aim for ambulant in-patients might be values in the range of 5–8mmol/l (90–144mg/100ml) and for in-patients confined to bed, values of 5–10mmol/l (90–100mg/100ml) would be acceptable.

Having made appropriate adjustments in the doses of insulins, A_1, B_1, A_2 and B_2 to bring the pre-meal blood glucose into the normal range, the next step is to check whether the post-prandial blood glucose is satisfactory – for example, in the range between 6·0–10·0mmol/l (108–180mg/100ml). However, values outwith this range cannot be improved by insulin dose adjustment if the pre-meal value is satisfactory. For example, if 2 hours after breakfast the blood glucose was 15·0mmol/l (270mg/100ml) and before lunch 5·0mmol/l (90mg/100ml) an increase in insulin A_1 to improve the reading after breakfast might induce hypoglycaemia before lunch. Instead, the carbohydrate content of breakfast could be reduced, more exercise encouraged 1–2 hours after breakfast, some of the breakfast carbohydrate transferred to a mid-morning snack, or switching to a quick-acting insulin such as Actrapid could be considered. In general, diabetics showing high glucose peaks after meals and then a steep decline towards the next meal run the greatest risk of hypoglycaemia (Chapter 18), especially if exercise is increased above average.

Some problems affecting diabetic control

Low renal threshold to glucose Most commonly seen in youngsters, a low renal threshold to glucose can occur temporarily in pregnancy (Chapter 12) or under the influence of the counter-regulatory anti-insulin hormones of stress. In particular, growth hormone, cortisol and glucagon influence renal plasma flow and clearance, favouring a lower threshold to glucose; as a consequence essential fuel is lost, making the patient more vulnerable to ketosis and aggravating the symptoms of uncontrolled diabetes. The carbohydrate content of the diet may have to be increased to counter the urinary loss and patients adjusting their insulin dose by urine tests may need to reduce the appropriate dose wherever tests show $\frac{1}{2}\%$ or better. Control by blood glucose monitoring is more helpful.

The honeymoon phase Some diabetics, shortly after diagnosis, may temporarily require very little or even no insulin for perhaps between two and six months. Such patients have often just mastered a complex four-insulin regime and as they watch the doses dwindle they naturally assume a miraculous cure. If the total daily dose of insulin is less than 20 units, patients can be controlled by a single daily injection of long-acting insulin before breakfast, or if the daily total is less than 0·1 unit per kg body weight, insulin may be stopped. Urine tests should be continued and insulin restarted on re-appearance of glycosuria.

Somogyi effect: the insulin dose paradox Some patients may waken with 2% glycosuria, slight ketonuria and significant fasting hyperglycaemia not – as might be expected – from lack of insulin, but because of unrecognised hypoglycaemia during the night. This effect, first described by Somogyi, is a result of the hyperglycaemic anti-insulin hormones mobilising glucose from the liver in response to hypoglycaemia (Chapter 18). Such patients need less rather than more insulin, so it is important to be constantly alert to this possibility. Worse still, patients may aggravate the situation by increasing their overnight insulin as a consequence of poor fasting blood or urine glucose values. The Somogyi effect is most likely to occur in any of the following circumstances:

1 severe carbohydrate restriction in an underweight patient;
2 vague headache, anorexia or nausea (chronic hypogly-caemia, Chapter 18);
3 marked weight gain suggestive of excess insulin dosage;
4 unexplained general increase in insulin daily requirements (especially in those using high purity insulins); and
5 hypoglycaemia at other times in the day.

Although occurring most commonly at night, the effect may happen at other times, and if it is suspected, a significant reduction in the dose of insulin will confirm the diagnosis. Thus, if on re-ducing the dose of overnight insulin either symptoms or 2% glycosuria improve *excess* insulin must have been the cause. Failure to recognise this effect often leads to situations of so-called 'brittle diabetes' characterised by wide swings in blood glucose. In general, insulin dosage should not be increased on the basis of a single high blood-glucose measurement: check to confirm whether there are other features of insulin lack, namely thirst, polyuria, nocturia and always at least think of the possibility of the Somogyi effect before arbitrarily increasing the insulin dose.

Insulin preparations

Early commercial insulin produced after its discovery in 1921 by Banting and Best was a relatively impure yet clear *soluble* preparation, lasting 6–8 hours from the time of injection. The first success in making a long-acting insulin came from the Nordisk laboratory in Copenhagen in 1935 by combining insulin, zinc and protamine; unfortunately, this long-acting *protamine zinc* insulin was not suitable for mixing in the same syringe with short-acting soluble insulin. However, Dr. Hagedorn, working at the Nordisk laboratory, produced in 1947 a crystalline protamine insulin also known as *Isophane* or NPH (*Neutral Protamine Hagedorn*) which can be mixed with the soluble kind.

The Lente insulins were produced by another Danish laboratory – Novo – in 1950. These prolonged-action insulins contain zinc in amorphous or crystalline form; the amorphous insulin zinc suspension – *Semi-Lente* is medium acting; crystalline insulin zinc suspension – *Ultra-Lente* is long acting; while a combination of 30% Semi-Lente and 70% Ultra-Lente is inter-mediate in action – *Lente*. If all this is confusing there is much more to follow!

Commercial insulin is made from beef and pork pancreas. As beef insulin has three amino-acids, and pork one, which differ from human insulin, these differences were at one time thought to be the main reason for the antigenicity of commercial insulin. It is now appreciated that certain impurities derived from the pancreas used in the commercial production of insulin also stimulate insulin-binding antibodies, so confirming their anti-genicity. Gel filtration of re-crystallised insulin followed by anion-exchange chromatography removes almost all detectable impurities. Virtually non-antigenic, neutral porcine insulin is now available in short, medium and long-acting forms which are the result of research in the previously mentioned Novo and Nordisk laboratories of Copenhagen. The Danes have the little pigs and the big know-how essential for the production of these purified insulins which may be described as high-purity, fractionated, monocomponents or single-peak – terms related to features of their production.

Does this mean that less-purified commercial insulin is obsolete? Time will tell. Meantime there are just not enough pigs to supply the world's needs for insulin and so far insufficient non-antigenic beef insulin is commercially available. Currently, there are three clear clinical indications for high-purity insulins: insulin resistance; lipoatrophy at injection sites; and allergic reactions to ordinary commercial insulin.

Table 10.2   Insulin preparations available in the United Kingdom*

Conventional beef insulin	*Purified pork alternative*
Soluble	Actrapid MC
	Leo Neutral
Neutral soluble, Nuso	as above

ISOPHANE INSULINS

Isophane NPH	Leo Retard

INSULIN ZINC SUSPENSIONS

Lente	Monotard MC
Semilente	Semitard MC
Ultralente	—
	(Ultratard MC is purified BEEF, and Lentard MC purified BEEF and PORK insulin)

OTHER INSULINS

Protamine zinc	—
Globin zinc	—

MIXTURES

Leo Mixtard: Neutral 30 % + Retard 70 %
Leo Initard: Neutral 50 % + Retard 50 %
Rapitard MC: Purified Pork neutral + Beef insulin
          zinc suspension.

All insulins are available in 40 and 80 units per cc strengths, but soluble also available in 20 and 320 units per cc strengths. Conventional beef insulins are made by British insulin manufacturers. MC (Monocomponent) insulins are made by NOVO, and Leo is made by NORDISK; both Danish manufacturers.

*Many of these insulins are available under different brand names in other countries.

These problems are discussed in the next section. Claims that the high-purity insulins might also diminish the diabetic's tendency to microangiopathy (Chapter 13) have not so far been founded on scientific evidence.

In summary, the various insulins currently available fall into the following groups:

soluble insulin,
prolonged-action protamine insulins,
prolonged-action insulin-zinc suspensions, and
high-purity porcine insulins, of short, medium and long actions. (See Table 10.2.)

The choice of insulin

In deciding which insulin or insulins will be most appropriate in a particular clinical situation, the following three main variables should be considered:

conventional or purified insulin;
single long-acting once-daily insulin; or
a twice-daily 2, 3 or 4 insulin system.

Conventional or purified insulin   There are several clinical situations where conventional insulin preparations are at a disadvantage and where the highly-purified insulins are clearly indicated.

Insulin allergy   During the first month of using conventional insulin, patients may develop itchy red lumps a few hours after the injection. These usually remit spontaneously within a few weeks and provided that the injection technique is otherwise satisfactory, there is no cause for concern. However, if persistent, the features will resolve quickly on switching to purified insulin. Similarly, if severe pain develops at injection sites even after using conventional insulin for several months or years a switch to high-purity insulin will resolve the problem. More generalised anaphylactic reactions to conventional insulin occur extremely rarely, but can be aborted by a similar change to purified insulin.

Lipoatrophy and lipohypertrophy at injection sites   Usually as a consequence of several years of injections using conventional insulin, lipoatrophy begins as shallow pits at injection sites and is more commonly troublesome or disfiguring in females. Although the cause is not known lipoatrophy is probably an immune reaction to conventional insulin because the lesion does not occur in patients treated from the outset with purified insulin. For the young female who wishes to be as attractive in a bikini as her friends, there is a good case for using purified insulin from the onset of diabetes. In those with established lipoatrophy, improvement will gradually occur after switching to purified insulin, indeed the pits can be encouraged to fill by injecting directly into the lipoatrophic areas.

Soft painless swellings at injection sites – lipohypertrophy – are caused by injecting insulin repeatedly into the same area. Unlike lipoatrophy, it is not associated with insulin impurities; instead it is an area of local lipogenesis stimulated by high insulin concentration and will not improve by switching to purified preparations.

Insulin resistance This is usually arbitrarily defined as a total daily insulin requirement in excess of 200 units for more than seven days. All patients treated with conventional insulin develop circulating anti-insulin antibodies to a greater or lesser degree. As a general rule – to which, of course, there are exceptions – the higher the insulin dosage, the more insulin will be bound to anti-insulin antibodies and the less 'free' insulin will be available. Although insulin resistance as defined above is extremely rare, lesser degrees where the patient requires in excess of 120 units of conventional insulin daily are more common. A switch to purified insulin in such cases leads to a dramatic fall in daily requirements. Again as a general rule *the greater the dose of conventional insulin, the greater the reduction in dosage on switching to purified insulin.* In order to prevent a dangerous fall in blood glucose patients receiving more than 120 units of conventional insulin should receive only half their usual dose on the first day of switchover.

Apart from allergy, lipoatrophy or insulin resistance, should patients be switched to purified insulin on other grounds? The 'purer is better' ideology might lead to the belief that all patients should have these insulins and also that they might prevent or delay the onset of the serious long-term complications. There is no evidence to support this contention – on the other hand, there are some other theoretical advantages of purified insulin. Since insulin antibodies cross the placental barrier (Chapter 12) there is a case for using purified insulin in pregnancy. There is also a theoretical case for using purified insulin when it is anticipated that the need is temporary, ie. during an intercurrent illness, or surgery in a patient normally controlled by oral agents (Chapter 11), or in gestational diabetes. Time will give a clearer answer.

Switching to purified insulin In general, patients need approximately 20% less insulin when switched from conventional preparations and, as mentioned above, the greater the dose, the greater the fall. As a rule of thumb, drop the dose by a percentage equal to half the dose. In other words if the dose is

> 40 units reduce by 20%
> 60 units reduce by 30%
> 80 units reduce by 40%, etc

The dose can then be further adjusted upwards or downwards in the light of changes in urine glucose (page 125) or *blood* glucose (page 129) the following day and subsequently.

Single long-acting daily injections When the Lente insulins were introduced (page 133) with once-daily injection in mind, simplicity for the patient rather than good diabetic control was the main consideration. Nevertheless, diabetics with some pancreatic reserve may be adequately controlled by daily long-acting insulin. Often the elderly (where strict control in the prevention of long-term complications is less important than relieving symptoms) can be managed on once-daily injections, which is simpler when insulin therapy is dependent on visits from a district nurse.

Patients diagnosed before puberty may be controlled in the early stages by daily injections, especially when there is partial recovery of pancreatic function. Likewise, some of those developing diabetes in middle life who are unresponsive to oral agents may achieve good control by once daily insulin. Whether using purified monocomponent Lente insulin (Monotard) or conventional Lente, the dose is best adjusted to the results of blood or urine tests obtained before the main evening meal when the insulin is at its peak effect. Poor control in the forenoon with high post-breakfast blood glucose values might be an indication to switch to a combination of short- and long-acting insulin taken together before breakfast (page 122, Fig. 10.3). Conventional insulins used this way are soluble plus isophane. Purified alternatives are Neutral plus Retard or Actrapid plus Monotard. But poor control in the evening associated with satisfactory fasting blood or urine tests indicates that the long-acting insulin cannot be increased without the risk of nocturnal hypoglycaemia. Twice-daily injections are then imperative unless the fault lies in excess carbohydrate intake during the evening.

Twice-daily, 4-insulin system This has already been described on page 124, with short-acting insulins A_1 and A_2 and medium acting insulin B_1 and B_2 (Fig. 10.4). Suitable combinations are shown in Table 10.3.

Table 10.3

	Short-acting, A	*Medium-acting, B*
Conventional insulin	Soluble	Isophane
Purified insulin	Actrapid	Retard
Purified insulin	Neutral	Retard
Purified insulin	Actrapid	Monotard
Purified insulin	Actrapid	Semi-tard

On your marks, get set, go!

For those who with nostalgia prefer such quaint measures as inches, yards, gills, pints, rods and perches, the current system of measuring units of insulin in relation to marks on the diabetic syringe should warm their hearts. Thus in Britain and Europe insulin is currently available in two strengths: 40 units per ml and 80 units per ml. The British Standard BS1619 diabetic syringe and its various plastic counterparts have *twenty marks* per ml (Fig. 10.7); hence, each mark equals 2 units of 40-strength or 4 units of

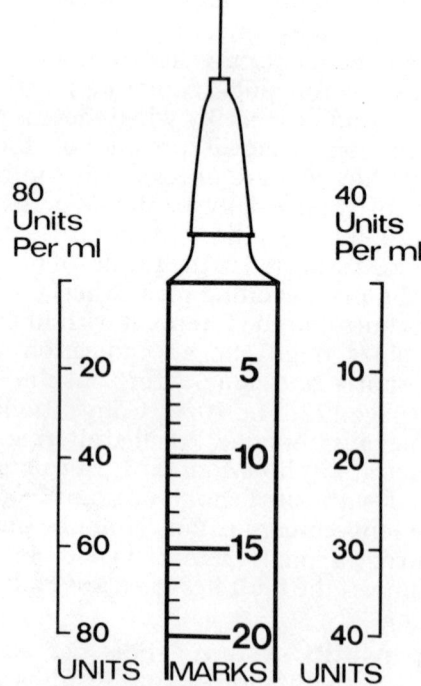

Fig. 10.7 Diabetic syringe 1 ml = 20 marks. Each mark of 80 strength insulin = 4 units and each mark of 40 strength insulin = 2 units

80-strength insulin. This is easy once the patient knows what to do, but very confusing to others, especially at times of emergency admission to hospital. The alternative American system of 100 units per ml with a syringe marked accordingly, ie. 1 mark = 1 unit is much simpler. Patients prefer this alternative and with improved manufacturing technology suitable syringes are now available which allow patients to draw up even small doses with accuracy.

Syringe care, injection technique and other practical aspects of drawing up insulin from the bottle are best explained and demonstrated by those experienced in patient guidance (Chapter 8, Fig. 10.8). Disposable needles are now available for all insulin-dependent diabetics up to the age of 16 years attending National Health Service hospitals in Britain.

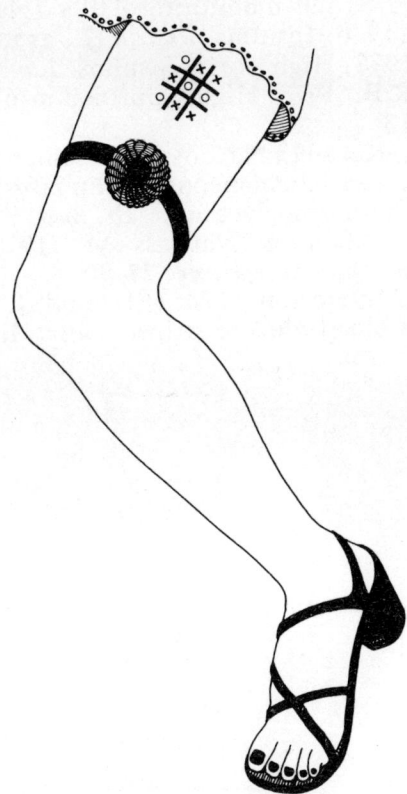

Fig. 10.8 Injection technique and 'noughts and crosses' – O for odd days and X for even days, thus alternating legs and varying site from time to time

Conclusion

Until better insulin delivery systems or such alternatives as islet-cell transplantation become available, patients (and doctors) will have to persevere with doing things the hard way. If this chapter has helped to make insulin therapy a little less painful for both patient and doctor it will have served its purpose.

Further Reading

1 Sonksen P.H., Judd S.L. & Lowy C. (1978) Home monitoring of blood glucose. *Lancet*, **i**, 729–732
2 Walford S., Gale E.A.M., Allison S.P. & Tattersall R.B. (1978) Self-monitoring of blood glucose. *Lancet*, **i**, 732–735
3 Editorial (1978) Self-monitoring of blood glucose. *Lancet*, **i**, 757
4 Turner P. (1976) Insulins. *Pharm. J.*, **217**, 583–584
5 Editorial (1977) High purity insulins. *Lancet*, **i**, 128–129
6 Tattersall R.B. (1978) Highly purified insulins. *Prescriber's J.*, **18**, 8–13
7 Pickup J.C., Keen H., Parsons J.A. & Alberti K.G.M.M. (1978) Continuous subcutaneous insulin infusion: an approach to achieving normoglycaemia. *Br. med. J.*, **i**, 203–207
8 Alberti K.G.M.M. & Nattrass M. (1978) Highly-purified insulins. *Diabetologia*, **15**, 77–80
9 Lawson, P.M., Kesson, C.M. & Ireland, J.T. (1979) Performance of blood-glucose strips. *Lancet*, **ii**, 742

CHAPTER 11

Oral Hypoglycaemic Agents and the Management of Milder Diabetics

Everyone wants the magic tablets. On learning of the diagnosis of diabetes, uppermost in the patient's mind is the question: will it be tablets or injections? And the likelihood is that it will be tablets, because oral therapy is now the mainstay of treatment for most maturity-onset diabetics. We have come a long way from the early faltering steps in the search for an alternative to insulin: today a galaxy of preparations is available – most of these being, in the strictly pharmacological sense, safe and remarkably free from toxic side effects. But lurking in the background there is now a suspicion that the indiscriminate use of some oral agents may aggravate the diabetic's tendency to cardiovascular disease (Chapter 13). This possibility was first highlighted in 1970 by the University Group Diabetes Program (UGDP) studies in America – a rigorously scientific if not very practical trial – which was interpreted to show a greater risk of cardiac death using oral as opposed to insulin therapy. Remember that the immediate aim of achieving good diabetic control by using tablets must be compatible with the long-term objective of avoiding the development of serious diabetic complications.

What are the indications for oral therapy? Of course, tablets are no alternative to insulin, and thus they have no place in the treatment of insulin-dependent or ketoacidosis-prone diabetics. At the other extreme of glucose intolerance many diabetics can be controlled easily and safely by diet alone. Tablets are for the solid middle ground. In a sense they do replace insulin because previously such patients – who could not be controlled by diet – needed small daily doses of insulin; for these diabetics, tablets are the greatest boon. But many patients need neither insulin nor tablets, yet they are often unwilling or unable to co-operate in adhering to a restrictive diet. Especially in middle age, enjoyment of food becomes a habit with little relationship to energy requirements. When patients' eating behaviour is incompatible with their metabolic problems too often we go for the soft option and give tablets to counter the symptoms of uncontrolled diabetes consequent upon calorie excess. Perhaps such an unholy alliance between patient and doctor may be excused so long as the treatment has no harmful effects, but unfortunately those oral agents most suitable for the overweight diabetic are the worst offenders in terms of side effects.

Oral hypoglycaemic agents are, in descending order of importance, of three groups: sulphonylureas, biguanides, and other kinds.

Sulphonylureas

Sulphonylureas are now the most widely used and effective oral hypoglycaemic agents. Their discovery in wartime was the result of astute clinical observation and subsequent research on a par with the best of military intelligence. In the wine-growing country of south-western France, wartime deprivation led to food shortage, hunger, malnutrition and frequent typhoid outbreaks. When a new sulphonamide derivative was introduced in 1941, Dr Marcel Janbon noticed that some of his patients with typhoid lost consciousness. He suspected hypoglycaemia due to malnutrition, but when three patients died of hypoglycaemia, his suspicion switched to the drug. With the aid of Dr Auguste Loubatières the hypoglycaemic effect of the drug was confirmed and subsequent research with other sulphonamide derivatives led to the development of the sulphonylureas.

Pharmacology and action   Loubatières showed that the main hypoglycaemic effect of the sulphonylureas is produced by stimulating the beta cells of the pancreas to release pre-formed insulin. Electron-microscopic studies have shown how the sulphonylureas stimulate the release of insulin granules from the beta cell cytoplasm – the so-called beta-cytotropic action. In other words, the sulphonylureas are to the failing pancreas as the hearing aid is to the failing ear. There must be some pancreatic beta-cell function, otherwise the tablets are as useless to the diabetic as the hearing aid is to the totally deaf. Sulphonylureas have also stimulated diabetologists into looking for other actions of the drugs. Although not as immediately dramatic as the beta-cytotropic effect, alternative effects are probably important in the long term since there is little proof that pancreatic stimulation is prolonged, yet the hypoglycaemic effect is sustained in the long-term. The following actions have been identified:

1 diminished hepatic glucose release by inhibition of glycogenolysis and gluconeogenesis;
2 alpha-cell vacuolisation and diminished glucagon release;
3 inhibition of glucose absorption from the gut; and
4 stimulation of the insulinotropic hormones such as gastric
   inhibitory polypeptide (G I P)* and secretin.

Confirmation of direct effects of the sulphonylureas on hepatic
and other functions has always been difficult because such actions
could equally be attributable to the insulin released by the beta-
cytotropic effect. Likewise, ideas about their direct or indirect
effect on glucagon have swung in and out of fashion. And it is
perhaps unwise to generalise. Each sulphonylurea has its own
special characteristics. More recently introduced potent sulphonylureas (glibenclamide and glipizide, Table 11.1) may not
only stimulate the beta cell to release insulin but also sensitise the
beta-cell system to the subtle normal insulin-releasing stimuli.

Adverse side effects Sulphonylureas rarely cause adverse side
effects. The most serious problem, especially with the more potent
and quick-acting preparation glibenclamide, is hypoglycaemia.
This is most likely to happen when sulphonylureas are used
without proper assessment of the need for them, or if the dose is
not sensibly adjusted in the light of the patient's response. Chronic
hypoglycaemia may often occur in the elderly especially if there is
failing renal function (Chapter 14) or loss of appetite.
   Allergic skin reactions, including photosensitivity, may occur in
about 2% of cases with any sulphonylurea, but more severe skin
reactions with exfoliative dermatitis are rare. Cross-sensitivity
with other sulphonylureas is usual. Distressing alcohol intolerance
affects about 5% of patients treated with chlorpropamide, and
sulphonylureas may occasionally cause nausea or other gastrointestinal side effects.

**Chlorpropamide and inappropriate secretion of anti-
diuretic hormone (ADH)** Chlorpropamide is the only sulphonylurea in which this adverse effect can be turned to advantage
in treating diabetes insipidus. A significant inappropriate ADH
effect with marked hyponatraemia occurs extremely rarely and
usually in elderly patients having had the drug for an extended
period. The effect can often go unnoticed mainly because otherwise stable diabetics rarely have their electrolytes checked.

* Also known as glucose-dependent insulin-releasing polypeptide.

Indications for sulphonylureas Check the section on assessment of severity of diabetes (Chapter 5). Note that sulphonylureas are most suited to those diabetics who remain hyperglycaemic or have symptoms of uncontrolled diabetes despite dietary precautions. Often in the few weeks before diabetes is diagnosed the patient will assuage the severe thirst with glucose-containing drinks so that the initial blood glucose may be artificially high. Remember Mrs. Sweet-tooth (Chapter 3) and how her symptoms settled with simple dietetic advice. Remember also that obese patients should not be given sulphonylureas: the drug will lower the blood glucose, relieve the symptoms and make the patient feel much better, but weight will be gained when it should be lost and the battle with the patient's appetite will also be lost.

Non-obese diabetics, previously controlled on diet, may require the addition of a sulphonylurea either temporarily or permanently if an intercurrent illness or other minor stress causes deterioration in control (Chapter 20).

Method of use Although several sulphonylureas are listed in Table 11.1, chlorpropamide, glibenclamide and glipizide are those most widely used. Chlorpropamide has the longest biological half-life and although the slowest to produce its full hypoglycaemic effect it is most suitable for once-daily prescription. Glibenclamide is the most powerful, while glipizide is intermediate in action. Whatever preparation is chosen continued assessment is best achieved by regular urine testing, as follows:

1 Teach the patient how to use the Clinitest or a similar urine testing procedure (Chapter 5, p.64).
2 Recommended that urine samples be obtained for testing on waking and two hours after the main evening meal twice or thrice weekly.
3 Advise the patient to interpret the Clinitest scale thus:

0	$\frac{1}{4}$	$\frac{1}{2}$	$\frac{3}{4}$	1	2 per cent
GOOD				BAD	

4 Prescribe the sulphonylurea in the starting dose indicated in Table 11.1.
5 Advise the patient to increase the dose of chlorpropamide by 125 mg (half a tablet) or of the other two preparations by 5 mg (one tablet) if the urine tests remain *bad* after 10 days of treatment. Advise that the dose be reduced to half a tablet if the tests are *good*.

Table 11.1   Oral Hypoglycaemic Agents: tablet size, duration of action, initial and maximal doses; main indications

Approved name	Proprietary name	Tablet size mg	Duration of hypoglycaemic effect (hours)	Initial dose mg	Maximal dose mg	Main indication
Sulphonylureas						
Chlorpropamide	Diabinese	100, 250	Up to 60	100–250	375	Non-obese maturity onset diabetic, single daily dose
	Melitase	100, 250	Up to 60	100–250	375	
Glibenclamide	Daonil	5	5–20	5	15	Most effective available, brisk action, quick relief of symptoms
	Euglucon					
Glipizide	Minodiab	5	5–12	5–10	20	Brisk action, ideal for elderly with impaired renal function
	Glibenese					
Tolbutamide	Rastinon	500	5–12	1,000	3,000	
	Pramidex					
Acetohexamide	Dimelor	500	12–24	500	1,500	
Tolazamide	Tolanase	100, 250	12–24	100–250	1,000	
Biguanides						
Phenformin	Dibotin	50 SR*	12–24	50	100	Overweight, adjunct to sulphonylurea
	Dipar	50 SR				
Metformin	Glucophage	500, 850	12—24	500–850	2,000	As above
	Metiguanide	500				
Other						
Fenfluramine	Ponderax	20	6–12	40		Obese maturity onset diabetics where biguanide unsuited
		60CAP**	12–24	60	120	

Notes: Glymidine (Gondafon), glibornuride (Gluteril) and gliclazide (Diamicron) are sulphonylurea-related agents.
* SR = sustained release capsule. Phenformin (Dibotin) is also available as 25 mg tablets
** CAP = sustained release capsule

In this way the patient can make sensible adjustments without too frequent clinical review. By comparing blood glucose values with the urine tests obtained at home the advice can be appropriately modified, especially if the renal threshold is abnormally high or low (Chapter 5). Using this method the dose of glibenclamide can be gradually increased to a maximum of 15 mg or glipizide to a maximum of 20 mg daily. Although higher doses are often recommended, the beta-cytotropic effect is not dose related; if control is inadequate at these doses it is usually better to consider adding a biguanide (page 146) rather than increase the sulphonylurea towards potentially toxic levels. The aim of good diabetic control is to:

abolish symptoms,

bring the two-hours post-breakfast blood glucose in the satisfactory range (Table 11.2) for the patient's age, and

bring the patient's weight into the normal range for his age and height (Appendix 1)

Once good diabetic control is established the patient should be advised to continue regular urine testing and adjust the dose of tablets – or seek medical advice – if there is any significant change in the results. Often in this way the patient can make a sensible temporary increase in dose during intercurrent illness or alternatively find that medication is unnecessary after a few months of treatment if the effective dose has been small.

Unlike insulin-dependent diabetes, the disorder in the milder patient is more stable and frequent *blood* glucose estimation is unnecessary. Because glucose tolerance deteriorates with each meal, hyperglycaemia (and the chance of glycosuria) is greater after meals and especially after the main evening meal. Satisfactory *urine* or *blood* glucose values 2–3 hours after meals and particularly after the main evening meal are good evidence that diabetic control is good throughout the remaining 24 hours of the day.

Biguanides

Pharmacology and side effects In the past twenty years, the biguanides phenformin, buformin and metformin have found a place in the management of non-insulin-dependent diabetics in two main circumstances: obesity, and as an adjunct to the sulphonylureas.

The pharmacological action of the biguanides is still disputed although there is evidence that they lower the blood glucose by

reducing glucose absorption from the gut,

increasing uptake of glucose into peripheral tissues, and

decreasing gluconeogenesis from alanine, pyruvate and *lactate.*

The main advantage of the biguanides in obese diabetics relates to the fact that, unlike the sulphonylureas, they do not stimulate the pancreas to produce insulin but instead enhance its peripheral action. Inappropriate hyperinsulinism in the portal circulation due to the use of sulphonylureas in the obese unfortunately stimulates triglyceride synthesis (Chapter 6) and further fuel hoarding. However, the wisdom of using biguanides has been questioned in recent years mainly because of their effects on hepatic gluconeogenesis with an inevitable rise in blood lactate concentration. This may be of little consequence in the otherwise healthy diabetic, but dangerous lactic acidosis (Chapter 4, p.55) could arise in those with renal or hepatic disease, alcoholism (a common feature of the obese patient's excess fuel intake) or in those suffering a myocardial infarct complicated by shock and poor tissue perfusion (Jack Spratt, Chapter 7). Biguanides are excreted by the kidney, hence renal impairment increases the blood concentrations of both the drug and lactate. Phenformin is also metabolised in the liver so that those with liver disease (or alcoholism) are more at risk of lactic acidosis with phenformin than with metformin.

Aware of the remote risk of lactic acidosis, doctors often consoled themselves with the thought that biguanides might be good for the diabetic's coronary arteries through their known *in vitro* effect on fibrinolysis. But the UGDP report put paid to that notion when long-term studies showed an enhanced cardiac mortality in those taking phenformin. Should phenformin or other biguanides be used at all? Aware of the hazard of lactic acidosis, the British Committee on the Safety of Medicines has issued a warning suggesting that the use of phenformin should be restricted. Several other countries, including the USA, have taken similar action. Apart from lactic acidosis, biguanides have other troublesome side-effects: they tend to cause nausea, vague indigestion and as well as malabsorption of glucose perhaps of other nutrients including vitamin B_{12}. Indeed, some doctors have used biguanides both in the obese diabetic and non-diabetic in the belief that these side effects might suppress the appetite and diminish nutrient absorption and storage. About 20% of patients taking metformin can be shown to malabsorb vitamin B_{12} although many fewer ever develop low serum levels of the vitamin or other more serious haemopoietic defects.

Indications for biguanides Biguanides may be considered in the management of the obese diabetic who remains symptomatic (thirst, polyuria) or hyperglycaemic (Table 11.2) despite dieting. They may also be added to sulphonylurea therapy if the latter does not produce adequate diabetic control or if the response deteriorates after an interval (secondary sulphonylurea failure). However, if weight loss, hyperglycaemia or symptoms are significant, insulin therapy (Mrs. Peabody, Chapter 3) should be considered sooner rather than struggling with oral agents. Since the

introduction of more powerful sulphonylureas, secondary sulphonylurea failure may be prevented by switching to
glibenclamide.

Table 11.2   Blood glucose values at different ages

Satisfactory (not ideal) values. Patients remaining more hyperglycaemic despite
diet should have oral agents (see Table 11.1). Consider reducing dose, or stopping
therapy when these values are reached, especially if significantly more hyperglycaemic initially.

| Age in years | Fasting blood glucose | | 2-hours post-breakfast blood glucose | |
	mmol/l	mg/100 ml	mmol/l	mg/100 ml
40–49	5– 7	90–126	8–10	144–180
50–59	6– 8	108–144	9–11	160–200
60–69	7– 9	126–162	10–12	180–215
70 upwards	8–10	144–180	11–13	200–235

Method of use   If a biguanide is to be used either in obesity or as
an adjunct to a sulphonylurea, the following guidelines should be
applied:

1 exclude patients with renal, hepatic or cardiac disease;
2 exclude patients with a history of alcoholism;
3 the dose of biguanide should be limited to 100 mg daily of
   phenformin or 2 g daily of metformin (Table 11.1);
4 the patient should be instructed to stop the drug during any
   intercurrent illness (a temporary switch to a sulphonylurea
   or insulin may be necessary if the patient is hyperglycaemic);
5 think of lactic acidosis in any serious intercurrent illness
   (Chapters 4, p.55; 7, p.98);
6 biguanides should be withdrawn if the patient successfully
   loses his excess weight;
7 biguanides should be withdrawn when patients reach 70
   years of age because of the enhanced risk of cardiac disease
   and renal impairment;
8 check the serum vitamin B_{12} level from time to time,
   especially when using metformin and certainly in any
   unexplained anaemia.

With these precautions, and especially with the limitations on
maximum dose, the diabetic should be able to perform urine tests
to adjust the dose of tablets and have intermittent blood glucose

estimations as described in the section on the sulphonylureas. Gastrointestinal side effects are often most troublesome on the introduction of biguanides, so it is sensible to start the patient on either one tablet of metformin or one capsule of phenformin (Table 11.1) at the main evening meal, adding a second tablet or capsule at breakfast (if necessary) after an interval of 10 to 14 days provided that nausea or other side effects have not arisen.

Other drugs

Several other drugs are mildly hypoglycaemic (Chapter 20, p.240) or may enhance the effect of the sulphonylureas (others may have adverse effects, Chapter 20). However, if obesity is the problem and the biguanides are either contra-indicated or considered risky, a good alternative is fenfluramine.

Fenfluramine Fenfluramine (Ponderax), although primarily used as an appetite suppressant, is as effective as phenformin in lowering the blood glucose in obese hyperglycaemic diabetics. Besides reducing hyperglycaemia by appetite suppression, there is evidence that fenfluramine enhances peripheral glucose uptake, and especially where biguanides are contra-indicated, or if they cause troublesome nausea, diarrhoea or other side effects, it is a safer alternative. If diet adherence is the major problem and the patient is unable to control his appetite, fenfluramine is probably the sensible choice in the first instance. A starting dose is 40 mg of tablets or one 60 mg sustained-capsule daily, increasing to a maximum of 120 mg of either preparation after a short interval.

Conclusion

The initial assessment of patients should take account of recent intake of concentrated carbohydrate and their weight in relation to the correct value for age and height. Those who are close to their correct weight and remain hyperglycaemic despite a modest carbohydrate intake are most likely to benefit from a sulphonyl-urea. For those having distressing symptoms glibenclamide is quick acting, while chlorpropamide is slower in taking effect but is simplest for once-daily prescription in the long term. Biguanides may be added with caution in those who fail to respond adequately to sulphonylureas provided that renal or hepatic disease and other contra-indications have been excluded. Sulphonylureas should be avoided in the obese (except in the short-term to relieve distressing symptoms); again, biguanides should be used with caution if diet has failed, while those who cannot restrict their appetites may be treated more appropriately with fenfluramine.

Whatever therapy is chosen, drug dosage should be kept under regular review in the light of the patient's response and diet compliance. Those doctors swayed by the results of the UGDP study into believing that oral agents are bad for the coronary arteries in the long-term would have to give serious consideration to the problem of switching satisfied patients from oral agents to insulin. On the other hand, insulin should be introduced, without hesitation, for those diabetics unresponsive to oral agents.

Further Reading

1 Shen S-W. & Bressler R. (1977) Clinical pharmacology of oral antidiabetic agents (first of two parts).*New Engl. J. Med.*, **296**, 493-496

2 Shen S-W. & Bressler R. (1977) Clinical pharmacology of oral antidiabetic agents (second of two parts). *New Engl. J. Med.*, **296**, 787–793

3 Clarke B.F., Campbell I.W. (1977) Comparisons of metformin and chlorpropamide in non-obese, maturity-onset diabetics uncontrolled by diet. *Br. med. J.*, **ii**, 1576–1578

4 Editorial (1977) Biguanides and lactic acidosis in diabetics. *Br. med. J.*, **ii**, 1436

5 Editorial (1975) Oral hypoglycaemics in diabetes mellitus. *Lancet*, **ii**, 489–491

6 Chalmers T.C. (1975) Settling the UGDP controversy. *J. Am. Med. Ass.*, **231**, 624–625

7 Jarrett R.J., Keen H., Fuller J.H. & McCartney M. (1977) Treatment of borderline diabetes: controlled trial using carbohydrate restriction and phenformin. *Br. med. J.*, **ii**, 861–864

8 Nattrass M. & Alberti K.G.M.M. (1978) Biguanides. *Diabetologia*, **14**, 71–74

9 Luft, D., Schmülling R.M. & Eggstein M. (1978) Lactic acidosis in biguanide-treated diabetics. A review of 330 cases. *Diabetologia*, **14**, 75–88

10 Kesson C.M. & Ireland J.T. (1976) Phenformin compared with fenfluramine in the treatment of obese diabetic patients. *Practitioner*, **216**, 577–580

CHAPTER 12

Special Problems: Diabetes in Childhood and Pregnancy

Diabetes in childhood

Onset of diabetes in the early formative years, especially if before school age, is a frightening experience for the hapless parents who thereafter carry an added burden of responsibility in watching their child grow up. Fortunately, childhood diabetes is relatively uncommon; precise figures of its *prevalence* are difficult to obtain partly because, in the varied data available, different age limits have been set for the period of childhood. Estimates range between one in 1200 and one in 6,000 of children up to the age of 17 years. The register sponsored by the British Diabetic Association (Chapter 4, p.41) showed an overall annual *incidence* of new cases of one in 12,000. However, Figure 12.1 drawn from the same data also shows that the majority of childhood diabetics develop the disorder around puberty and that before the age of 5 years diabetes is therefore extremely rare. Not that this is of any comfort to the parents or to the doctor faced with the responsibility of diabetic

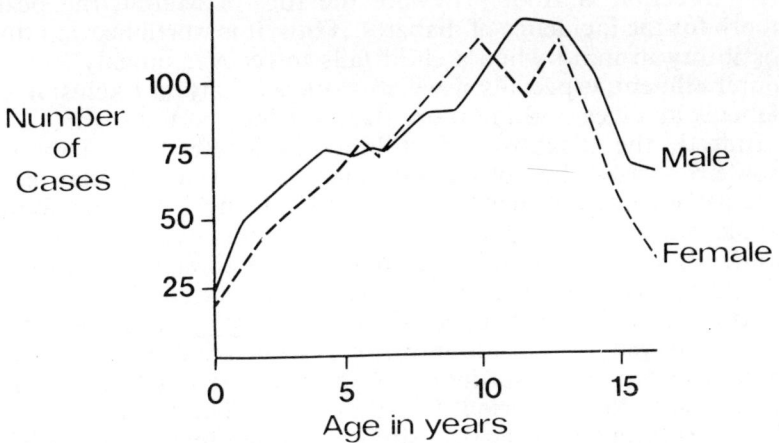

Fig. 12.1 Age at diagnosis in male and female children. See Register of Newly Diagnosed Children (page 41)

151

care. The genetics of childhood diabetes has already been discussed (Chapter 4, p.42) in relation to HLA status which in childhood may confer susceptibility to diabetes. The interface between certain HLA alleles and genes involved in immunity is rapidly coming into sharper focus yet particular virus infections which switch the unlucky child from good health to florid diabetes have not been identified with certainty. But Figure 12.2, again

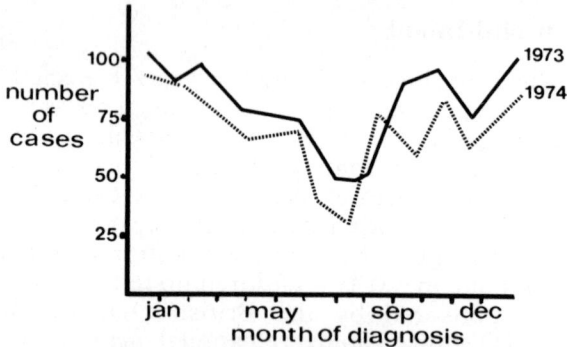

Fig. 12.2 Month of diagnosis of diabetes in childhood. Majority of cases diagnosed in winter with sharp increase in September from summer low and peak in spring months

based upon the Childhood Register of the British Diabetic Association, also shows that the season of diabetes is winter when most infection is afoot – beware the Ides of March, the peak month for the incidence of diabetes. Thus, it is worth bearing this possibility in mind when a child fails to recover quickly from a winter ailment, especially if weight-loss is a feature. Exclusion of diabetes involves nothing more than a urine test for sugar.

Indeed, the diagnosis of childhood diabetes is usually no problem – it is the subsequent management which may give parents and others such headaches. Essentially, the metabolic problem in terms of glucose-insulin homeostasis is no different from other insulin-dependent diabetics, although the insulin dosage and the pace of events is on a different scale. Usually, the onset is abrupt, with features of the melting down of flesh and limbs, and polyuria of around 4 weeks' duration. Occasionally, there is evidence of disordered metabolism extending back over a considerably longer period with the affected child having grown significantly taller than other siblings. Sometimes such children initially have a relatively mild disturbance of carbohydrate metabolism, tempting the doctor to start treatment with a sulphonylurea. This is justified only if there is a strong family history of *mild* diabetes suggestive of mild maturity-onset diabetes of youth (MODY) as in the case of Susan (Chapter 3, p.30); see also genetics, Chapter 4, p.43), for otherwise a sulphonylurea at this stage only strains the already failing beta cells. Indeed, there is a school of thought supporting the view that if childhood diabetes could be predicted with greater certainty, long-term insulin-dependence might be prevented if exogenous insulin or other support could be given to tide the beta cell through the acute phase of immunological insult. Management of the child concentrates on three aspects:

> insulin,
> diet, and
> growth, development, diabetic control and life style.

Insulin   Both in ketoacidosis (Chapter 7) and ordinary circumstances, the general principles of insulin therapy (Chapter 10) apply, although smaller children require smaller doses. Fortunately, youngsters' kidneys are more efficient than those of adults in sorting out electrolyte imbalance and in excreting H^+ ions, provided that fluid intake is maintained, and if a child is still drinking well at diagnosis, intravenous fluids are unnecessary. If he is dehydrated, acidotic or unable to drink, fluids are essential, when intravenous saline and insulin, with the addition of potassium chloride as soon as there is clinical improvement, is the basis of management. Because of the renal efficiency, bicarbonate is rarely necessary. Instead of fluid at the rate of 1 litre per hour, a four-year-old might receive 250 ml per hour and a ten-year-old 500 ml per hour. Insulin, if added to the infusion, may be given via an infusion pump at the rate of 0·1 unit/kg body weight per hour after an initial dose of 0·2 units/kg body weight. If added directly to the intravenous saline, put 0·4 units/kg into the first bottle and 0·2 units/kg to each hourly bottle thereafter. Those preferring an hourly *intramuscular* régime may safely use the same doses of insulin as given by infusion pump. Doses of insulin and methods, including potassium replacement, are summarised in Table 12.1.

The child usually recovers quickly and as soon as significant improvement in the vital functions is evident or the arterial pH is above 7·2, the drip can be slowed to half the initial rate. Although intravenous fluids may have to be continued longer in the context of simultaneous infection or other illness, it is otherwise usually possible to stop the drip after 12 hours. Thus on the first day after admission a routine insulin régime may be planned for the long term.

Table 12.1 Intravenous therapy in childhood: a guide to insulin, saline and potassium replacement

Age in years	Approximate weight in kilograms	Initial dose of insulin (units)	Hourly dose of insulin* (units)	Intravenous normal saline volume per hour (ml) †	Intravenous potassium mmol/hour**
2	13	2·5	1·2	200	2·5
4	15	3	1·5	250	3
6	20	4	2	300	3
8	25	5	2·5	400	5
10	30	6	3	500	7
12	38	8	4	600	9

* The hourly dose of insulin may be given intravenously via an infusion pump or as an hourly intramuscular injection. If insulin is added directly to the intravenous infusion of saline the dose should be doubled (see text).

† The volume of saline per hour should be *halved* after the first 4 hours, or as soon as there is significant clinical improvement (see also Chapter 7). Switch to 5% dextrose once blood glucose falls below 15 mmol/l or 270 mg/100 ml.

** Add potassium *after* the initial hourly infusions of saline, or from outset if the child is passing urine freely.

Routine insulin therapy   Before puberty, children usually require remarkably small doses of insulin, often show significant recovery in pancreatic function after the initial insult, and seem to need less insulin than adults at night. A once-daily régime of insulin given before breakfast may, therefore, be suitable, especially initially whilst the patient and the parents settle down to their new way of life. For the girl who later wants to look as attractive in a bikini as her non-diabetic friends, purified insulin, which will not cause lipoatrophy at injection sites, is preferable and indeed has much to commend it in all newly diagnosed youngsters. Either a single long-acting insulin (Monotard) or once daily short + medium to long-acting (Actrapid + Retard) insulin (Chapter 10, p.134) may be suitable. An appropriate initial dose of insulin for a child with a good appetite might be 0·4 units/kg body weight of both short and long-acting insulin or 0·8 units/kg body weight of long-acting insulin alone; thereafter, the dose can be adjusted according to the results of urine tests (Chapter 10) in order to minimise blood tests, though the occasional confirmatory blood sample (best obtained by pricking the ear lobe) may be obtained as necessary. At this stage, so long as the child is thriving, strict control in terms of fine-tuning of the blood glucose (Chapter 10, p.129) is more than parents and child can cope with, and should be deferred until full recovery of weight-loss and the early hurdles of adjustment to diabetes are over.

More important at this stage is establishing good insulin injection technique and an understanding of the time actions of the insulins being used. Whether the initial education is given in hospital or on an out-patient basis depends on the facilities available locally. An experienced health visitor often learns more about family background and other aspects concerning co-operation and capabilities in the home environment. Whether the child learns to inject, or the parents (or both), depends on age and aptitude. Usually a child of six years or more can inject success-fully from the outset. Sterile disposable needles make the tech-nique virtually painless and are now available freely to all diabetic children under the age of 16 years attending National Health Service hospitals and diabetic clinics in Great Britain. Older children, particularly those developing diabetes at puberty or after, are best controlled on a twice-daily, four-insulin technique from the outset (Chapter 10, p.123) and most children diagnosed in the early years should be switched to the more advanced régime whenever control is inadequate on a simpler one.

Diet Initially the child may be profoundly underweight, and nothing more than limitation of concentrated carbohydrate may suffice until a specialist dietician discusses with the parents the previous pattern of eating and food habits. An unduly restrictive régime punctuated by sugar snacks to counteract hypoglycaemia doesn't encourage confidence. Because so many children are accustomed to being pampered with sugar goodies, it is hard for them to understand why their first successful injection cannot be rewarded with their favourite confectionery. Taking account of family circumstances, religious and personal preferences, allergies and any particular dislikes, dietetic advice involves two principles:

the child must have as much fuel as its non-diabetic brother in order to grow and develop normally, and

the carbohydrate should be evenly distributed throughout the daily meals and snacks.

Thus a ten-year-old might have 160 g carbohydrate per day (see carbohydrate exchanges, Appendices 3 & 4) distributed as approximately 25% at each of the three main meals and the remaining 25% as mid-morning, mid-afternoon and evening snacks (10 g carbohydrate may be added to or subtracted from the 160 g daily total for each year of age above or below 10 years). Although sugar foods and drinks are discouraged, ice-cream, fresh fruit, jelly and plain cakes or biscuits should be allowed. Extra fuel should be added to cover additional exercise and the dietary allowance generously increased for the growing active adolescent. Distribution of the carbohydrate can be modified in the light of subsequent diabetic control and particular times of either hyperglycaemia or hypoglycaemia.

Growth, development, diabetic control and life style

When diabetics attend the out-patient clinic, there is a natural tendency to look backwards over health and diabetic control since the previous visit. However, the growing child or adolescent often has anxieties about the future – the prospect of a new school, a new sporting activity, a future career; thus, *forward planning* should be an important aspect of the hospital visit. Many of the problems are discussed in Chapter 22. Adolescents probably need more medical skill (and time) than other diabetics, and clinics specially geared to the young are usually more successful than crowding such patients into a busy routine. By the age of 14–15 years, the adolescent is usually ready to begin monitoring his blood glucose at home (Chapter 10).

Adolescent patients, and their parents, need encouragement and guidance in coping with various hurdles, and the better they understand diabetic self-regulation, the greater the likelihood of success. Indeed, those with a good grasp of the principles of insulin-glucose homeostasis not only adjust their insulin and fuel intake to their varying activities but also can cope successfully with intercurrent ailments. Illness may strike suddenly, yet by taking small supplements of their quick-acting insulin plus easily palatable substitutes for the normal diet (Appendix 6) youngsters can avoid calling for medical help. Nevertheless, 'hot-line' access to the hospital diabetic clinic for advice by telephone can be a great asset. And if you are at the receiving end of the line? The key question is whether the child is still able to take food or fluid. If there is anorexia or vomiting the patient will require intravenous fluids and cannot be left at home.

Adolescents have to learn the facts of life. Diabetics have to learn the facts of diabetic life and usually respond with enthusiasm when even the complex aspects of diabetes are explained to them (witness the success of 'Dr. Robert's Corner' in *Balance*, the newspaper of the British Diabetic Association). When denied proper education, the co-operative muddle along as best they can. Those who cannot co-operate are usually suffering from a disrupted family life or social circumstances which prevent sensible eating or a reasonably ordered existence, while those who will not co-operate are often using diabetes to work out their adolescent hang-ups (Chapter 22) – yet once they mature they may prove to be the most reliable patients.

For those denied education, diabetes is an awesome hardship; for those who seek to be manipulative it can be turned into a powerful weapon against parents (and doctors), and for those taught diabetic self-control, diabetes is a challenge to which the majority respond with remarkable zeal.

Further Reading: Childhood Diabetes

1 Baum J.D. & Smith M.A. (1976) The diabetic child. *Hosp. Update*, **4**, 159–167
2 Craig J.O. (1977) *Childhood Diabetes and its Management.* London: Butterworth
3 Editorial (1977) Sex and juvenile diabetes. *Br. med. J.*, **i**, 595
4 MacGregor M. (1977) Juvenile diabetics growing up. *Lancet*, **i**, 944–945
5 Farquhar J.W. (1977) Diet and the diabetic child. *Br. med. J.*, **i**, 285–286
6 Editorial (1978) Diabetic complications in childhood. *Br. med. J.*, **i**, 942
7 Tattersall R. (1978) Highly purified insulins. *Prescribers J.*, **18**, 8–13

Diabetes and pregnancy

Amongst the childbearing population at large, pregnancy is usually medically uncomplicated and has a successful outcome for the vast majority of mothers (the perinatal mortality rate is about 2% in the UK). The pregnant diabetic has always fared much worse than others in terms of maternal morbidity and mortality, abortion rate and perinatal mortality. Fortunately, with better diabetic and obstetric care there has been a steady improvement in recent years so that most well-organised centres now expect a fetal mortality rate in the region of 5% or better. What went wrong in the past? We now know that poor control of insulin-glucose homeostasis created a quite inappropriate environment in which to nurture offspring and that the essence of improving the lot of the diabetic mother and her fetus involves fine-tuning of blood glucose control (Chapter 10, p.129) besides close co-operation between physician, obstetrician and paediatrician.

Even in the non-diabetic, pregnancy strains insulin-glucose

homeostasis, and glycosuria is a common finding on the ante-natal inspection. So at the outset it may be instructive to examine some aspects of carbohydrate metabolism in the normal pregnancy, particularly since these have a direct bearing upon the management of the known diabetic.

The effect of pregnancy on carbohydrate metabolism In pregnancy the fasting blood glucose tends to be lower than in the non-pregnant state and after a glucose load the peak blood glucose is reached later and may be higher, these changes being most pronounced in the third trimester. Some women, especially those under 21 years of age, show only a slight rise of blood glucose from fasting – implying efficient insulin-glucose homeostasis. Deterioration in glucose tolerance in the last trimester is attributed to increasing production of *placental lactogen* (HPL) which has growth-hormone-like activity. High levels of FFA (Chapter 6) may also contribute to insulin resistance, although normally the healthy pancreas responds by raising the insulin output.

Insulin is important to the growth of the fetus but maternal insulin does not reach the fetal circulation (nor does the exogenous insulin of the pregnant diabetic cross the placenta, although antibodies to insulin do so). Although insulin is probably present in the fetal pancreas and plasma by the age of 11 weeks, the pancreatic islets do not recognise glucose as a stimulus before 32 weeks. Maternal glucose passes to the fetal circulation by facilitated diffusion, the fetal blood glucose usually being lower than that of the mother. However, abnormal elevation of the maternal blood glucose stimulates the fetal pancreas with two main consequences which adversely affect the perinatal mortality: fetal macrosomia and neonatal hypoglycaemia.

Maternal hyperglycaemia stimulates hyperplasia of the fetal islets which directly contribute to fetal growth due to hyperinsulinism. The fetal macrosomia or typical big baby of the poorly-controlled diabetic not only has excessive weight, particularly of fat and protein, but is unduly likely to suffer traumatic birth by vaginal delivery. As soon as the large baby with its super-charged islets leaves the maternal environment of hyperglycaemia there is a serious risk of neonatal hypoglycaemia with consequent brain damage.

These two fundamental aspects of fetal abnormality are the main reasons for diagnosing diabetes during pregnancy, and aiming to control diabetes perfectly during pregnancy. Thus *glycosuria* in pregnancy always should be evaluated with care even though pregnancy raises the glomerular filtration rate and lowers the renal threshold to glucose. Because of the effect of pregnancy upon the renal threshold many cases of glycosuria will have no abnormality of glucose tolerance. Nevertheless, a 50 g oral GTT should be carried out in any of the following circumstances:

persistent glycosuria,
if there is a family history of diabetes,
obesity,
a history of previous stillbirth or perinatal death (especially if post-mortem examination showed pancreatic hyperplasia or fetal malformation),
a history of a previous 10 lb (4·5 kg) offspring, and
a history of a previous abnormal GTT in pregnancy.

The GTT should be interpreted according to the criteria in Chapter 5, p.66. If the GTT is normal in early pregnancy but glycosuria persists, it is usually wise to repeat the test at 32 weeks' gestation. Those found to have abnormal glucose tolerance during pregnancy should have a GTT six weeks (or later) after delivery. Remember that the term *gestational diabetes* (Sally, Chapter 3) is reserved for those who are diabetic during pregnancy but who have normal glucose tolerance thereafter. However, gestational diabetes is often the forerunner of permanent diabetes – about 50% develop the disorder within seven years of the pregnancy.

Management of the established diabetic With improved ante-natal management of the established insulin-dependent patient, there is no evidence that pregnancy adversely affects the long-term prognosis for the diabetic (Chapter 21). However, proliferative retinopathy (Chapter 15) and nephropathy (Chapter 14), especially when complicated by hypertension, may be adversely affected by pregnancy. Thus for the unfortunate few having developed such complications in the childbearing years, therapeutic abortion is advisable both because of the effect on the maternal prognosis and also because of the unlikelihood that the pregnancy will nurture a viable fetus. Unfortunately, many diabetics default from regular follow-up in adolescence (Chapter 22, p.256), and the first opportunity of re-appraisal of general health and diabetic control may therefore arise in pregnancy.

For those without diabetic complications *perfect diabetic control* should be established (see fine-tuning of blood glucose, Chapter 10). Provided that a twice-daily injection, four-insulin system is followed (Chapter 10, p.123) it is usually relatively easy to establish good diabetic control in the pregnant patient who has a special incentive to be co-operative. For those already well-experienced in self-regulation by *urine* glucose testing this is a good opportunity to teach home monitoring of *blood* glucose (Chapter 10, p.129).

Poorly-controlled patients or those unable fully to co-operate in self-regulation should be admitted to hospital, but those able to control their disorder by home monitoring of blood glucose need not be admitted until 36 weeks' gestation unless there is some other obstetric indication at ante-natal visits.

Remember that the renal threshold to glucose falls in pregnancy. Some patients may lose such large quantities of glucose that the relative starvation stimulates gluconeogenesis and ketogenesis especially overnight. Ketonaemia may have an adverse effect upon the fetus and should be avoided by augmenting the carbohydrate intake especially at the late evening or bedtime snack and first thing in the morning (a daily increase in carbohydrate of 50 g, ie. five 10 g exchanges or more, may be necessary, Chapter 9).

Especially in the last trimester, insulin requirements rise progressively usually by at least a third and often to double the normal quantity, due mainly to the growth-hormone-like effect of placental lactogen. Conversely, falling insulin requirements in late pregnancy or the sudden onset of hypoglycaemia may be the first warning of placental insufficiency.

Obstetric management   In the well-controlled diabetic there is no increase in the incidence of pre-eclampsia or hydramnios. In the past the pregnant diabetic was induced at 36 weeks partly on account of fetal macrosomia but also because of the increasing risk of placental insufficiency, but improved diabetic control and better methods of fetal monitoring especially from the 32nd week of gestation now make delivery at 38 weeks safe and preferable. Premature delivery increased the likelihood of *respiratory distress syndrome* (R D S) – a major cause of neonatal death in the past. Maturing fetal lungs produce phospholipids, especially lecithin, which reduce surface tension by acting as surfactants. Lecithin production usually increases from about 34 weeks' gestation. By measuring the lecithin/sphingomyelin ratio in a sample of amniotic fluid, fetal lung maturity can be assessed particularly in those instances where early induction of labour or caesarean section is indicated before 38 weeks' gestation. In non-diabetics a lecithin/sphingomyelin ratio of less than 2·0 suggests lung immaturity and a high risk of R D S. Unfortunately for the infant of the diabetic mother, a ratio greater than 2·0 is not a guarantee against R D S. Probably the most significant factor in reducing the risk of R D S in diabetic pregnancies is the enhanced opportunity of continuing a viable feto-placental unit in the diabetic for 38 weeks' gestation as a result of improved control.

Fetal and placental function can be assessed by various methods (Table 12.2), although most are of prognostic significance and are no substitute for better diabetic management. Salbutamol (Chapter 20, p.239) used by intravenous infusion to diminish uterine contractions in premature labour, may cause a sharp rise in insulin requirements in some patients probably due to its effect in stimulating lipolysis and glycogenolysis.

Table 12.2   Assessment of the fetoplacental unit. In addition to the usual antenatal routines the following tests are usually carried out from 32nd week till delivery

System	Test	Time
Fetal growth	Biparietal diameter by ultrasound	Weekly
Fetal skeletal maturity	X-ray	at 36 weeks
Fetal lung maturity	Lecithin/sphingomyelin ratio in amniotic fluid	at 37 weeks or 48 hours before delivery
Placental function	Plasma placental lactogen	As indicated obstetrically
Fetoplacental unit	24-hour urinary oestriol	As indicated obstetrically

Management of labour   The decision to deliver naturally or by Caesarian section depends upon obstetric rather than medical criteria. Patients having reached 38 weeks' gestation are more likely to have a successful vaginal delivery. Indications for Caesarian section include primigravida over 35 years of age, malpresentation, unstable lie, severe pre-eclampsia or dispropor-tion. Otherwise *surgical induction of labour* is the method of choice.

On the morning of induction a 5% dextrose infusion with insulin added directly or via an infusion pump as in the manage-ment of elective surgery (Chapter 20, p.236) is begun in place of the usual morning subcutaneous insulin and breakfast. An infu-sion rate of one litre per six hours is preferable while the blood glucose is maintained in the 4 to 6 mmol/l (72–108 mg 100 ml) range. Should Caesarean section prove necessary, it can be undertaken at any time using this glucose/insulin infusion al-though the dose of insulin should be halved on delivery. Insulin requirements usually drop sharply as soon as the placenta is delivered and unless there are post-partum complications, the insulin dosage on the following day should be reduced to the levels before pregnancy or if in doubt by at least a third.

Obstetric management following surgical induction depends upon local facilities, local custom and the availability of monitoring equipment. Recording the fetal heart rate and maternal uterine contractions can give a good indication of fetal hypoxia.

A long labour should be avoided for the sake of the fetus. Thus if the second stage is not reached within eight to ten hours with oxytocin infusion, Caesarian section should be effected. In general, the Caesarian section rate in diabetics is higher than in non-diabetic pregnancies.

Paediatric management Because of the higher risk of neonatal complications the paediatric medical and nursing team should be present at delivery. The main problems affecting the infant of the diabetic mother are:

> hypoglycaemia,
> polycythaemia,
> hypocalcaemia,
> hyperbilirubinaemia,
> respiratory distress syndrome, and
> congenital malformation.

Improved diabetic control in pregnancy has diminished these problems, with the exception of congenital malformation which is now the commonest single cause of death. There is an approximately *threefold* increased risk of major and minor congenital malformations affecting the infants of diabetic as opposed to non-diabetic mothers. Congenital heart and neural tube defects are most common, although sacral agenesis – a rare abnormality in others – is much more frequently seen in the infants of diabetic mothers.

It has been postulated that poor diabetic control at conception or at organogenesis during the first trimester of pregnancy may be of importance, so there is a good case for planning the pregnancy and establishing good diabetic control at that stage.

Conclusion

With the exception of those unfortunate diabetics having vascular complications when pregnancy should not be encouraged, the outlook for the pregnant diabetic today is significantly better than in previous times. Nevertheless, the young married couple seeking advice should be encouraged to have their family preferably before the mother is 25 years of age and to limit their offspring to two, or at most three. Sterilisation is advisable thereafter. The need for good diabetic control during pregnancy should be explained, while the poorly-controlled should be advised to defer pregnancy. There is no contra-indication to the use of the contraceptive pill (Chapter 20) in the young diabetic. Unless there is a particularly strong family history of diabetes the prospective parents can be reassured about the unlikelihood of diabetes in their offspring. The need for greater vigilance during pregnancy and the possibility of extended spells in hospital for those unable or unwilling to co-operate in home monitoring of blood glucose should be emphasised. The mother-to-be should also be advised that she is unlikely to be able to breast feed her baby due to a combination of factors which include defective lactation in pregnant diabetics and the lethargy of the infant born prematurely.

Further Reading: Diabetes and Pregnancy

1 Editorial (1976) Hyperglycaemia and hypoglycaemia during pregnancy. *Lancet*, **ii**, 889–890
2 Essex N. (1976) Diabetes and pregnancy. *Br. J. hosp. Med.*, **15**, 333–344
3 Stowers J.M. (1975) Special features of diabetic pregnancies and their progeny. In *Complications of Diabetes*. (Ed. H. Keen & J. Jarrett). London: Edward Arnold, 205–219
4 Soler N.G. (1978) Hyperinsulinism and respiratory distress in infants of diabetics. *Lancet*, **i**, 1054
5 Editorial (1978) Neonatal hypoglycaemia and nesidioblastosis. *Lancet*, **i**, 193–194
6 Sutherland H.W. & Stowers J.M. (1978) *Carbohydrate Metabolism in Pregnancy and the Newborn*. Berlin: Springer Verlag.

CHAPTER 13

Vascular Disease in Diabetes: Atheroma, Angiopathy and Other Disorders

Vascular disease is a major killer. We are all increasingly prone to sclerose, to clot, to develop arrhythmias or to have vascular tubing that wears out one way or another. On the basis of current mortality rates in England and Wales one man in eight could be expected to die from vascular disease before reaching retiring age and one in eleven from coronary artery disease alone. The odds are worse in Scotland. But for diabetics they are far worse. In whatever country, here, Europe, or elsewhere, death from de-generative vascular disease is about twice as great in diabetics as in non-diabetics; moreover diabetic females tend to fare as badly as men.

Alarmists proclaim that vascular disease has reached epidemic proportions. If this is an over-statement it is at least nearer the truth so far as diabetics are concerned. Because of this special susceptibility, identification and control of factors which might either cause or aggravate atheroma in diabetics are of particular importance. Two approaches are possible: one is to study the underlying structural changes in the blood vessels, the other is to identify and examine risk factors – measurable associates such as hypertension, for example – having some adverse bearing on pathology. Either way we are in checkmate. Structural change is best seen at death so that early features are difficult to study, whilst risk factors tend to be correlated with clinical events. But coronary heart disease is a chronic, often symptomless, condition with acute manifestations only in the late stage: sometimes sudden death occurs without any warning symptoms. Therein lies the dilemma for the student of vascular disease: freedom from symptoms cannot be equated with clean coronary arteries.

Pathogenesis of atheroma

Normal muscular and elastic arteries have three distinct layers

(Fig. 13.1). The inner layer or intima is composed of a continuous sheet of endothelial cells forming a barrier to the plasma, and an internal elastic lamina separating the intima from the media. Sandwiched between the endothelium and the elastic lamina is a connective tissue matrix containing occasional smooth-muscle cells. These cells are worth watching. One of the effects of ageing (which may be accelerated in diabetes) is a gradual proliferation of smooth-muscle cells and because this process underlies the atheromatous lesion it is of fundamental significance.

The media (Fig. 13.1) or middle layer consists of diagonally orientated smooth muscle cells, variable amounts of collagen, small elastic fibres and mucopolysaccharides. Unlike the intima, the morphology of the media does not alter with age. The adventitia, or outer layer, consists of fibroblasts intermixed with smooth-muscle cells.

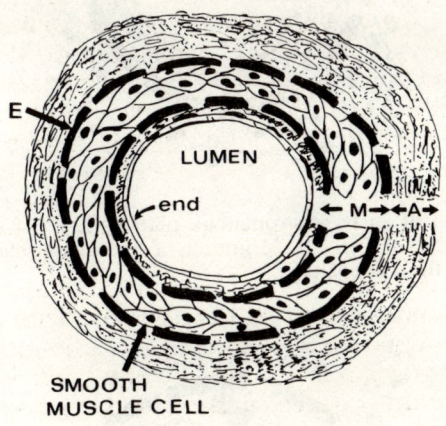

Fig. 13.1 Diagram of muscular artery, showing intima with endothelial cell (end) barrier to vessel lumen. Media **M** composed of smooth muscle cells separated by inner and outer layers of elastic laminae **E**. Outer connective tissue adventitia **A**

Three lesions of varying significance are recognised in atheroma: fatty streaks, fibrous plaques and complicated lesions.

The fatty streak is a focal accumulation of smooth-muscle cells containing and surrounded by lipid. Present in the aorta of almost every child from the age of ten, the lesions gradually increase in size and distribution thereafter, but are probably relatively unimportant, being neither a forerunner of other lesions nor a cause of clinical abnormality. The fibrous plaque is the hallmark of advancing atheroma; consisting of intimal lipid-laden smooth-muscle cells, it elevates the intimal surface causing protrusion into the lumen (Fig. 13.2).

The serious running sore of atheroma, however, results from disruption of the endothelial barrier at the site of the fibrous plaque causing the complicated lesion where the plaque is altered by haemorrhage, cell necrosis, mural thrombosis and calcification (Fig. 13.3).

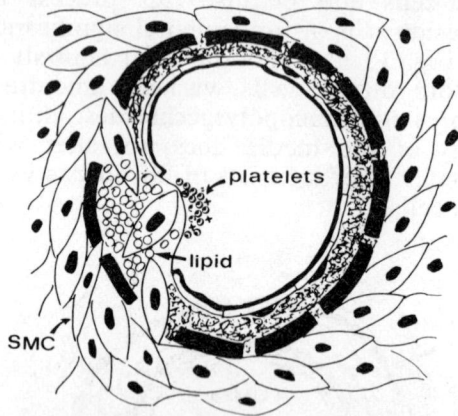

Fig. 13.2 Diagram of early atheromatous plaque. Loss of endothelial lining favouring aggregation of platelets. Migration of smooth muscle cells (SMC) into intima containing lipid deposits

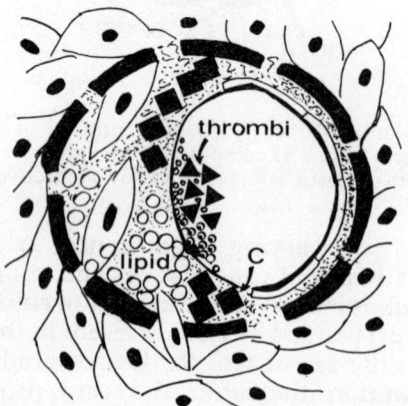

Fig. 13.3 Diagram of more advanced atheromatous plaque markedly occluding the vessel lumen and complicated by thrombus, lipid, calcification **C** and fibrosis

The key to atheroma probably lies embedded in factors causing smooth-muscle cell proliferation and endothelial damage.

Recent research has shown that the replication of smooth-muscle cells may be genetically determined; perhaps this is the basis of the long-recognised concept of the inheritance of poor tubing. Endothelial damage may be caused by the shear-stress of hypertension, hyperlipidaemia, or hormonal and metabolic factors influencing vascular tone. Focal desquamation of the endothelial barrier opens the way to platelet aggregation besides deposition of lipids both within the cells and into the surrounding connective tissue matrix. Platelet and other mitogenic factors aggravating smooth-muscle proliferation have yet to be clearly identified, but the recent discovery that cells of the smooth-muscle type have a surface receptor activated by lipoproteins forges a new link between the fundamental pathological process of atheroma and one of the recognised risk factors.

Atherogenic risk factors

In the general population the important atherogenic risk factors are:

> hypertension,
> high serum cholesterol with low HDLs,
> cigarette smoking,
> diabetes mellitus, and
> stress.

Such additional factors as age, sex and family history of atheroma cannot be controlled; moreover, the female diabetic forfeits some of the relative immunity enjoyed by the non-diabetic members of her sex. Most attention is focused on hypertension, cholesterol and smoking because they are amenable to control, whereas it is difficult to get to grips with stress which is less easy to quantify and which anyway tends to be dismissed as an unfortunate fact of life.

Diabetes and atheroma

Is diabetes just another risk-factor in the atheroma saga, or is there a more fundamental relationship? We move onto slippery ground where it is easy to lose one's bearings. Consider insulin, for example. If diabetes is an atheroma risk, perhaps insulin deficiency (a feature of diabetes) may play some part. Nothing illogical so far, but are diabetic patients insulin-deficient? After all, obese diabetics are characterised by having excessive plasma-insulin values;

likewise, insulin-dependent patients frequently experience prolonged periods of insulin excess whether sufficient or not to induce frank hypoglycaemia, and zealous efforts to lower the blood glucose by increasing insulin dosage or by inappropriate use of sulphonylureas may further aggravate hyperinsulinism. Insulin-induced hypoglycaemia may stimulate a catecholamine response with potential adverse haemodynamic effects in the susceptible.

There is good experimental evidence that hyperinsulinism drives lipid metabolism towards atherogenesis: high insulin levels stimulate the incorporation of cholesterol and other lipids into the atheromatous plaques of vessel walls. Insulin can be shown to inhibit arterial-wall lipase, thus preventing local plasma lipid clearance; to stimulate proliferation of intimal smooth-muscle cells; and in excess also to stimulate hepatic lipid synthesis (Chapter 6); so there is good experimental evidence (yet to be proven in man) that insulin is atherogenic. However, a complex situation can arise in diabetics because insulin deficit could lead to mobilisation of fatty acids from adipose tissue and by inhibiting the fat-clearing enzyme lipoprotein lipase, allow lipids to remain in the plasma. Diabetics may be in double trouble so far as lipids are concerned, either having too much lipid swilling in the circulation when hyperglycaemic and lacking insulin or being exposed to lipogenesis in the vessel wall at times of insulin excess. What about HDLs to keep the coronary arteries clean (Chapter 6)? Studies in non-diabetic populations have shown that high levels of HDL's are protective against coronary artery disease and that those with vascular disease have low levels of HDLs. Although some studies have shown low HDL values in diabetics, recent evidence suggests that this might not hold for all diabetics[5].

Indeed, the blood lipid pattern in diabetes, discussed in Chapter 6, is another elusive subject. Remember that plasma lipids are usually measured in the fasting state, so that the finding of normal values in many diabetics may be a poor index of what happens throughout the remainder of the 24 hours and an even worse index of lipid-sludging in atheromatous vessel walls. Even if we lack precise methods of measuring the lipid status in diabetics, we certainly do not lack clues worthy of further examination.

What about clotting? There is evidence of a tendency to a hypercoagulable state in diabetes, with increased platelet adhesiveness, an increased tendency to spontaneous aggregation and of a heightened sensitivity to such aggregating agents as ADP, adrenaline and collagen[6]. Moreover, diabetic patients' platelets can be unusually active in synthesising a prostaglandin-E-like material. Increased levels of the platelet-specific protein beta-thromboglobulin (B-TG) in diabetics have been reported by some workers and contradicted by others. Unfortunately, platelet technology is laborious and highly vulnerable to subtle changes in patients' blood between venepuncture and test-bench. Nevertheless, enhanced atheromatous lesions in diabetics may well relate to metabolic factors which one day might be effectively controlled by pharmacological platelet agents (there is no shortage of claims to fame in this field, but few agents manage to stay the course). Elevated fibrinogen levels and diminished fibrinolytic activity are other tricky aspects of the coagulation story and fibrin deposition certainly has an important rôle in certain specific diabetic renal lesions (Chapter 14). Poorly-controlled diabetics, especially those who are dehydrated and hyperosmolar (Chapter 7), tend to be in a hypercoagulable state with increased blood viscosity at high and low shear rates. Thus abnormal platelet function, diminished fibrinolytic activity and altered blood viscosity may all have adverse effects on the diabetic vascular endothelium. Little wonder that the complicated atheromatous plaque is more marked and extensive in the diabetic.

Mis-directed therapy may also be harmful, the atherogenic effect of excess insulin having already been mentioned. Especially in the past, strict low-carbohydrate diets (Chapter 9) were high-fat 'atherogenic' diets. Perhaps one of the least expected results, however, was the controversial outcome of the American trial aimed at minimising diabetic complications in patients undergoing various treatments using oral hypoglycaemic agents, placebos or insulin (UGDP Study, Chapter 11). The authors were surprised to find an excess cardiovascular mortality in the groups of patients treated with oral hypoglycaemic agents. As all the patients in the study were mild diabetics and oral hypoglycaemic agents were not really necessary, those who undertook the trial were rigorously scientific (if not very practical) in their methods. But it would be quite unscientific to extrapolate from these findings that oral hypoglycaemic agents are similarly harmful in other more hyperglycaemic diabetics.

Before becoming too despondent, however, it is worth noting that vascular disease is not an inevitable accompaniment of diabetes and the fact that many diabetics escape such insults is a clear incentive to search out its cause in those less fortunate. But diabetics have another problem: the disorder is complicated by its own exclusive form of disease in capillaries and arterioles (diabetic microangiopathy). The discovery of this lesion was made by a brilliant young Hamburg pathologist at odds with the world about him: let him now take the centre of the stage!

Diabetic microangiopathy

In 1934 Paul Kimmelstiel sailed westwards to start a new life in the United States of America. In his pocket were some microscope slides which were to upset dramatically a diabetic world still basking peacefully in the aftermath of the discovery of insulin. In New York, Kimmelstiel faced a hard-headed board of examiners which he had to convince of his competence to work in America. He demonstrated his slides, which showed curious hyaline masses in the glomeruli of eight patients who had died of renal failure and with well-reasoned argument attributed the lesions to diabetes mellitus because seven of the eight patients were known to have had the disorder. Although Kimmelstiel had difficulty in convincing the Americans he was allowed to stay, and with the assistance of Clifford Wilson published his work in the *American Journal of Pathology* in 1936. As a result, sceptical pathologists turned to their microscopes to examine the diabetic kidney with a new zeal. Within the following decade there was a flurry of publications, not only confirming Kimmelstiel's work, but also describing other capillary and arteriolar lesions in diabetes. Next, it was the turn of the eye. In the retina, capillary and other small-vessel disease peculiar to diabetes and characterised by microaneurysms, bleeding and often rapid progression to blindness was being increasingly noted.

By now it was becoming apparent that the survival conferred on diabetics by insulin had been bought at a high premium. The fact that the renal and retinal lesions were peculiar to diabetes led the Danish physician Knud Lundbaek to postulate in 1954 the now-well-recognised concept of a specific blood-vessel disease in diabetes (diabetic angiopathy): 20 years after Kimmelstiel's pioneer work angiopathy was an established fact of diabetic life (and death). Its cause is one of the major unsolved problems of diabetes, although the curious hyaline lesion first seen in the glomerulus by Kimmelstiel remains its untarnished hallmark.

Clinical details of the major sites of diabetic angiopathy are described later: kidney disease, in Chapter 14; the eye, in Chapter 15; and the foot, in Chapter 17.

The fundamental aspects of possible significance in the pathogenesis of diabetic small-blood-vessel disease are also discussed in the section on the kidney (Chapter 14), but in the meantime a brief examination of the effects of diabetes mellitus on the capillaries may serve as a useful introduction to a complex subject.

The normal capillary wall has a foundation of basement membrane ground substance separated from the vascular lumen by endothelium (Fig. 13.4). Abnormal thickening of the basement membrane is the characteristic lesion in diabetes. Basement membrane belongs to the collagen group of glycoproteins. In the past decade intense efforts have been made to identify metabolic abnormalities in basement membrane synthesis in diabetes. One interesting and crucial result has emerged: hyperglycaemia

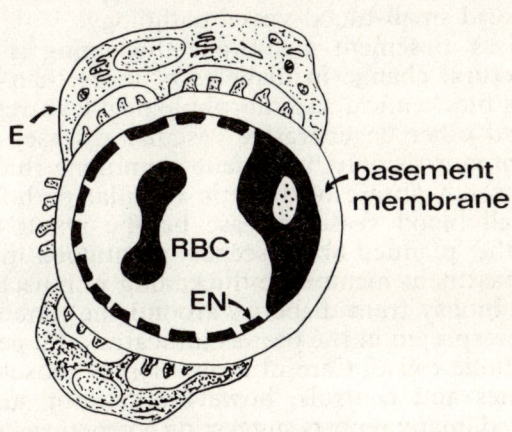

Fig. 13.4 Diagram of glomerular capillary cut in cross section showing the basement membrane and a red blood cell (RBC) within lumen to represent the scale. Inner endothelial lining **EN** and outer epithelium **E**

favours increased synthesis of basement membrane glycoprotein[9]. Before rushing to the conclusion that this is the essential link between poor diabetic control (hyperglycaemia) and diabetic microangiopathy, caution is necessary on two counts:

1 The clinical and pathological features in the diabetic glomerulus and retina cannot be explained on the basis of basement membrane thickening alone.
2 In the experiment diabetic animal, hyperglycaemia induces increased basement membrane thickening, but even at levels of hyperglycaemia which would be intolerable to patients, more advanced diabetic lesions are rarely seen.

Additional factors of pathogenic significance are growth hormone and fibrin deposition.

As will become apparent in the clinical sections (Chapters 14 & 15), growth hormone adversely influences basement membrane thickening and retinopathy. Growth hormone injections accelerate basement membrane thickening in the experimental diabetic animal,[12] while in diabetic patients pituitary ablation diminishes glomerular capillary basement membrane thickening. Growth-hormone-deficient diabetic dwarfs seem to be protected from angiopathy[10]. Fibrin deposition becomes increasingly apparent as basement membrane thickening progresses and is probably the essential component which converts basement membrane disease from a relatively muted accompaniment of diabetes into more florid small-blood-vessel pathology.

Nevertheless, basement membrane thickening is the characteristic structural change in diabetes of more than a few years duration. Its biochemical and morphological features are, unlike atheroma and other degenerative vascular disease, exclusive to diabetes. Not surprisingly 'basement membrane thickening' has become the catch-phrase of diabetic vascular pathology. Could diabetic small blood vessel disease be the result of a *genetic* influence – the 'planned obsolescence' mentioned in Chapter 8? Reports of basement membrane thickening in muscle capillaries obtained by biopsy from diabetics around the time of diagnosis have been interpreted in the past as indicative of a genetic rather than a metabolic cause. Careful evaluation of muscle capillaries from diabetics and controls, however, has not sustained this view[11]. Indeed, many reports suggesting a genetic cause now look slightly shop-soiled in the light of our better understanding of the genetics of diabetes. Moreover, in spite of genetic differences between juvenile-onset and maturity-onset diabetes, both groups may develop indistinguishable renal and retinal vascular lesions. At present there is no evidence of increased frequency of any particular H L A phenotypes (Chapter 4) in relation to the presence or absence of diabetic retinopathy.[13]

The relationship between atheroma and diabetic angiopathy

Could diabetic small-blood-vessel disease be an additional factor in precipitating the increased tendency to atheroma in diabetics? This is a perfectly reasonable question without a clear answer. The suggestion has been made that diseased nutrient capillaries of arteries might aggravate atheroma, but, as indicated earlier, atheroma results from intimal damage consequent upon factors disturbing the interface between the blood and the vascular endothelium. Perhaps small-blood-vessel disease in the myocardium might aggravate cardiac ischaemia but again there is no definite evidence to support this. On the other hand, diabetic renal disease due to angiopathy (Chapter 14) causes hypertension and hypercholesterolaemia – both atheroma risk factors. Remember that hyperinsulinism was thought to be atherogenic and that hyperglycaemia favoured increased basement membrane synthesis (diabetic angiopathy). How can we reconcile these two apparently contradictory extremes with the clinical state of our unfortunate diabetic patients simultaneously corroded by both types of vascular disease? Remember the normal ebb and flow of the blood sugar in which wide fluctuations are avoided (Fig. 13.5) – perhaps

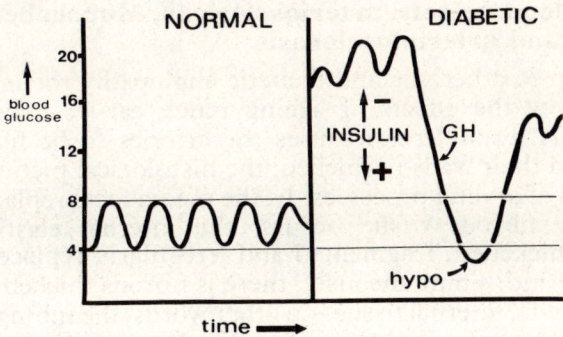

Fig. 13.5 Diagram comparing normal blood glucose range (4-8 mmol/l, 72-144mg/100 ml) and poor controlled diabetic hyperglycaemia (insulin −) a steep fall in blood glucose (insulin +) with growth hormone release (GH), hypoglycaemia (hypo) and rebound. Not to scale

the problem for diabetic blood vessels is that wide fluctuations are not avoided. The upswings of hyperglycaemia favour basement membrane thickening while the downswings of hyperinsulinism may aggravate atheroma (Fig. 13.5). But the wide fluctuations, by stimulating growth hormone and cathecholamine release besides upsetting blood lipids, may compound the problem by adding factors known to accelerate both basement membrane thickening and atheroma (Table 13.1).

Table 13.1   Adverse effects of hyperglycaemia and hyperinsulinism

Hyperglycaemia	*Hyperinsulinism*
Basement membrane thickening	Growth hormone secretion
Elevated blood lipids	Catecholamine release
Abnormal blood viscosity	Vessel-wall lipogenesis
Abnormal platelet function	Proliferation of smooth-muscle cells

Diabetics are alone in begetting small-blood-vessel disease because the upswings of hyperglycaemia and the wide oscillations of blood glucose are peculiar to diabetes. Although sharing atheroma with the non-diabetic population, diabetic angiopathy may not only increase such risk factors as hypertension and hypercholesterolaemia but hyperinsulinism may add its special burden. It is the blood glucose see-saw that seems to do the damage in diabetes.

Ageing blood vessels: arteriosclerosis, Monckeberg's sclerosis and arteriolosclerosis

In addition to atheroma and diabetic angiopathy the large blood vessels show the effects of ageing much earlier than in non-diabetics. Arteriosclerosis causes the arteries to be firmer than normal and their walls to thicken, the histological picture being a compound of several processes. In the media focal replacement of muscle by fibrous tissue occurs, the internal elastic lamina becomes thickened, fragmented and irregularly replaced by fibrous tissue and, simultaneously, there is fibrous thickening of the subendothelial internal tissue – in other words, the tubing becomes thicker and less elastic. Monckeberg's sclerosis is the name given when *calcification* is added to the above process of fibrous change: the tubing becomes thicker and rigid.

The ageing process in arterioles – arteriolosclerosis – seen especially in the kidney and eye (Chapters 14 and 15) is similar to the change seen in hypertensive non-diabetics. However, the process occurs more frequently in normotensive and hypertensive diabetics.

With these burdens added to the previously mentioned atheroma and angiopathy, it becomes easier to understand why vascular disease is regarded as the major physical illness affecting diabetics today. As civilisation progressed, malnutrition and its henchman infection gave way to the diseases of ageing – vascular degeneration and cancer. Whereas there is no sound evidence of more cancer among diabetics, vascular disease they have in abundance. This special relationship with the major killer suggests that a better understanding of the metabolism of blood vessels may be the key to helping the 1% of the population who are known diabetics besides the ninety and nine who are not.

Further Reading

1   Ross R. & Glomsett J.A. (1976) The pathogenesis of atherosclerosis. *New Engl. J. Med.*, **295,** 369–375; 420–423

2   Editorial (1976). Prevention of coronary heart disease. *Lancet*,
    i, 783–785
3   Jarrett R.J. & Keen H. (1975). Diabetes and atherosclerosis. In
    Complications of Diabetes (Ed. H. Keen & R.J. Jarrett)
    London: Edward Arnold, 179–203
4   Editorial (1977). The monoclonal theory of atheroma. *Br. med.
    J.*, **i**, 1371–1372
5   Reckless J.P.D., Betteridge D.S., Wu P., Payne B. & Galton
    D.J. (1978) High-density and low-density lipoproteins and
    prevalence of vascular disease in diabetes mellitus. *Br. med.
    J.*, **i**, 883–886
6   Editorial (1978) Platelets, beta-thromboglobulin and diabetes
    mellitus. *Lancet*, **i**, 250–251
7   Alberti K.G.M.M. & Hockaday T.D.R. (1975) The bio-
    chemistry of the complications of diabetes mellitus. In
    Complications of Diabetes (Ed. H. Keen & R.J. Jarrett)
    London: Edward Arnold, 221–263
8   Editorial (1977) Pathogenesis of diabetic microangiopathy. *Br.
    med. J.*, **i**, 1555–1556
9   Spiro R.G. (1976) Search for a biochemical basis of diabetic
    microangiopathy. *Diabetologia*, **12**, 1–14
10 Winegrad A.I. & Greene D.A. (1978) The complications of
    diabetes mellitus. *New Engl. J. Med.*, **298**, 1250–1251
11 Williamson J.R. & Kilo C. (1977) Current status of capillary
    basement membrane disease in diabetes mellitus. *Diabetes*,
    26, 65–73
12 Osterby R., Jensen E.B., Gundersen H.J.G. & Lundback K.
    (1978) Growth hormone enhances basement membrane
    thickening in experimental diabetes. *Diabetologia*, **15**,
    487–489
13 Möller E., Persson B. & Sterky G. (1978) H LA phenotypes
    and diabetic retinopathy. *Diabetologia*, **14**, 155–158

CHAPTER 14

The Diabetic Kidney

Overheard on the Ward Round:

Junior doctor: 'We admitted an interesting diabetic problem yesterday. Hypoglyacaemia due, I think, to hypothyroidism.'
Consultant (a man of few words): 'Tell me more.'
Junior doctor: 'She is a 54-year-old who has been diabetic for 20 years. There has been vague ill health for the past year, her insulin dose has been falling, yet she was admitted to the Casualty Department following hypoglycaemia while shopping. She looks pale and puffy. Of course, the serum thyroxine result is not yet available but there is a normochromic normocytic anaemia and the serum cholesterol is quite elevated.'
Consultant (greets the patient): 'Does the urine look frothy when you leave a sample to test for sugar?'
Patient: 'Funny you should ask, I had noticed that for some time now.' (The consultant examines the optic fundi, the junior doctor looks puzzled – he often does. They move away from the bedside.)
Consultant: 'Diabetic nephropathy.'
Junior doctor: 'But the blood urea is only 8·2 mmol/l (50 mg/100 ml).'
Consultant: 'Diabetic nephropathy is an insidious process which is easily missed. The falling insulin requirement relates to its diminished clearance. Insulin is protein-sparing, often the urea is only moderately elevated. The appearance, the anaemia and the hypercholesterolaemia are all characteristic of renal disease and from what the patient said, you'll find albumin in the urine.'

Kidney damage in diabetes is often overlooked. Perhaps the more dramatic presentation of such other complications as ketoacidosis (Chapter 7), visual loss due to retinopathy (Chapter 15) or lower-limb gangrene (Chapter 17) blunt the awareness to the slow and silent progress of renal impairment. Yet, as Paul Kimmelstiel first demonstrated (Chapter 13, p.170), the glomeruli and renal arterioles are major targets for structural damage in diabetes. There is a close correlation with diabetic retinopathy, but the retinal lesions are readily detected with the opthalmoscope whereas renal involvement may cause few clinical features until it is well advanced.

Diabetic nephropathy

This is a useful general term embracing the various glomerular, arteriolar and infective lesions which can occur in the kidney. To understand how these lesions develop the following stages have to be examined:

1 *thickening* of the glomerular capillary basement membrane,
2 increased *permeability* of the basement membrane,
3 increased *fibrin* deposition in the basement membrane,
4 *glomerulosclerosis* (as first noticed by Kimmelstiel),
5 *renal ischaemia*: arteriolar lesions, and
6 pre-disposition to infection: *pyelonephritis*.

1 Thickening of the glomerular capillary basement membrane Electron microscopy, by sharpening the focus on glomerular capillaries (Fig. 14.1), has shown that excess of basement membrane material in the capillary wall is characteristic of diabetes.

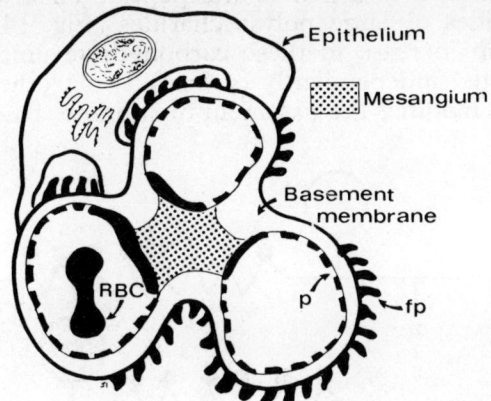

Fig. 14.1 Diagram of glomerular capillary lobule. 3 capillaries cut in cross section, **RBC** within the lumen of one to show the scale. Note the outer epithelium with its system of foot processes **fp**, the pores **p** in the endothelium and the central mesangial zone. Basement membrane is synthesised in the epithelial cytoplasm and removed by proteases in the mesangium

Moreover, recent biochemical studies and animal experiments have shown two fundamental features:

(a) there is a direct correlation between the degree of hyperglycaemia and the amount of basement membrane thickening,[3] and
(b) biochemical evidence shows that insulin lack will increase the incorporation of carbohydrate into basement membrane glycoprotein[2].

D.T. M

In other words *poor diabetic control* and *basement membrane thickening* go hand in hand. This bond between the metabolic disorder and a structural lesion in small blood vessels is of fundamental significance and worthy of closer study. Basement membrane is normally synthesised by the *epithelial* cells (Fig. 14.1), turns over slowly but continuously and is removed by the proteases of the *mesangial* cells[4] (Fig. 14.1). Unlike other glomerular diseases, in diabetes the epithelium remains intact, synthesis is unimpeded and may indeed be stimulated by high growth-hormone levels[5]. But mesangial function is poor, the mesangial cells gradually disappear and basement membrane removal is impaired and in this way basement membrane accumulates in the diabetic glomerulus.

Biochemically, basement membrane belongs to the collagen group of glycoproteins although no collagen fibres are visible in its amorphous structure. There is a high content of carbohydrate (10%) which is attached to the peptide chains as either small disaccharides or large polysaccharides (Fig. 14.2). In diabetes there is an increase in these carbohydrate units which can be incorporated independently of insulin – in other words hyperglycaemia modifies the basement membrane structure. However,

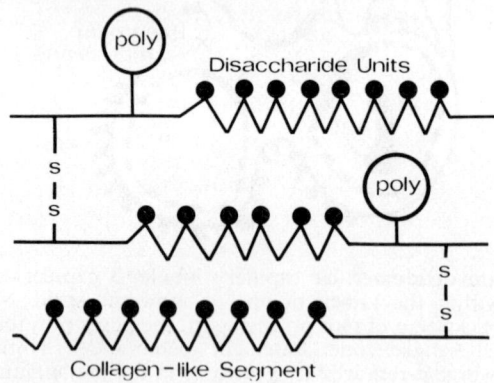

Fig. 14.2 Diagram of glycoprotein structure of basement membrane. Small disaccharide units attached to irregular 'collagen-like' segment. Large polysaccharide units **poly** attached to polar segments joined by disulphide **s-s** bridges

as bulky carbohydrate units increase, protein cross-linkages diminish, so we may visualise the diabetic basement membrane as in Figure 14.3.

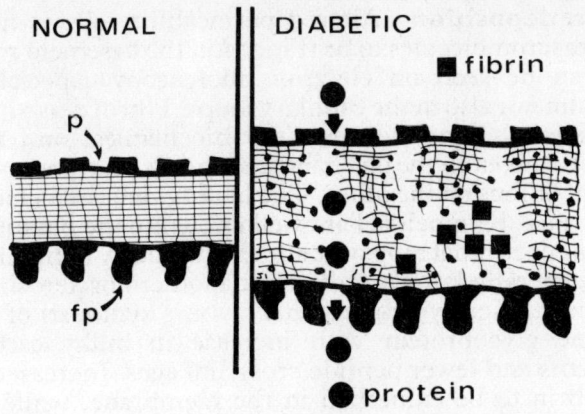

Fig. 14.3 Diagram of normal and diabetic glomerular capillary basement membrane separating the endothelium with its pores **p** and the epithelium with foot processes **fp**. Altered glycoprotein structure of thickened diabetic basement membrane with increased bulky carbohydrate components and loss of cross-linkages allowing proteinuria and fibrin deposition. Although drawn from electron micrographs in which proteinuria and fibrin can be seen, the glyco-protein structure is beyond the resolution of the electron microscope

2 **Permeability of basement membrane** Although thickening advances slowly but steadily during periods of poor diabetic control, the alteration in its structure (Fig. 14.3) makes the membrane more porous; thus *albumin* transit increases as the membrane thickens and changes in composition. Remember, however, that the epithelial cells remain intact (see above) and so much of the escaping albumin may be trapped in the epithelium, allowing many patients to reach quite advanced glomerular damage without albuminuria necessarily being present (this is a complex subject affected by subtle changes in electrical charge, exercise, perfusion pressure and other factors). Upsets in diabetic control will tend to aggravate albuminuria and improvement may diminish it, although this does not mean that the fundamental structural lesion is changing; certainly albuminuria usually means trouble in the kidney, but freedom from albuminuria can be misleading.

Altered permeability has other consequences. All sorts of antigens or antigen-antibody complexes may be trapped in the basement membrane to lead the immunologist astray. Immuno-fluorescence may demonstrate exciting things, but these are usually secondary to the altered permeability rather than of primary significance.

3 **Fibrin deposition** Altered permeability allows fibrinogen-derived macromolecules to be trapped in the basement membrane. *Fibrin* can be seen on electron microscopy especially in the mesangium but also in the capillary loops. Fibrin deposition forges a fundamental bond between the biochemical and functional defect of diabetes on the one hand and the ultimate more-advanced structural lesions on the other. The latter glomerular changes, first noted by Paul Kimmelstiel are well known to the pathologist who today examines renal biopsy or autopsy tissue by light microscopy, and are generally known as diabetic glomerulosclerosis.

To summarise, hyperglycaemia favours synthesis of basement membrane glycoprotein with increase in bulky carbohydrate components and fewer peptide cross-linkages. Increased porosity allows fibrin to be enmeshed in the membrane, while defective mesangial cell function diminishes basement membrane turnover (Fig. 14.4).

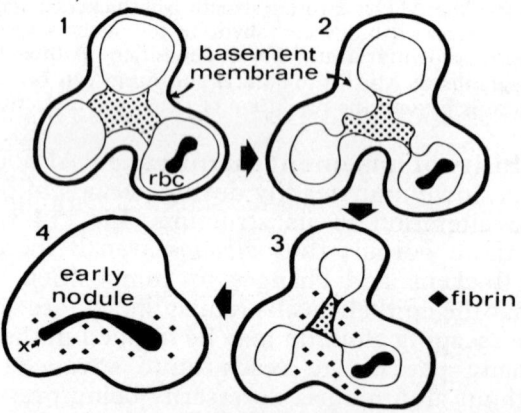

Fig. 14.4 Diagram of the evolution of the diabetic lesion from the normal lobule **1**, to increased basement membrane accumulation **2**, loss of mesangium and fibrin deposition **3** and ultimate occlusion of the lobule **4** with fibrin deposition and fibrinoid material **x** finally occluding the vascular space. Stage 3 is equivalent to *diffuse*, and stage 4 to early *nodular* glomerulosclerosis (see below)

4 **Glomerulosclerosis** Diabetic glomerulosclerosis is the general term for a group of four lesions, which often co-exist: diffuse, nodular (Kimmelstiel-Wilson), exudative, and hyalinisation. Whether they represent variants of one pathogenic process or arise independently is uncertain, although their common end point is glomerular hyalinisation.

Diffuse glomerular lesion The degree of renal failure and nephrotic syndrome correlate best with this lesion which begins with thickening of the whole circumference of the wall of peripheral capillaries of the glomerular tuft. With increasing severity, the lesion becomes diffuse within the glomerulus and generalised in the kidney (colour plate). Further progression leads to narrowing of the capillar lumina and eventually to complete hyalinisation of the glomerulus.

Nodular glomerular lesion The nodular lesion is the most reliable way of diagnosing diabetic nephropathy by light microscopy. Within an affected glomerulus, which may be normal in size or slightly enlarged, nodules occupy the centres of single or multiple peripheral lobules. The fully developed lesion may be an almost spherical, homogeneous, vacuolated fibrillar or lamellar mass often having a patent or distended capillary running over its surface. The main diagnostic features are that the nodule is focal, peripheral, centrilobular and acellular (Colour Plate I.1).

Exudative glomerular lesion The exudative lesion is the least specific of the glomerular changes in diabetes, occurring also in various non-diabetic disorders associated with renal failure. The lesion usually consists of rounded or crescentic deposits of either homogeneous or vacuolated intensely accidophilic material without nuclei, representing various proteins and fibrinoid which have leaked into the glomerular lumen.

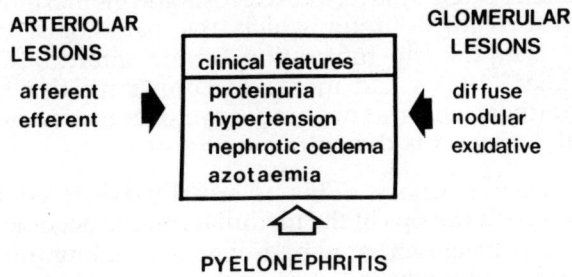

Fig. 14.5 Diabetic nephropathy. Clinical features and various glomerular, arteriolar and infective lesions

Glomerular hyalinisation As a consequence of the above lesions, increasing numbers of glomeruli become completely hyalinised in advanced cases. There may be shrinkage of the glomerular tuft, or periglomerular fibrosis with thickening of Bowman's capsule by connective tissue fibrils.

5 Renal ischaemia *Arterial lesions* Although atheroma is more common in diabetes, there is no evidence of its increased incidence in the larger renal vessels of diabetics.

Arteriolar lesions Hyaline lesions affect both the afferent and efferent arterioles in diabetes. Although similar to the fibrinoid lesion of the hypertensive kidney, normotensive diabetics often have more marked arteriolar disease than hypertensive patients.

Tubular lesions Various lesions may be found in the tubules of diabetics, but few are of specific significance and in general they are secondary to glomerulosclerosis, ischaemia, pyelonephritis or longstanding electrolyte disturbance.

The 'Armanni-Ebstein lesion' or 'glycogen nephrosis', first described in 1877, consists of glycogen-laden vacuoles in the tubules of the cortico-medullary region and was a common post-mortem finding in the pre-insulin era; it is now occasionally found in those who die following uncorrected hyperglycaemia, acidosis and dehydration.

6 Interstitial Tissue: predisposition to infection: pyelone-phritis *Urinary tract infections* Several factors may predispose the diabetic to urinary tract infection, including the effect of diabetic autonomic neuropathy (Chapter 16, p.207) on the bladder favouring stasis, the possibility of catheterisation still being used in ketoacidosis, and the probability that infection is more likely to occur in renal tissue affected by arteriolosclerosis and glomerulosclerosis. However, the features upon which the pathologist diagnoses infection – lymphocytic infiltration of the intertubular tissue, periglomerular fibrosis and increased connective tissue – could result from either ischaemia or chronic pyelonephritis, and thus the histological diagnosis is difficult.

Renal Papillary Necrosis This is usually triggered by acute infection in which the tips of the medullary tissue become necrotic. The lesion may be execerbated by ischaemia leading to sloughing papillae with profuse haematuria and ureteric obstruction, but with improved antibiotic therapy it is becoming rare in diabetics except where there has been analgesic abuse – now one of the main causes of papillary necrosis.

Evolution of diabetic nephropathy

There is no reliable evidence that glomerular capillary basement membrane lesions precede the onset of juvenile diabetes[1]. The initial progress of the ultrastructural defects is slow and even after 20 years of insulin-dependent diabetes the basement membrane may be only slightly more than double its normal thickness, when early-to-moderate diffuse glomerulosclerosis will be evident on light microscopy.

Impaired basement membrane turnover leads to its accumulation in the mesangium where phagocytic function becomes increasingly defective. Thus, various proteins clog up this central stalk of the lobule and as *fibrin* is increasingly deposited in the more permeable membrane the structure of the glomerulus is permanently altered and damaged. Although these processes affect glomeruli diffusely, increase in the mesangial area reduces the vascular and urinary space within the glomerulus with adverse haemodynamic consequences favouring occlusion of peripheral lobules and nodule formation. Whether the associated arteriolar lesions result from the haemodynamic effects of glomerular damage, or are a further factor accelerating glomerular injury is uncertain. Many of the features in the interstitial tissue which resemble healed chronic peylonephritis may be secondary to ischaemia; nevertheless the diabetic kidney is particularly vulnerable to infection in the late stages of disease. Multiple and variable factors (infection, electrolyte disturbance, intercurrent illness or misguided treatment) may hurry the patient towards advanced nephropathy and renal failure. Moreover, the diabetic has no immunity to other diseases which might affect the kidney.

Clinical features
The following are the main clinical features:

> proteinuria,
> peripheral oedema,
> renal failure,
> normochromic anaemia,
> hypertension, and
> pyelonephritis.

None of the above is specific to diabetes and, to make matters more difficult for the clinician, patients are often found to have quite advanced renal disease (either on renal biopsy or at post-mortem) without the above features being evident. The patient's vitality is sapped insiduously away, yet chronic deterioration in kidney function may be difficult to detect.

Proteinuria Although generally regarded as the classic sign of diabetic nephropathy, effective monitoring of filtered protein by the healthy glomerular epithelium (page 179) may diminish excretion in the early stages so that assessment on the basis of proteinuria may be unrealistic. Nevertheless, if proteinuria is present, it is reasonably reliable evidence of diabetic glomerulosclerosis provided that cardiac failure, pyuria or ketoacidosis are excluded. In patients over 60 years of age, proteinuria is most commonly due to cardiac failure. Since proteinuria is often initially intermittent, a 24-hour urine collection for total protein estimation is the best guide to severity. Tests of differential protein clearance do not clarify the diagnosis.

Oedema Often due to other causes – for example, occurring temporarily after any upset in diabetic control (Chapter 20, p.241) or because of cardiac disease – oedema in diabetic glomerulosclerosis is most marked at the stage when the glomeruli are diffusely affected before hyalinisation develops. At this stage, proteinuria may be in the region of 6·0 g/24 hours and the blood urea only marginally elevated. With marked or prolonged proteinuria, the plasma proteins (especially albumin) will be low; simultaneously the serum cholesterol and ESR become elevated.

Renal failure The glomerular filtration rate falls with increasing histological abnormality, but measurement of endogenous creatinine clearance may be unreliable because hyperglycaemia, glycosuria, albuminuria and ketoacidosis are sources of error in creatinine determination. Although the blood urea is the simplest and most reliable index, the protein-sparing effect of insulin may give more optimistic values than in other types of renal failure. Thus the blood urea is often in the range of 8–12 mmol/l (50–75 mg/100 ml) only rising steeply in the terminal stage of disease. (As a clinical guide to severity, multiply the blood urea by 1·5 in insulin-dependent diabetics.) Occult pyelonephritis, with impaired tubular function and poor H^+ ion excretion may contribute to acidosis or make the treatment of ketoacidosis more difficult.

Anaemia Normochromic, normocytic anaemia, mainly due to failure of erythropoiesis is common once the blood urea exceeds 20 mmol/l (120 mg/100 ml) and is unresponsive to haematinics, although iron and folate deficiency should be excluded, especially if the patient's diet is protein restricted. Transfusion gives only a temporary benefit.

Hypertension Renal arteriolar lesions precede hypertension, patients with diabetic nephropathy are often normotensive, but the finding of typically arteriosclerotic hypertension is good evidence of renal and more widespread vascular disease.

Pyelonephritis Particularly when found in males, diabetic nephropathy and autonomic neuropathy may be the underlying cause.

Diagnosis

Because the clinical features of diabetic nephropathy are essentially non-specific, accurate diagnosis depends upon percutaneous renal biopsy. Where this is impractical, the ophthalmoscope is the most useful alternative, for if specific diabetic retinopathy is evident, diabetic nephropathy is a certain accompaniment.

Prevalence Without reliable diagnostic methods, assessment is difficult. Long duration of juvenile-onset insulin-dependent diabetes is the most important factor. After 20 years duration, some degree of nephropathy will be evident on biopsy, whereas in late-onset diabetes, nephropathy may be present at diagnosis or appear within a few years.

Management

There is no specific remedy for diabetic nephropathy. The usual principles for patients having renal disease apply, but water balance and the other functions of the kidney must be watched with greater care and special attention given to diet, drugs and insulin therapy.

Asymptomatic patients Diabetics with asymptomatic proteinuria (or only histological evidence of glomerulosclerosis) require no special measures, although drugs excreted by the kidney should be used with greater caution – this applies particularly to sulphonylureas, biguanides and to insulin. Unexplained hypoglycaemia or diminishing insulin requirements, especially in the long-standing diabetic, may be the first evidence of nephropathy.

Heavy proteinuria and oedema The diabetic diet should be

modified to contain 80–100 g protein per day, preferably of animal origin and ideally an extra white of egg or two per day because increasing protein from meat sources tends undesirably to increase the salt load. Diuretics should be given to control oedema, in resistant cases large doses of powerful agents such as frusemide (Lasix) 40 to 80 mg, although occasionally up to 500 mg daily under careful supervision may be necessary. The effect of thiazide diuretics on body potassium may adversely affect glucose tolerance, although this can be avoided with amiloride (Midamor) or spironalactone (Aldactone).

Uraemia Wide fluctuations in the blood sugar make diabetic control difficult. Protein restriction is unwise in the presence of continued proteinuria. All drugs should be used with extreme caution. Anaemia, anorexia, neuropathy, lower-limb trophic ulceration, failing vision from retinopathy, silent myocardial infarction and infection may all add to the patient's troubles (see late diabetic syndrome, Chapter 21, p.251). Acidosis usually relates to impaired renal function (see Anion Gap, Chapter 7, p.91); indeed, ketoacidosis is rare in patients with advanced diabetic nephropathy, but hyperosmolar coma is more common.

Dialysis and transplantation Regular haemodialysis is technically possible although access to the circulation or maintenance of a shunt may be affected by poor peripheral vessels. The results are usually less good than in other conditions, although recent reports have been more favourable. However, the general condition of the patient may not justify the burden placed on limited resources. Similar restrictions apply to renal transplantation which has also given poorer results than in non-diabetics, except when the donor is a HLA-identical sibling.

Pituitary ablation Although introduced in the empirical treatment of diabetic retinopathy, improvement in the glomerular capillary basement membrane lesion can be expected if pituitary ablation is undertaken at an early stage. On the other hand, advanced arteriolar lesions or hyalinisation will not improve. Moreover, pituitary destruction will have an initial adverse effect upon renal plasma flow and GFR, and so the operation is ill-advised if the creatinine clearance is less than 60 ml/minute.

Prognosis

Patients with clinical features of diabetic nephropathy, or histological evidence on biopsy of Kimmelstiel-Wilson nodules, exudative lesions or glomerular hyalinisation, have a poor prognosis. The outlook will also be affected by the presence or absence of other specific or non-specific complications (see the *late diabetic syndrome*, Chapter 21, p.251). In established uraemia, death may often result from some other vascular episode, but even patients with only slightly impaired renal function should always be managed with caution. Once the serum creatinine exceeds 200 μmol/l (2·3 mg/100 ml) the patient's days are numbered[7] unless freedom from other complications makes renal transplantation feasible before the creatinine exceeds 600 μmol/l (7 mg/100 ml).

Further Reading

1 Cameron J.S., Ireland J.T. & Watkins P.J. (1975) The Kidney and renal tract. In *Diabetic Complications* (Ed. H. Keen & R.J. Jarrett) London: Edward Arnold, 99–150

2 Spiro R.G. (1976) Search for a biochemical basis for diabetic microangiopathy. *Diabetologia*, **12**, 1–14

3 Fox C.J., Darby S.C., Ireland J.T. & Sönksen P.H. (1977) Blood glucose control and glomerular capillary basement membrane thickening in experimental diabetes. *Br. med. J.*, **ii**, 605–607

4 Ireland J.T. (1978) Basement membrane. In *Diseases of Connective Tissue* (Ed. D.J. Gardner) *J. clin. Path.*, **31** Suppl., 59–66

5 Osterby R., Jensen E.B., Gundersen H.J.G. & Lundbaek K. (1978) Growth hormone enhances basement membrane thickening in experimental diabetes. *Diabetologia*, **15**, 487–489

6 Editorial (1978) End-stage diabetic nephropathy. *Br. med. J.*, **ii**, 1175–1176

7 Jones R.H., Hayakawa H., Mackay J.D., Parsons V. & Watkins P.J. (1979) Progression of diabetic nephropathy. *Lancet*, **i**, 1105–1106

CHAPTER 15

Diabetes and The Eye

Eyesight is a precious commodity. Ophthalmologists exist to maintain its value when disease or injury threatens. In diabetes most attention and interest focuses upon retinopathy, but diabetic patients cannot be properly assessed and advised about treatment unless their visual problems are approached in an orderly and comprehensive way. There is little point in generating excitement over a few microaneurysms when the patient's problems are due to refractive errors.

This chapter is aimed at clinicians providing general diabetic care so that most effective use may be made of ophthalmological services both in terms of assessment, and treatment to prevent or delay blindness. Whether the patient complains of visual loss or is found on ophthalmoscopy to have retinal disease, the clinician must be aware of the broad indications for therapeutic intervention or the advisability of an expert opinion. The absence of definite signs could mean that more sophisticated testing is required. Until otherwise proven, the patient is the best judge of defective vision and diabetics complaining of visual symptoms should always be referred for an ophthalmologist's opinion. However, as treatment is increasingly being recommended *before* visual loss, the clinician must be aware of early warning signs of danger.

The following aspects are considered:

   clinical features of diabetic eye disease,
   assessment of the diabetic patient,
   management, and
   aetiology of diabetic retinopathy.

Because the fundamentals of the aetiology of diabetic retinopathy are complex, they can be better understood after considering the various clinical features and methods of management.

At the outset, however, the reader should appreciate that assessment of the diabetic patient is best conducted in an orderly fashion; the examination should therefore begin with the external eye and proceed carefully through to the optic nerve head.

Clinical features in diabetes

Examination of the following systems can be a valuable prelude to a detailed view of the retina:

lids and conjunctiva,
eye muscles,
anterior uvea,
lens, and
intra-ocular pressure.

Lids and conjunctiva Often the previously undiagnosed diabetic presents with recurrent styes or blepharo-conjunctivitis. At one time it was thought that variations seen in the conjunctival vessels – small microaneurysms and capillary dilation – were diagnostic of diabetes, but in the diabetic such features are difficult to distinguish from inconsequential vascular anomalies which are also seen in non-diabetics. Moreover, difficulties in grading conjunctival vessel permutations have combined to remove conjunctival vessel examination from the list of possible diagnostic procedures in diabetes.

Eye muscles When a patient over 40 years of age presents with an external ocular palsy, diabetes will be found to be the underlying cause in 25–30% of cases (Chapter 16). The sixth nerve is usually involved but partial third palsies also occur; combinations of these or other muscle palsies are uncommon. Histology shows involvement of the vasavasorum in the diabetic vascular process. Nevertheless, nearly all patients recover within three or four months and recurrences are rare.

Anterior uvea Rubeosis iridis – new vessel formation of the iris – will only develop in diabetic patients having advanced retinal disease. In diabetics the lesion is usually bilateral, whereas rubeosis following a central retinal vein occlusion in the non-diabetic is unilateral. Rubeosis may not always be evident on naked eye examination and is best detected by careful slit-lamp observation. The lesion carries a poor prognosis because the patient is likely to develop secondary glaucoma. Also, the abnormal vessels, if cut at surgery, may bleed excessively.

Lens In general, diabetics are liable to develop simple senile cataracts about 10 to 15 years earlier than in the non-diabetic population, and every ophthalmologist has imprinted in his memory the knowledge that diabetes and cataracts go together. Thus it is always a wise precaution to exclude diabetes when any patient presents with cataract. The majority of diabetic lens opacities are identical to those regarded as 'senile cataracts' (Table 15.1).

Table 15.1   Cataracts in diabetes

Non-specific	Senile
	Cortical
	Nuclear
	Combined cortical and nuclear
Specific	Young adult
	Hyperosmolar (reversible)

The management of 'senile' cataracts is similar to those occurring in non-diabetics: the best glasses are fitted until vision drops below the level required for day-to-day living (approximately 6/60 distance vision and N10 near print). Cataract extraction is slightly more hazardous, while the prevalence of post-operative inflammation and haemorrhage is higher: nevertheless, the vast majority of diabetics do well following cataract extraction.

Two other forms of cataract may present in diabetics (Table 15.1). In young adults, rapidly progressive, initially granular opacities scattered throughout the lens can spread in a matter of months to cause dramatic visual loss. This form of cataract involves surgery at a time in the patient's life when the operation is technically more difficult because of the firmness of the suspensory ligaments of the lens and leads to the possibility of vitreous loss which may cause such long-term complications as retinal detachment and glaucoma. The advent of phacoemulsification of the lens, however, may prove to be a better way of dealing with this problem.

Finally, patients developing a severe hyperosmolar state (Chapter 7) may develop sudden dramatic swelling of the lens and milky flocculant opacities; the lens capsule may become corrugated and vision rapidly deteriorates. This is the one form of cataract in diabetes which is reversible with rehydration and correction of the metabolic upset.

Intra-ocular pressure   The majority of diabetic patients are in the older age groups in which chronic simple glaucoma is common. Thus, even in the absence of rubeosis iridis, the intra-ocular tension should be checked before dilating the pupil to examine the optic fundi.

The retina

Do not rush to classify the retinal findings: rather, collect and collate all the available clues in an orderly way. And beware – what can be seen with the ophthalmoscope may be only the tip of the iceberg. The following retinal changes may be seen in the diabetic eye:

> venous dilation and beading,
> microaneurysms, 'blot' haemorrhages, A/V shunts,
> arteriolar constriction, microinfarcts, soft exudates,
> superficial and preretinal haemorrhages,
> hard exudates, and
> neovascularisation.

Venous dilation in segments can be the first sign of diabetic retinal disease. Observer error is common, but a run of alternating dilations and constrictions – beading appearance – can be diagnostic (Colour Plate I.2).

Microaneurysms, micro- 'blot haemorrhages', arteriovenous shunts   Sacular formation of either the venous side of capillaries, or less often of the terminal arterioles, leads to the development of microaneurysms. These small, round, often isolated or alternatively clustered dark red areas are well-nigh impossible to separate from small 'blot' haemorrhages contained in the deeper layers of theretina. Fluorescein follow-through of the retinal circulation may help in distinguishing between them if the aneurysms are perfused (Colour Plate II.3). When capillaries dilate into arterio-venous shunts, fluorescein can outline the features clearly.

Arteriolar constriction microinfarcts, soft exudates   Occlusion of an arteriole feeding several retinal capillaries leads to an infarct that can be seen with the ophthalmoscope. Before this stage, multiple retinal capillary infarcts may be present, but these are not visible with the ophthalmoscope and can be seen only by fluorescein angiography. With the ophthalmoscope alone it is not always possible to distinguish small infarcts which give rise to focal ischaemic swellings or 'soft exudates'; these have a fluffy greyish-white appearance with indistinct edges and have assumed greater importance now in relation to treatment (Colour Plate II.3).

Superficial and pre-retinal haemorrhages   Where the constraints of connective tissue are minimal, bleeding spreads in streaks or fan-wise in the superficial layers of the retina. Pre-retinal or sub-hyaloid haemorrhages develop a linear appearance as they gravitate into the shape of shallow boats (Colour Plate II.4). Some of these haemorrhages may burst through into the vitreous.

Hard exudates   Hard or waxy exudates which have distinct edges and a yellow or white colour result from the extravasation of lipids and plasma proteins into the retinal layers. Although they may vanish spontaneously, it is doubtful whether the areas that they covered are ever again viable. Hard exudates can be found anywhere in the retina but produce dramatic effects upon vision when concentrated around the posterior pole and especially over the fovea (Colour Plate II.5). Fluorescein leakage may frequently be demonstrated in the region of hard exudates, indicating further ischaemic damage. When such leakage leads to macular oedema the patient is described as having *diabetic maculopathy* – an appearance which may be difficult for the amateur to recognise with the ophthalmoscope. Hard exudates (which are easily recognised) are the clue to this possibility.

The presence of any of the above features constitutes non-proliferative diabetic retinopathy.

Neovascularisation, fibrous tissue formation   New vessels forming in the diabetic eye may remain flat within the retinal tissue – intra-retinal microvascular abnormalities (IRMA). IRMA also include dilated capillaries and arteriovenous shunts. When the vessel formation is *pre-retinal* it is definitely *neovascular*. Secondary fibrous tissue development may lead to fronds of tissue spreading across the retina or into the vitreous, and these carry a high risk of intravitreal haemorrhage, contraction and retinal detachment (Colour Plates III. 6; III. 7).

The presence of these signs constitutes proliferative diabetic retinopathy (Table 15.2).

Table 15.2   A classification of diabetic retinopathy

Non-proliferative	A	*Mild background*
		Venous dilation
		Microaneurysms
		Blot haemorrhages
		Arterio-venous shunts
		Soft exudates
		Hard exudates
	B	*Maculopathy*
Proliferative	A	Slow
	B	Florid
	C	Advanced

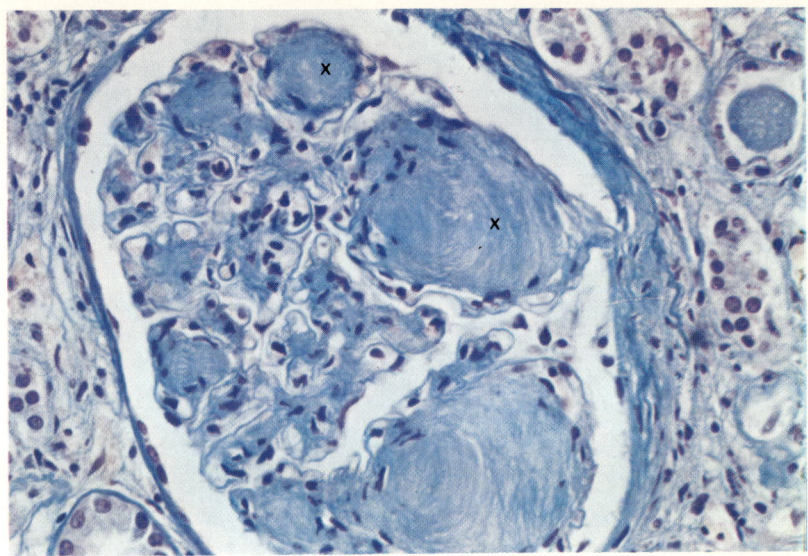

1 Diffuse and nodular diabetic glomerulosclerosis. Glomerulus containing large and small peripheral, acellular nodules **x**. Remainder of capillary loops show diffuse thickening of the capillaries.
Martius scarlet-blue stain × 300

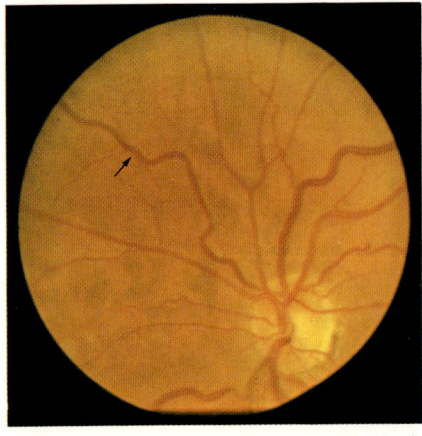

2 Early diabetic retinopathy. The veins show calibre variation known as 'beading' (one area arrowed)

PLATE II DIABETES TODAY

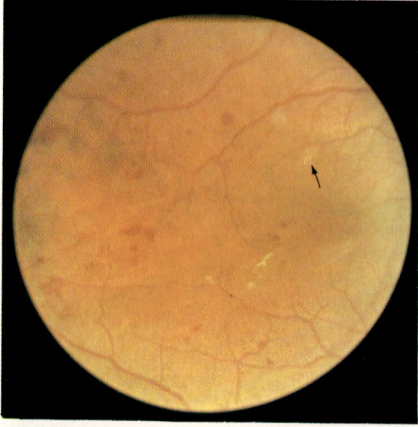

3 Scattered areas of microaneurysms and blot haemorrhages. Note the indistinct edges of the soft exudates (arrowed)

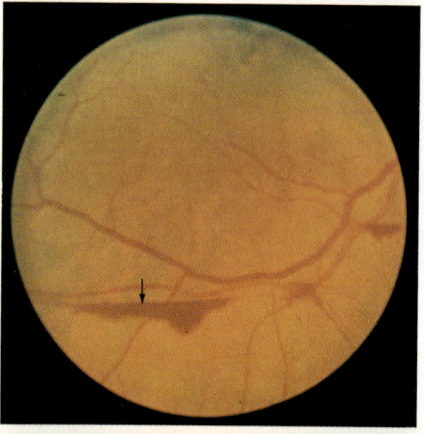

4 Pre-retinal haemorrhages. The blood gravitates to show a sharp upper border (arrowed)

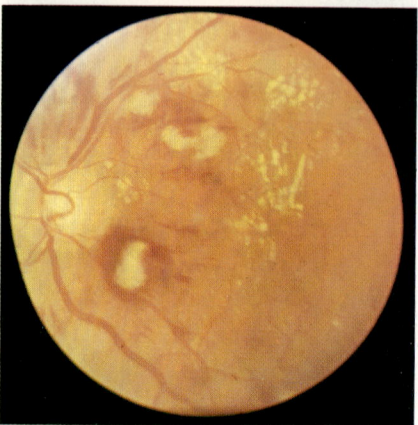

5 Haemorrhages and hard and soft exudates. Some of the haemorrhages are more superficial and fan out over the retina. There is macular oedema

Plates III and IV will be found between pages 208, 209

If the proliferation is rapid with startling visual loss and complications, the retinopathy is said to be *florid*. Lesser degrees of neovascularisation or discreet and relatively static lesions may be regarded as *slow*. *Advanced* neovascularisation mainly involves the vitreous.

The vitreous

It follows from the above that the vitreous may contain:

    haemorrhage of short or long duration,
    proliferating neovascular tissue,
    proliferating tissue plus fibrosis or traction bands, and
       retinal detachment.

Haemorrhage causes both structural and biochemical changes within the vitreous gel which are the subject of intensive study as a result of which it has been suggested that primary vitreous alteration may occur at the vitreo-retinal interface in some diabetics.

Although in Table 15.3 a possible method of classification into non-proliferative and proliferative retinopathy has been made, it should be appreciated that this is both empirical and incomplete. Nevertheless, it attempts to take account of the limitations of resolution of the ophthalmoscope and the limitations of the less expert observer.

Assessment of the diabetic patient

The following aspects should be considered:

    the age of patient,
    corrected vision,
    intra-ocular pressure,
    fundus examination, and
    fields of vision.

Age Very few adolescents present with diabetic retinopathy, although unfortunately nearly all acquire it in due course. Approximately 70–80% are quoted as having retinopathy after 20 years of insulin-dependent diabetes. Conversely some 10–15% of those who develop diabetes in middle age will be found to have retinopathy at diagnosis or may even present on this account (remember Mr. Puff, Chapter 3). Moreover, the vast majority of diabetics who develop retinopathy of a sufficient degree to cause marked impairment of vision are elderly and their difficulties may be compounded by refractive errors, involutionary sclerosis and hypertension. Present evidence suggests that the rate at which any patient accelerates towards diabetic retinopathy is in part affected by the degree of metabolic control (Chapters 8; 13). So far as the juvenile-onset diabetic is concerned, control in the first 10 years of diabetes seems crucial. Paradoxically, it is at this time of their diabetes that least thought is given to the possible ravages of retinopathy.

Corrected vision Hyperglycaemia can cause osmotic changes within the lens which produce *myopia*. Obversely, temporary *hypermetropia* may occur as the previously-untreated diabetes is brought under control, which can be particularly distressing for the elderly patient who is unable to read because the reading correction becomes inadequate. Even well-controlled diabetics may suffer transient variations. Thus it is important to make sure that all diabetics have the best possible spectacle correction. However, the undiagnosed diabetic may consult an optician, being unaware of diabetes as the cause of myopic changes. The glasses prescribed will be useless when the correct diagnosis is made and the hyperglycaemia controlled by diabetic treatment. These patients should wait perhaps for three months of improved control before having a further change of glasses.

Intra-ocular pressures Since the majority of diabetics are elderly, a small percentage will have chronic simple glaucoma (CSG). According to some authorities, CSG is said to be more common amongst diabetics than non-diabetics. If a patient has rubeosis iridis (page 189) tensions should be measured at least four times a year because of the high risk of secondary glaucoma in this group.

Fundus examination Provided that there is no tendency to angle-closure glaucoma (this can be clarified at the first visit to the ophthalmologist by examination of the angle of the anterior chamber), always dilate the pupils for an adequate examination of the fundus, otherwise vital evidence may be missed. The lower nasal quadrant may develop retinopathy before other areas and may be seen only through a dilated pupil. Suitable mydriatrics are cyclopentolate and/or phenylephrine. For the specific purpose of comparison from visit to visit or for classification by internationally accepted standards, photography is necessary. Furthermore, fluorescein angiography is essential for a full understanding of a retinopathy because it displays areas of non-perfusion, leakage, aneurysms, shunts and neovascular tissue which may not be seen by routine ophthalmoscopy.

Fields of vision   In a few patients without visible retinopathy, loss of segments of the field of vision can be demonstrated. The methods required are accurate, but useful only for research purposes. On the other hand, recording of larger field defects, caused for example by plaques of hard exudates, is necessary in the evaluation of the response to treatment. Both static and kinetic visual field estimations are desirable in these circumstances. Other tests of visual function – colour vision for example – have been advocated from time to time but, again, these have been mainly developed for research purposes. In practice, the patient remains one of the best judges of visual function.

The management of diabetic eye disease

General aspects, control and cigarette smoking   The effect of poor diabetic control on vascular disease has been discussed in Chapters 8, 13 and 14 and is further examined in relation to retinopathy at the conclusion of this chapter. Several studies have shown that cigarette smoking has an adverse effect upon diabetic retinopathy and those at risk should be advised appropriately. Control of arterial blood pressure may also delay the progress of diabetic retinopathy.

Hard exudates   Clofibrate (Atromid-S) appears to increase the rate of absorption of hard exudates. It may do so by lowering the blood lipids and favouring the uptake of lipid from tissue sites, leaving retinal macrophages free to attack the lipid deposits. Improved visual acuity is unlikely to occur because the 'cleared' areas are composed of non-functioning neuronal tissue. Nevertheless, if clofibrate is used on a long-term basis, further damage may be prevented. The best results are obtained in those having early exudative retinopathy, particularly where the macular area has so far been spared but is under threat of extension of exudation from the peri-macular region.

Anti-platelet agents   Although increased platelet adhesiveness can be demonstrated in poorly-controlled diabetics (Chapters 13; 16), other diseases in which platelet stickiness occurs are not characterised by retinopathy. Nevertheless, some authorities believe that blockage of terminal arterioles leading to retinal infarction and some forms of haemorrhage are due to altered platelet behaviour in diabetes. Claims of benefit from prolonged treatment with aspirin have been made, but the investigation of other agents more capable of reducing platelet stickiness *in vivo* should be pursued.

Maculopathy – light coagulation When oedema covers the fovea, permanent loss of central vision is threatened. Fluorescein angiography may show leaking points or unsuspected neovascular tissue, both of which may be responsive to coagulation therapy. Close to the macula the argon laser is easier to use because it creates smaller burns, only requires the presence of retinal red blood cells for a successful 'take' and can be more accurately centred using a slit-lamp-beam technique.

If a single area of leakage is not detectable, a horse-shoe-shaped barrage of treatment around the macula (avoiding the maculo-papillary bundle) can be very successful in reducing foveal disease.

Neovascular tissue, proliferation, fibrous tissue, sub-hyaloid haemorrhage and light coagulation Isolated flat areas of intra-retinal neovascularisation may be coagulated by *xenon* or *argon* techniques (Colour Plate III.8). Some experts believe that coagulation of arterio-venous shunts should be avoided because they protect hypoxic areas of the retina. However, even with clear fluorescein pictures it is not always possible to be dogmatic about the distinction between shunts and early neovascular tissue and there must be many instances of mistaken coagulation of shunts that lead to no apparent damage. Forward-projecting neovascular tissue should be coagulated as soon as possible to prevent intra-vitreal haemorrhage.

Extensive sheets of I R M A or projecting neovascular tissue may be attacked either by attempting local extermination or by peripheral barrage of the retina. The latter technique has gained in popularity since follow-up trials have demonstrated its efficacy. Theoretically, peripheral ablation reduces the total need for oxygen in the retina allowing maximal usage by the remaining areas. Hypoxia may be a stimulant to neovascularisation (see page 00). Certainly, a dramatic reduction in central new vessels may result from this treatment; in particular, new vessels on or near the optic disc may be discouraged successfully. Alternatively, disc vessels may be eradicated by *argon* laser coagulation. The *xenon* arc is unsuitable in this situation because retinal pigment must be present before a reaction can occur.

Fluorescein angiography should be advised in patients having extensive fibrous plaques or sub-hyaloid haemorrhages because these areas may have underlying neovascular tissue waiting for coagulation.

Pituitary ablation Pituitary ablation is the treatment of choice in young (especially under the age of 35 years) insulin-dependent diabetics who develop *florid* retinopathy.

Extensive neovascularisation, particularly when arising from the disc or progressing rapidly with recurrent bleeding into the vitreous and associated with considerable background retinopathy, is the main criterion for selection. Massive fibrosis will not respond. The patient must be fit for the procedure and able to cope with diabetic self-regulation, especially the added complexities of post-operative endocrine replacement therapy. Definite contraindications are impaired renal function, poor cardiac function or the presence of significant autonomic neuropathy (Chapter 16). Remember that there is a further reduction in renal plasma flow and glomerular filtration after pituitary ablation (page 186), thus those with a GFR lower than 60 ml/minute are unlikely to enjoy post-operative success. Modern techniques of transphenoidal pituitary surgery make the procedure straightforward in the hands of the expert neurosurgeon. Currently a combination of pituitary ablation and pre-operative photocoagulation is successfully reversing *florid* retinopathy in those unfortunate (and relatively rare) youngsters who develop this form of retinopathy which in the past rapidly progressed to blindness.

Urokinase and vitreous surgery Urokinase is the treatment of choice in *massive* uncomplicated intra-vitreal haemorrhage. 25,000 Ploug units are injected directly into the centre of the vitreous through a small opening in the sclera 6 mm from the limbus in the supero-temporal quadrant of the eye. B-scan ultrasonography of the vitreous should be carried out beforehand to detect possible 'fibrous' tissue or a detached retina. Glaucoma should also be excluded because raising the intra-ocular pressure in these patients could be dangerous. Provided that appropriate precautions are taken, urokinase is a safe, reliable, simple and cheap method of removing vitreous haemorrhage. First used in clots more than six months old, there is now evidence that urokinase may be injected safely much earlier and that it accelerates natural clot resolution. The shorter the time that blood lies in the vitreous cavity the better because it is toxic to the retina and induces 'fibrous' tissue formation.

Vitreous surgery is useful in those patients having developed traction bands or opaque vitreous membranes and may be used as a prelude to retinal detachment surgery. However, the technique is not for amateurs, it takes time to learn and even in expert hands may be complicated by vitreous loss, haemorrhage and detachment of the retina.

Retinal detachment This is the final insult to the retina produced by repeated haemorrhage, traction bands, proliferating tissue and hole formation. Detachment is more serious in diabetics than in others and despite vigorous surgery, loss of sight may be the outcome.

Aetiology of diabetic retinopathy

Although the precise causes of diabetic small-blood-vessel disease in general, and of diabetic retinopathy in particular, still elude us, the following is a list of some of the main factors of importance:

1 capillary basement membrane thickening (Chapter 14, p.177),
2 accumulation of sorbitol (Chapter 16, p.203),
3 altered platelet stickiness, decreased fibronolytic activity, hypercoagulable state (Chapter 13, p.169),
4 poor diabetic control (Chapters 8, p.106; 13, p.173; 14, p.177),
5 excess growth hormone and other hormonal imbalance (Chapter 13, p.173),
6 genetic factors (Chapter 13, p.172),
7 breakdown of the blood-retinal barrier,
8 capillary non-perfusion/closure,
9 retinal hypoxia and neovascularisation,
10 central retinal artery perfusion pressure, and
11 open-angle glaucoma and diabetes.

As indicated above, items 1–6 have been discussed elsewhere. The remaining aspects are of particular significance in the eye and worthy of closer examination.

Breakdown of the blood-retinal barrier In discussing small-blood-vessel disease (Chapter 14, p.178), it was shown that hyperglycaemia (or insulin-lack) had several effects upon the basement membrane – increased thickness, increased carbohydrate, fewer cross-linkages and increased permeability.

Whether similar changes in the retinal vessels lead to small-vessel leakage and damage to the blood-retinal barrier is less certain. An additional feature which may be of particular importance in retinal disease, however, is degeneration and loss of capillary *pericytes*. Eosinophilic degeneration in the nuclei of pericytes is unique to diabetes. These cells, which are functionally similar to the glomerular *mesangial* cells (Chapter 14), may be responsible for maintaining normal basement membrane turnover and regulating vascular permeability. However, the effects of pericyte loss, in relation to breakdown of the blood-retinal barrier, remains speculative.

Capillary non-perfusion/closure Capillary non-perfusion or closure may be the forerunner of microaneurysm formation. Changes in perfusion are first detected experimentally at the arteriolar end of capillaries where microaneurysms first appear. Whether the vessels are occluded by glial ingrowth or compressed by surrounding retinal tissue is uncertain. Retinal tissue ischaemia could lead to swelling and capillary compression, or alternatively the intra-ocular pressure gradient, which is lower in ischaemic segments, could lead to capillary non-perfusion. These changes seem to be patchy: areas of closure and non-perfusion may alternate with parts where there is increased flow in the capillary bed.

Retinal hypoxia and neovascularisation Besides diabetes, new vessel formation occurs in a variety of diseases in which there is retinal anoxia or hypoxia. The mechanism is obscure. However, the hypoxic state, the presence of some viable tissue and poor venous drainage may combine to stimulate a *vasoformative* factor similar to that produced by some malignant neoplasms. Certainly the reduction of tissue competing for scarce oxygen supplies, by photocoagulation of extensive areas of peripheral retina, often leads to a dramatic disappearance of the neovascular tissue. The rapid regression of new vessels after pituitary surgery suggests that *growth hormone* may influence the vasoformative process.

Central retinal artery perfusion pressure Hypertensive diabetics may have accelerated retinopathy and those suffering from unilateral carotid insufficiency frequently have less retinopathy on the side of the reduced arterial pressure. Conversely, high *intra-ocular* pressure reduces the chances of retinopathy in patients with glaucoma or ocular hypertension (see below). The opposite applies to those with a low intra-ocular pressure as, for example, after cataract surgery.

Diabetes and open-angle glaucoma According to some sources, there is a higher than normal prevalence of primary open-angle glaucoma in the diabetic population; the converse of more diabetics in patients with glaucoma also applies. The higher intra-ocular pressure in these patients has, as mentioned above, a protective effect with respect to the development of retinopathy. However, high intra-ocular pressure may lead to optic nerve damage and loss of visual fields and the ophthalmologist is often in a quandary about how energetically pressure should be reduced in the diabetic with glaucoma. Some cases of glaucoma can be recognised as a corticosteroid response in that the disorder is produced temporarily by the administration of corticosteroids. In general, there are more 'steroid responders' amongst the diabetic population, and those having this type of response may be protected, to some extent, from the development of diabetic retinopathy. Perhaps 'steroid responders' for glaucoma and mild diabetics share a common genetic linkage.

Conclusion

The retina provides an easily-seen mirror reflecting the state of the small blood vessels in diabetes. It shares with the renal glomerulus the unique distinction of being a prime site of vascular injury specific to diabetes. The glomerulus and retina also share the richest blood supply per cubic millimetre of tissue in the body, the former for the purpose of filtration, the latter because of the enormous oxygen demands of retinal tissue. Whereas both sites suffer from the abnormal metabolism of poorly controlled diabetes, they may do so in quite different ways. Metabolic changes in the retinal tissue consequent upon insulin lack may well lead to the local production of harmful metabolites (lactic acid and sorbital, for example) and to tissue swelling causing secondary changes in capillaries as a consequence of *compression*. Further ischaemia would be a stimulant (via hypoxia) to *neovascularisation*.

Prevention of retinal disease in diabetes again relates to good diabetic control.

The ophthalmoscope can be used to assess whether or not poor diabetic control is having a visible effect upon diabetic small blood vessels and both in terms of evaluating the patient's wellbeing and the possible need for eye therapy, routine ophthalmoscopy is therefore essential. As regular examination of every patient would require an army of ophthalmologists, those responsible for diabetic care must learn the rudiments of eye examination. The ophthalmologist can assist in developing training programmes. Perhaps a satisfactory working schedule for the ophthalmologist would be:

1 examination of new diabetics within a year of diagnosis, for base line assessment,
2 an annual examination of juvenile-onset diabetics from 10 years of diabetes onwards,
3 annual examination of all patients with mild background retinopathy,
4 urgent examination of all patients experiencing a disturbance of vision.

So long as diabetic retinopathy heads the list of the medical causes of blindness, some diabetics who would have benefited from earlier treatment will inevitably be overlooked. Both education and ophthalmologists are needed to overcome the visual insults of diabetes.

Further Reading

1 Kohner E.M. & Dollery C.T. (1975) Diabetic retinopathy. In *Complications of Diabetes* (Ed. H. Keen & J. Jarrett) London: Edward Arnold, 7–97
2 Palmberg P.F. (1977) Diabetic retinopathy. *Diabetes*, **26**, 703–709
3 Editorial (1978) Vitreous haemorrhage. *Br. med. J.*, **i**, 940

CHAPTER 16

Diabetic Neuropathy

Catch a diabetic by the Achilles tendon and the chances are that it will not be painful. For most diabetics, peripheral nerve damage is a mild symptomless disturbance leaving the patient blissfully unaware of any defect. That is where the danger lies. Loss of sensory function in the lower limbs leads to minor foot damage passing unnoticed, with the result that trophic change may progress to serious ulceration and the risk of gangrene without the patient being aware that anything is amiss. Although this chronic painless peripheral neuropathy in the lower limbs is the most common lesion in diabetics, others may be acutely distressed especially by pain in bed or at rest and, indeed, nerve damage may arise in a variety of clinically distinct forms:

> symmetrical sensory neuropathy,
> acute painful neuropathy,
> diabetic amyotrophy,
> mononeuropathies,
> mixed motor and sensory neuropathy, and
> autonomic neuropathy.

Like many other aspects of diabetes, there is uncertainty about the aetiology of neurological dysfunction. Structural or functional changes are difficult to correlate with those biochemical disturbances so far demonstrated in peripheral nerves. Besides, the defects in peripheral nerve function associated with diabetes are more complex than in most non-diabetic types of neuropathy. The characteristic functional defect found on electro-physiological testing is *delayed nerve conduction* while histologically the structural change seen in peripheral nerve is patchy loss of myelin segments otherwise known as *segmental demyelination*. Each segment of nerve has a myelin sheath arising as an outgrowth of the Schwann cell (Fig. 16.1), thus demyelination may be due to a defect in the Schwann cell, or secondary to axonal disease. In the early stages the axons remain, so that remyelination and recovery is possible. In more advanced cases, however, the axons disappear and so prevent remyelination and return to normal nerve conduction.

Biochemically the fatty acid composition and synthesis of myelin can be shown to be abnormal in diabetes, but it is difficult to correlate these changes with the patient's metabolic status; in particular, there is no specific relationship to altered lipid metabolism. Chronic hyperglycaemia can be shown to alter metabolism in peripheral nerve with diversion of glucose into the *sorbitol-fructose* pathway (Fig. 16.2). Whether accumulation of sorbitol causes nerve damage remains uncertain. This is an important issue, however, because confirmation of adverse effects would be a clear

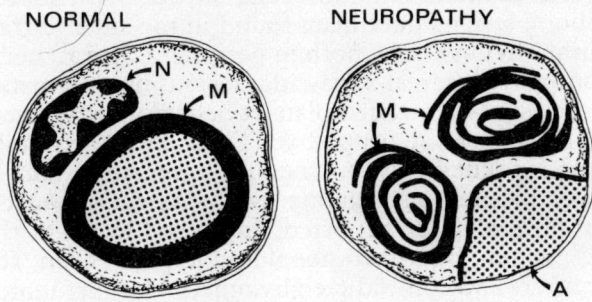

Fig. 16.1 Cross-section diagram of normal and damaged sural nerve as seen on electron micrograph of biopsy. Normal axon cylinder surrounded by medullary sheath **M**, embedded in cytoplasm of a Schwann cell with its nucleus **N**. In neuropathy the medullary sheath **M** is disrupted and fragmented while the axon cylinder **A** has been displaced to the periphery of the cell

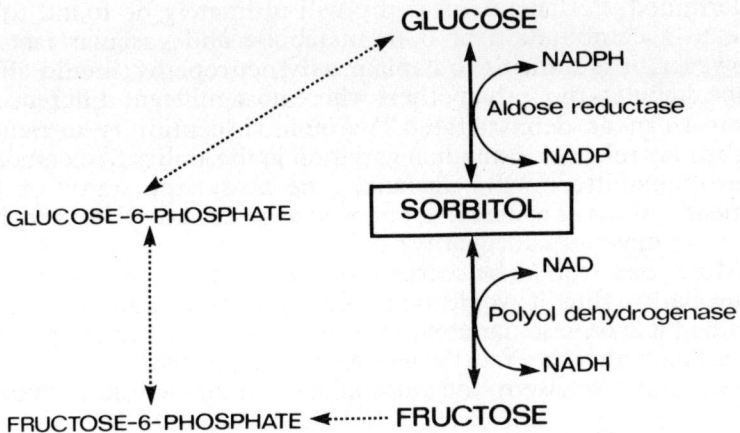

Fig. 16.2 Pathways of sorbitol metabolism. Swelling of tissue may be caused by accumulation of sorbitol or by changes in the redox state of NAD and NADP which also affects the water content of cells

indication for improving diabetic control or perhaps using aldose reductase inhibitors (Fig. 16.2).

Arguments continue about the fundamental cause of diabetic neuropathy, the two major theories being (a) metabolic and (b) vascular. The symmetrical distribution of diabetic peripheral neuropathy, the relationship to alteration in diabetic control and the demonstrated correlation in experimental diabetes between abnormal nerve conduction and hyperglycaemia all favour a metabolic cause. On the other hand, several vascular abnormalities have been demonstrated in relation to diabetic neuropathy. Thrombotic lesions have been found in the small intraneural and perineural blood vessels, both in peripheral (sural) nerve biopsies and at autopsy. Interest in vascular lesions has intensified with the demonstration of abnormal platelet behaviour in diabetic patients having peripheral neuropathy. Thus increased adhesiveness, increased tendency to spontaneous aggregation, and heightened sensitivity to such aggregating agents as ADP, adrenaline and collagen have all been reported. Increased levels of the platelet-specific protein beta-thromboglobulin have been reported by some workers and contradicted by others[6]. Unfortunately, platelet technology is both difficult and tedious; moreover, in vitro results can be affected significantly by what happens to the patient's blood between venepuncture and laboratory. Untreated or badly controlled diabetics will have a hypercoaguable state favouring platelet aggregation and thrombosis, but whether this is a direct cause of neuropathy or a passive concomitant remains to be determined. Perhaps neuropathy will ultimately be found to be due to a combination of both metabolic and vascular factors. However, it is difficult to explain why neuropathy should affect some diabetics more than others where no significant difference in control can be demonstrated. Variable susceptibility to neuropathy may relate to individual variation in the ability to metabolise neurotransmitters[4]. For instance, the acetylator status of the patient may act as a marker for neuropathy (fast acetylators are less likely to develop neuropathy).

Much has still to be learned about the aetiology of diabetic neuropathy, thus it would be premature to speculate how much biochemical or vascular abnormalities lead to the subtle upsets in ionic flux which generate the altered action potentials in peripheral nerves and give rise to the varying and variable clinical features.

Clinical features

Symmetrical sensory neuropathy This is the commonest

form of diabetic neuropathy found in the long-standing diabetic who may be unaware that anything is amiss. The most constant early findings are impaired vibration and deep pain sensation distally in the legs and feet with some distal impairment of cutaneous sensation. Although the majority of cases are mild, such patients are at constant risk of developing trophic ulceration of the feet (Chapter 17). Some patients also progress to a more severe syndrome with predominant lower but also some upper limb sensory loss in a 'stocking and glove' distribution. The gait becomes ataxic as a consequence of loss of afferent proprioception, giving rise to the description 'pseudo-tabes'.

Acute painful neuropathy Either at the time of diagnosis or following an episode of ketoacidosis in the long-standing patient, some diabetics develop an acute neuropathy with intense distal parasthesiae. Persistent aching or burning discomfort down the front of the legs and in the feet at rest or in bed at night are characteristic. Sometimes the pain is brief and lancinating, similar to tabetic lightning pains. Rest pain is the diagnostic feature which distinguishes diabetic neuropathy from the claudication of lower-limb ischaemia.

Diabetic amyotrophy In diabetic amyotrophy the features are proximal instead of distal and patchy rather than symmetrical: thus pain and wasting of proximal muscles are typical. Most commonly the quadriceps are involved although the proximal muscles in the upper limbs are sometimes affected. Similar to painful neuropathy, the amyotrophy is most common either at diagnosis of diabetes or following an episode of poor control. The affected muscles are acutely tender to the touch, while loss of motor function and pain cause weakness and immobility to the point where the patient may be bedridden. Whether amyotrophy is primarily a myopathy related to the metabolic disturbance or secondary to a neurological lesion remains uncertain. Fortunately, with energetic treatment – analgesics and active physiotherapy – amyotrophy carries a much better prognosis than most other forms of neuropathy and complete recovery is usual.

Mononeuropathies Isolated cranial nerve lesions, especially involving the 3rd and 6th nerves to the external ocular muscles (Chapter 15) but also affecting the 5th, 7th and 8th cranial nerves are more frequent in diabetics than in the general population. Diabetes should always be excluded, therefore, in any patient presenting with an isolated cranial nerve lesion. In diabetes isolated lesions may also arise where pressure palsies are known to occur, such as at the lateral popliteal nerve head, or where the nerve may be trapped, such as the median nerve in the carpal tunnel at the wrist. Both cranial and peripheral palsies tend to resolve spontaneously and are rarely recurrent.

Mixed motor and sensory neuropathy Some patients with the more acute sensory neuropathy associated with burning pain and parasthesiae may also develop symmetrical motor involvement with marked distal weakness and muscle wasting. The small muscles of the feet and lower limbs waste symmetrically, leading to foot drop. Such severe involvement of muscles is rare, however; it is much more common for long-standing diabetics gradually to develop wasting of the intrinsic muscles of the foot which causes a claw-foot deformity (Chapter 17) with dropping of the metatarsal heads and clawing of the toes.

Autonomic neuropathy Involvement of the autonomic nerves usually arises in the long-standing diabetic who also has evidence of peripheral neuropathy. Autonomic neuropathy is a common accompaniment of the late diabetic syndrome (Chapter 21) and thus because of the associated renal involvement and presence of other serious complications carries a poor prognosis. However, careful questioning or examination will often reveal some evidence of autonomic impairment at an earlier stage. One particularly distressing aspect for the diabetic patient is *hypoglycaemic unawareness* (Chapters 10 and 18) in which the usual warning signals of a falling blood glucose – agitation, sweating, palpitations – are lost; the unfortunate patient may wake up in a hospital casualty department wondering how it all happened. A panorama of autonomic symptoms and signs have been described in diabetic patients and can be classified as follows:

> cardiovascular,
> gastrointestinal,
> genito-urinary: impotence and bladder dysfunction,
> sudomotor: altered sweating, and
> vasomotor.

Cardiovascular Tachycardia and absence of sinus arrhythmia are the result of autonomic cardiac denervation. More serious, however, is the risk of dysrhythmia and spontaneous cardiac arrest. The response to beta blockers may be impaired (Chapter 20) with the result that such drugs may fail to slow a tachycardia or relieve angina. Postural hypotension can be severely incapacitating for the diabetic. Always remember to take the diabetic's blood pressure both standing and lying. A fall in systolic pressure in excess of

20 mmHg on assuming the erect posture is characteristic of autonomic neuropathy (provided that sodium depletion is excluded).

Gastrointestinal features Defective oesophageal motility and sluggish gastric emptying, although rarely associated with dysphagia, may cause vague abdominal distension, anorexia and occasional vomiting. Simultaneous erratic changes in blood glucose make diabetic control difficult. The diagnosis of altered motility is often difficult to establish because of the intermittent nature of the features and radiological confirmation of delayed gastric emptying is rarely possible, although a dilated stomach can usually be demonstrated. Constipation is a common feature of autonomic involvement, although diarrhoea – the so-called 'diabetic diarrhoea' – is much more distressing. Frequent bowel motions, usually more troublesome at night and associated with faecal incontinence if there is sphincter incompetence, are the characteristic features. Other possible causes of diarrhoea should always be excluded, although the finding of a lax anal sphincter on rectal examination supports the diagnosis.

Autonomic involvement of the gallbladder may occasionally be seen radiologically, when at cholecystography it is found to be both enlarged and poorly contracting.

Genito-urinary: (*a*) *Impotence* Although poor diabetic control may cause temporary impotence, up to 50% of diabetic males over the age of 45 develop a more permanent impotence due to diabetic neuropathy. Although libido remains normal and evidence of endocrine dysfunction in terms of abnormal plasma gonadotrophin or testosterone levels is absent, proving that impotence is due to autonomic neuropathy is often difficult. Impotence may be one of the earliest symptoms of diabetic neuropathy and when other features of peripheral or autonomic damage are absent the diagnosis is based on the circumstantial evidence of diabetes if psychological factors can be excluded. Sometimes impotence is preceded by retrograde ejaculation due to involvement of the sympathetic nerve supply to the bladder neck, although patients may be unaware of this defect. It is the parasympathetic damage causing failure of erection which disturbs patients and their partners.

(*b*) *Bladder dysfunction* Autonomic involvement of the sacral nerves leads to loss of bladder sensation resulting in urinary frequency, urgency, hesitancy, dribbling and incomplete bladder emptying. There may be varying amounts of residual urine, or in more advanced cases an atonic painless distension of the bladder. These defects unfortunately predispose to urinary tract infection and pyelonephritis'(Chapter 14). Such dysfunction must also be given careful consideration by the renal transplant surgeon (Chapter 14).

Sudomotor dysfunction   Altered sweating. The characteristic defect is loss of the sweating function in the lower body and a compensatory increase in the upper half – 'diabetic anhydrosis'. Gustatory sweating (facial sweating during eating) has recently been described in diabetics having autonomic neuropathy. The profuse facial sweating, in the territory of the superior cervical ganglion, may be mistaken by both patients and doctors as being of hypoglycaemic origin.

Vasomotor   Loss of vasomotor response to heating and cooling can be distressing. In the late diabetic syndrome (Chapter 21) altered sympathetic tone may not only give a bounding dorsalis pedis or posterior tibial pulse but also aggravate pitting oedema due to altered vascular permeability. It has often been wondered why patients may have good peripheral pulses and digital ischaemia (Chapter 17); it is possible that vascular shunting in patients having altered vasomotor function may be the explanation.

Diagnosis of neuropathy

Clinical awareness and taking the trouble to remove the patient's shoes and stockings are the basis of diagnosis in the asymptomatic case. Careful examination of the feet (Chapter 17) may reveal all, and when no abnormality is detected sensory testing – including squeezing the Achilles tendon – may suffice to confirm that neuropathy is present. Vibration sense may be diminished below the knee and more impaired at the ankle. Joint position sense is impaired at the toe but only rarely in the upper limbs. The ankle jerk is frequently absent.

Remember that neuropathic pain is characteristically *rest pain* – especially agonising in bed at night. This pain, in its more florid form, may be associated with distressing parasthesiae so severe that contact with bedclothes may be unbearable. Severe pain, the associated insomnia, depression and anorexia lead to a pathetic picture well described as neuropathic cachexia.

Ask the male diabetic about impotence. Always consider the possibility of autonomic neuropathy (particularly if there is evi-

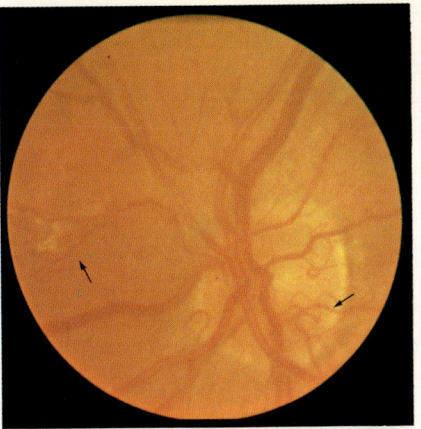

6 Flat neovascular tissue (arrowed) IRMA (Intra-retinal microvascular abnormalities)

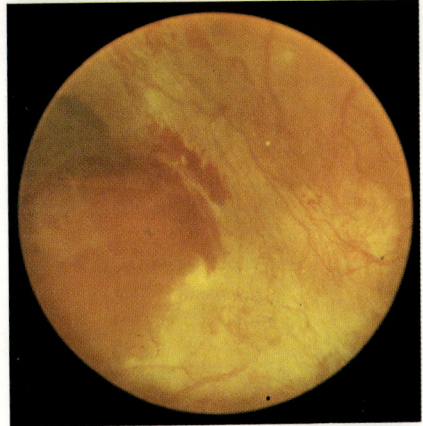

7 Raised fronds of neovascular tissue, haemorrhage and fibrous tissue

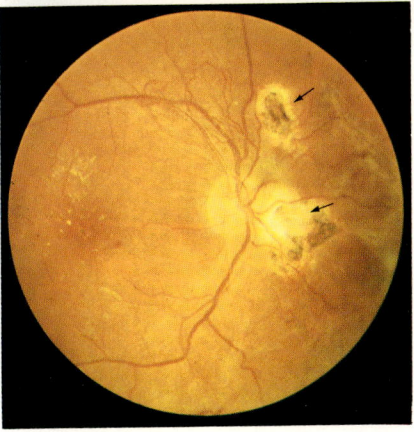

8 Areas of xenon light coagulation (arrowed) beside the optic disc and patches of neovascular tissue requiring treatment

Plates I and II will be found between pages 192, 193

PLATE IV DIABETES TODAY

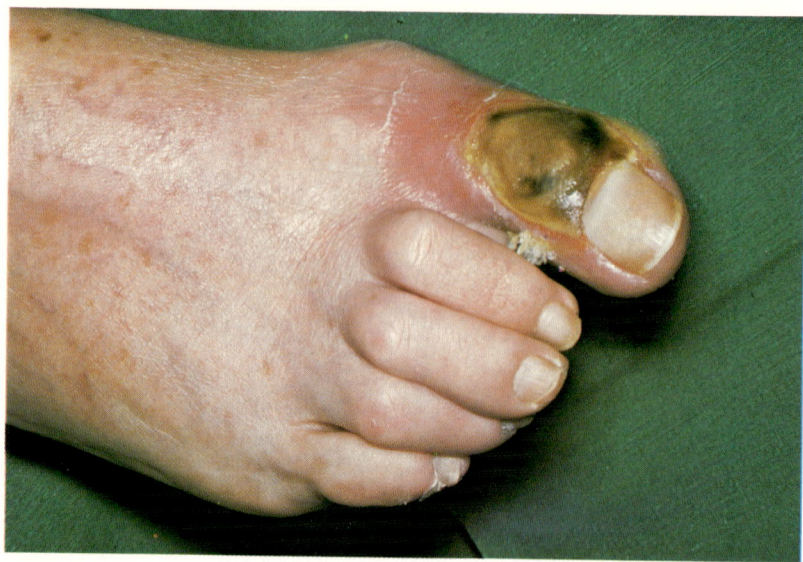

9 Ulceration of great toe due to neuropathy, ischaemia and infection. Note claw-like deformity of remaining toes

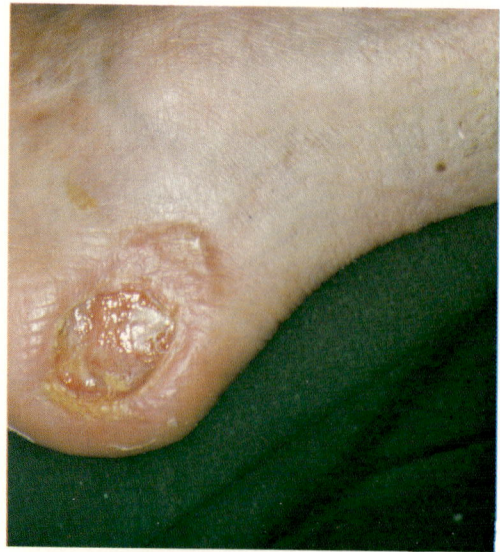

10 Trophic ulceration of the heel due to diabetic neuropathy; an easily-neglected painless lesion

To face page 209

dence of peripheral neuropathy) in diabetics with vague indigestion, anorexia or constipation, and if there is diarrhoea, especially if troublesome at night, assess anal sphincter tone.

Remember that diabetics are susceptible to the whole panorama of other non-diabetic disorders, and in atypical cases always consider such other possibilities as carcinomatous neuromyopathy. Moreover, other conditions affecting nerve function, for instance cervical spondylosis or alcoholism, may cause more acute neurological features in diabetics who are more vulnerable to nerve damage. In cases of doubt the following investigations may be considered:

> tests of motor and sensory nerve conduction velocity,
> nerve biopsy,
> muscle biopsy, and
> tests of autonomic function.

1 Tests of motor conduction velocity in diabetics tend to show a reduction, even in those without clinical evidence of neuropathy, when compared with non-diabetics. In diabetics with clinical neuropathy, the velocities are significantly reduced.

2 Examination of nerve biopsy tissue by light and electron microscopy is diagnostic, but the procedure is rarely justified clinically.

3 Examination of muscle biopsy tissue shows loss of the normal chess-board appearance of the muscle bundles with shrinkage of individual muscle fibres due to neurogenic muscle atrophy, but again this procedure is rarely necessary for clinical management.

4 Various simple tests help to confirm autonomic neuropathy:

(a) Postural hypotension   A fall in systolic blood pressure in excess of 20 mmHg on assuming the erect posture is abnormal.

(b) Blood pressure during sustained handgrip   A pressure rise of less than 10 mmHg on sustained handgrip is abnormal.

(c) Valsalva manoeuvre   Comparison of the R-R interval on an ECG tracing during and after the valsalva manoeuvre in which the patient blows through a mouthpiece and maintains 40 mmHg for 15 seconds will show abnormality in baroreceptor reflex function.

(d) R-R interval variation   On standing, normal subjects show a rapid increase in heart-rate followed by a relative bradycardia maximal after about 30 beats. By measuring the R-R interval on an ECG at beats 15 and 30 and expressing the results as the R-R interval at 30 divided by the R-R interval at 15, normal subjects have a ratio of 1·1 or greater whereas those with autonomic

neuropathy have ratios around unity or less. This recently described simple test can easily be incorporated into the ECG routine in cases where autonomic neuropathy is suspected[7].

Management

In general, treatment is disappointing, there being no known remedies. Attempts to improve diabetic control are hindered by the altered gastric motility of autonomic neuropathy while the stress of severe pain tends to cause insulin resistance. The asymptomatic patient with sensory neuropathy (and all others with neuropathy) need sensible advice about foot care (Chapter 17).

Relief of pain and other unpleasant sensory symptoms can be difficult. Membrane-stabilising preparations such as carbamazepine (Tegretol) or phenytoin sodium (Epanutin) relieve symptoms in about 50% of cases, but phenytoin can aggravate insulin resistance (Chapter 20). Simple analgesics are of limited value while more powerful drugs may create risks of addiction or diminish mobility by excessive sedation. Indeed, mobility should be energetically encouraged if muscle wasting and further deterioration is to be avoided. Sedation should be aimed at giving a good night's sleep: chlorpromazine (Largactil) or diazepam (Valium) are particularly helpful. Often the pain causes fear of cancer or other anxieties which are relieved by explanation of the real cause and reassurance that the pain will gradually resolve.

Unfortunately the other features of sensory and autonomic neuropathy do not improve. Impotence is permanent (even if intermittent initially) so false hopes should not be raised. Again, sympathetic discussion and explanation is remarkably helpful ". . . if it's just my diabetes, then I don't mind . . ." is the characteristic response of the stoical diabetic accustomed to other hardships.

Treatment of the other effects of autonomic neuropathy is limited to attempting to relieve some of the more distressing symptoms. Postural hypotension is difficult to control, sympathetic blocking agents for hypertension should be avoided. Fludrocortisone (Florinef) may be of some help, but should be used with caution in those who also have diabetic nephropathy. Supportive leg bandages or 'G' suits are sometimes necessary, although graded exercises under the guidance of a physiotherapist or sleeping with the head of the bed on blocks may often help to encourage the disheartened back to their feet. The anorexia and distension of altered gut motility may respond to small doses of thioridazine (Melleril). When other causes of diarrhoea have been excluded, codeine phosphate, ephedrine or such atrophine derivatives as Lomotil may be necessary to improve bowel control. Patients with autonomic neuropathy should be warned about hypoglycaemic unawareness and if undergoing surgery the anaesthetist should be carefully advised of the risks of cardiac arrest and respiratory problems in the presence of autonomic neuropathy.

Prognosis

Although mononeuropathies and acute painful neuropathies carry a good prognosis diabetics having chronic sensory and autonomic neuropathy are constantly at risk of developing various problems. Those with retinopathy and visual loss cannot use their eyes to compensate for blunting of lower-limb proprioception, and unfortunately many diabetics with neuropathy have other complications. Once autonomic neuropathy is widespread, and especially in those having postural hypotension, the prognosis for life is poor, usually because of associated renal disease and other life-threatening complications. Moreover, there is a constant risk of lower-limb trophic ulceration or worse . . . (Chapter 17).

Further Reading

1 Thomas P.K. & Ward J.D. (1975) Diabetic neuropathy. In *Complications of Diabetes* (Ed. H. Keen & R.J. Jarrett) London: Edward Arnold, 151–178
2 Campbell I.W. (1976) Diabetic autonomic neuropathy. *Br. J. clin. Pract.*, **30**, 153–156
3 O'Malley B.C., Timperley W.R., Ward J.D., Porter N.R. & Preston F.E. (1975) Platelet abnormalities in diabetic peripheral neuropathy. *Lancet*, **ii**, 1274–1276
4 McLaren E.H., Burden A.C. & Moorhead P.J. (1977) Acetylator phenotype in diabetic neuropathy. *Br. med. J.*, **ii**, 291–293
5 Editorial (1977) Painful diabetic neuropathy. *Br. med. J.*, **ii**, 349
6 Editorial (1978) Platelets, beta-thromboglobulin and diabetes mellitus. *Lancet*, **i**, 250–251
7 Ewing D.J., Campbell I.W., Murray A., Neilson J.M.M. & Clarke B.F. (1978) Immediate heart-rate response to standing: simple test for autonomic neuropathy in diabetes. *Br. med. J.*, **i**, 145–147
8 Editorial (1978) Diagnosis of autonomic neuropathy. *Br. med. J.*, **ii**, 910–911

CHAPTER 17

The Diabetic Foot

Elderly diabetics and those with evidence of other complications are liable to develop faulty undercarriages. Three elements are responsible for serious foot problems: neuropathy, ischaemia and infection.

Either neuropathy or ischaemia may consort with infection to produce tissue damage, although frequently all three unite in an unholy alliance, which if not promptly recognised and treated, may erupt into gangrene. Neuropathy and ischaemia are not easily amenable to treatment and because in their presence infection is more difficult to control, prevention is better than cure. Hence the importance, not only of recognising early warning signs of trouble, but also of educating the patient about foot care (and footwear). Much can be done by sensible management of early lesions; thus the *chiropodist* plays a central rôle, both in terms of prevention and of treatment of foot problems. Indeed, despite an ever-increasing population of ageing diabetics at risk, the incidence of gangrene and the need for amputation is declining as a direct consequence of the enlightened involvement of chiropodists in diabetic care. Instructions in foot care to diabetic patients usually include advice to examine the feet carefully every day. Perhaps it is not unreasonable, therefore, to expect those responsible for diabetic patients to know how to examine the diabetic foot – and even to do so at least occasionally, whether or not symptoms are present. Indeed, serious problems arise so often in the context of painless neuropathy that all too often medical advice is sought too late.

The various clinical lesions depend upon whichever of the three major elements – neuropathy, ischaemia or infection – is predominant; thus at the outset it is useful to examine the influence of each upon the diabetic foot.

Neuropathy

Although diabetic neuropathy (Chapter 16) mainly causes trouble through blunting of deep pain sensation, defective motor and other sensory functions, as well as autonomic neuropathy, all predispose to foot problems. Weakness of the small muscles of the foot leads to

212

clawing, especially of the 3rd, 4th and 5th toes, due to the unopposed pull of the long muscles of the foot. As a result weight distribution is disturbed, the metatarsal heads become prominent giving rise to callosities which are the forerunners of penetrating ulcers. Autonomic defects in bone nutrition can be seen on radiology, the characteristic x-ray appearances being resorptive changes with thinning of the metatarsal and phalangeal shafts and loss of differentation between cortex and medulla. Other x-ray features are disruption of the articular surfaces and disorganisation of the joints (Charcot's joints), fractures, fragmentation and dislocation, particularly of the metatarsophalangeal joints.

Ischaemia

The diabetic is vulnerable to ischaemia in several ways (Fig. 17.1).

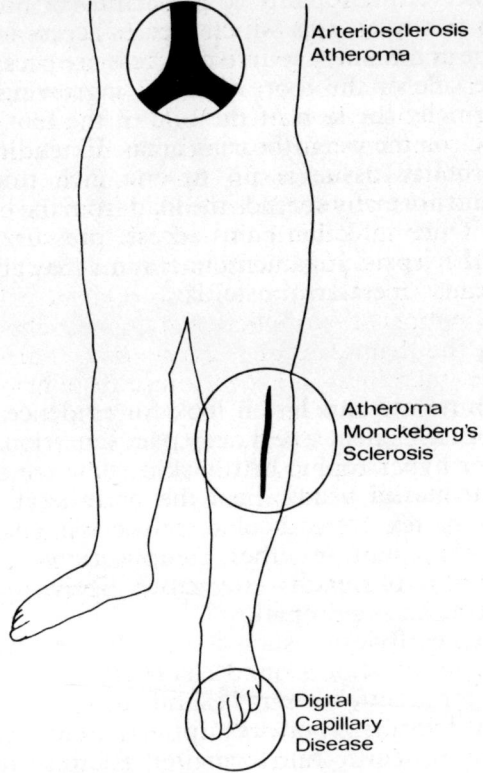

Arteriosclerosis
Atheroma

Atheroma
Monckeberg's
Sclerosis

Digital
Capillary
Disease

Fig. 17.1 Diagrams of lesions in large, medium or small vessels which may individually or collectively aggravate peripheral ischaemia

Large-vessel disease (arteriosclerosis and atheroma) may affect the blood supply to the leg, and medium vessel disease (chiefly atheroma but also Monckeberg's sclerosis) may cause claudication with features no different from those seen in non-diabetics except that atheroma tends to extend more distally into smaller vessels. But in addition, diabetics are prone to their own unique variety of digital capillary disease besides having an increased predisposition to large and medium-vessel pathology. Thus when the peripheral pulses are intact, diabetics may have ischaemic toes due to capillary disease – and when the pulses are absent the foot is even more vulnerable to ischaemia as a consequence of vascular lesions at so many levels.

Infection

In the presence of neuropathy or ischaemia (or both) the foot is constantly at risk to trauma which creates access to smouldering infection. The commonest source of access are pressure sores and callus on the sole of the foot, bunions, ingrowing or badly cut toenails. Normally the skin of the sole of the foot is supple and relatively thick on the weightbearing areas. Extending beneath the skin the fibrofatty tissue is up to one inch thick under the calcaneum, and normally spreads the load from the bones to a wide surface area. Once infection gains access, pressure spreads both the load and the sepsis. Ligamentous trauma may allow spreading infection to cause metatarsal osteitis.

Assessment

In those with no obvious lesion look for evidence of peripheral neuropathy or ischaemia; assess deep pain sensation and vibration sense; look for hypertrophic brittle skin, claw toe deformity and prominent metatarsal heads. Feel the peripheral pulses, assess ischaemia by the texture and colour of the skin and by poor hair growth. Take account of other complications: diabetics with retinopathy or nephropathy are more likely to have digital capillary disease and neuropathy.

If there is an early lesion such as a small penetrating ulcer at a pressure point or infection around a nail bed, the above assessment is even more important, but x-ray examination should be included to assess bony deformity, bone resorption and to exclude evidence of osteomyelitis or sequestrum formation. Radiological evidence of calcification in the arteries of the foot is a further warning of a poor blood supply.

Management

Those without obvious lesions but having evidence of either neuropathy or ischaemia need careful advice about footwear and cleanliness. Often going off on holiday wearing new shoes causes immense damage due to the lack of pliability of the new footwear and unaccustomed exercise. 'My feet are killing me!' is the anguished cry of the footweary traveller, who with normal proprioception, avoids foot trouble. The diabetic may not feel a thing; yet his feet may kill him! Sensible shoes should fit in such a way that the heel of the foot is retained in the heel seat while leaving the toes room to function. A lacing shoe or one with an adjustable strap fastening over the instep prevents the foot from moving forward in the shoe and gives the toes freedom. Low-fronted fashion shoes are not for diabetics. Tight socks, stockings or garters are also out: soft woollen socks are in. Diabetics should avoid walking barefoot, avoid extremes of temperature (no hot water bottles for cold feet) and cut their toe nails carefully transversely.

Those with neuropathy or ischaemia should have the benefit of regular expert chiropody and not attempt to cut their own toe nails. They should be warned against the use of medicated cornplasters, paints and other patent remedies usually containing acids which do more harm than good to early neuropathic or ischaemic lesions. The chiropodist may advise the sparing application of lanolin cream or emulsifying ointment to dry skin or for a moist skin surgical spirit followed after drying by dusting with talcum powder.

And those with penetrating ulcers, toe sepsis or other evidence of more serious pathology? (Colour Plate IV.9, 10) *Complete rest* to the foot is the basis of management. Even in the presence of marked cellulitis, rest, raising the limb and antibiotics may transform a clinical picture that seemed hopeless. Surgery is only required urgently in two situations:

> drainage of a large fluctuant abscess, and
> in pure ischaemia without neuropathy, where major artery surgery, as in the non-diabetic, may be effective in large-vessel occlusion.

Otherwise management is conservative in the first instance. The extent of the underlying pathology should be assessed by radiology, although bone lesions may not show on the x-ray for two or three weeks so that if a lesion fails to respond to rest and antibiotics the x-ray should be repeated after an interval. During rest, care should be taken to prevent the development of pressure sores on the heels of both the good and the bad legs. Padded canvas slings may be helpful. Local applications to septic areas should be confined to *eusol* soaks or *Debrisan* beads which absorb pus, fluid and bacterial toxins without adhering to the wound surface or damaging the more viable edges of the lesion. Cultures from neuropathic ulcers commonly yield both aerobic and anaerobic bacteria. When there is gas formation, anaerobes are usually associated with coliforms so that the chosen antibiotic should cover this mixed flora. A dangerous extension of gas-forming infection should be suspected in soggy tissue, or radiology may show gas shadows extending towards the leg in which case urgent surgery becomes necessary.

Failure to respond to rest and antibiotics may warrant carefully planned surgery in the following instances:

1 to debride a deep ulcer with evidence of underlying necrotic infected bone which must be removed;
2 to remove an ischaemic infected toe;
3 infection spreading into the metatarsals from a septic toe in the neuropathic foot may respond to a ray excision in which a deep wedge is created on removal of the affected toe (Fig. 17.2) and the wound left open to granulate;

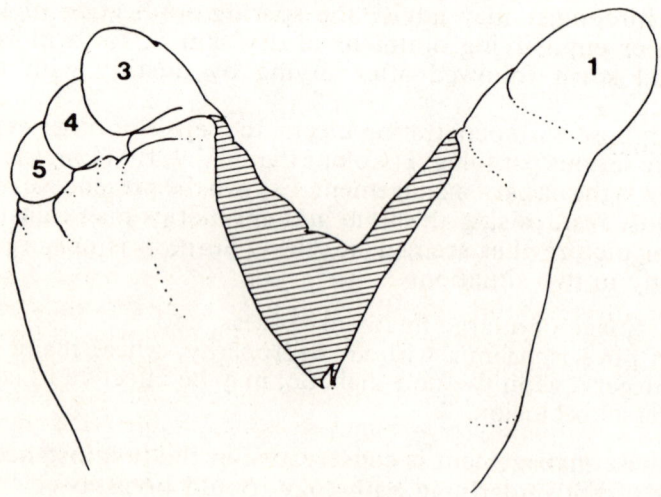

Fig 17.2 Ray excision of gangrenous second toe because of infection spreading into metatarsal bone

4 gangrene of one or more toes with evidence of poor blood supply to the remainder of the foot warrants below-knee amputation – although diabetic lesions are often painless, rest pain is evidence of serious ischaemia warranting amputation;

5 amputation may also be necessary in patients who have failed to respond to a more limited procedure – those whose blood supply is so compromised that below-knee amputation is unlikely to be successful, carry a poor prognosis.

Apart from the above exceptions, well-intentioned surgeons should not rush to operate. Well-demarcated dry gangrene of one or more toes without pain or other evidence of ischaemia in the remainder of the foot may be left to separate spontaneously during conservative management. When surgery is necessary, tourniquets should not be used, sutures should be used only sparingly (or not at all) and flaps designed to fall together without tension.

Whether treated conservatively or with the aid of surgery, healing is always slow and many weeks of patience may be necessary. Convalescence and long-term care depends upon the availability and co-operation of expert chiropody. Once healing is established, the chiropodist may provide specially-constructed shoes to give protection to pressure areas or other deformities. Such shoes can be vacuum formed and padded to give protection and accommodate any bulky deformity. More permanent surgical shoes can be made, if necessary.

Prognosis

A successfully-treated cellulitis in a previously neglected foot often has a salutary effect and the subsequent co-operation in foot care may give the patient many years without further serious trouble. On the other hand, the patient who develops a serious trophic ulcer despite sensible foot care from the outset is unfortunately subject to the law of diminishing returns. If much has already been done in terms of care and protection then there is little more to offer. Such patients usually have advanced neuropathy and ischaemia, and other serious diabetic complications may also be life-threatening. Nevertheless, for the vast majority of older diabetics or those with early neuropathy much foot trouble can be prevented by sound advice, foresight and the use of chiropody.

In summary, corn plasters are out and sensible shoes are in. The feet should be examined carefully (doctor) and if you do not like what you see give the patient's feet a rest, use systemic antibiotics and get a good chiropodist. The surgeon's knife is rarely necessary in the first instance except when there is ischaemic pain – but then the patient will let you know.

Further Reading

1 Meggitt B. (1976) Surgical management of the diabetic foot. *Br J. hosp. Med.*, **16**, 227–232
2 Swallow A.W. (1976) Chiropody for the diabetic foot. *Br. J. hosp. Med.*, **16**, 235–238
3 Editorial (1977) Diabetic feet. *Br. med. J.*, **i**, 338
4 Editorial (1977) Diabetic foot ulcers. Lancet, **i**, 232–233
5 Levin M.E. & O'Neal L.W. (1977) *The Diabetic Foot.* Saint Louis: C.V. Mosby

CHAPTER 18

Hypoglycaemia

Believe it or not, the brain is a heavy consumer of fuel. Normal cerebral function depends upon a steady supply of oxygen and glucose; indeed, the brain soaks up much of the hepatic glucose output during fasting. Whenever the blood glucose falls below 2.0 mmol/l (36 mg/100 ml) cerebral function may become grossly erratic to the point of unconsciousness or, even worse, irreversible brain damage. Not surprisingly, the body has developed several defence mechanisms to counteract a falling blood glucose; these sensibly include 'hot-line' neural connections between the brain and the pancreatic islets. From our knowledge of carbohydrate metabolism we know that there are two key factors in hypoglycaemia:

inappropriately excessive *insulin* in the blood, and
lack of *glucose* supply.

Thus in hypoglycaemia the neural and hormonal defences are concerned with quickly switching off insulin release and mobilisation of glucose into the blood. Catecholamines and glucagon stimulate hepatic glycogenolysis to augment glucose production and can back up the process by adding in gluconeogenesis, if necessary. This safety mechanism may fail the patient when catecholamine release is defective or in liver disease where there is impaired ability to release glucose or when the circulation is swamped with inappropriately excessive amounts of insulin. Thus we can identify the following main causes of *fasting hypoglycaemia*:

1 mismanaged diabetic control with insulin or oral agents;
2 insulinoma, or other tumours whose secretions mimic the action of insulin;
3 liver disease;
4 impaired catecholamine action: B_2 receptor blockade;
5 increased sensitivity to insulin: hypopituitarism, Addison's disease; and
6 alcohol and other drugs affecting the liver.

Inappropriate or mismanaged treatment of the diabetic is the commonest (and most easily preventable) cause of fasting hypoglycaemia which is most likely to occur in two circumstances:

lateness for, or missing meals, and
increased exercise diverting glucose to muscle.

The features of hypoglycaemia can also be induced in the non-
diabetic following feeding – *reactive hypoglycaemia*. The most
typical example of the latter is post-gastrectomy reactive hypoglycaemia where glucose from the meal is delivered to the small
bowel and portal system so quickly that the beta cells respond too
vigorously in releasing insulin and, having no further glucose to
dispose of, there can be inappropriate hyperinsulinaemia in the
post-prandial period. Unfortunately, in addition to true reactive
hypoglycaemia, a whole rag-bag of vague symptoms are often
attributed to this cause, but hypoglycaemia, like anaemia, requires
laboratory confirmation to establish the diagnosis. Many patients
are given and swallow iron or have injected more exotic haematinics for 'anaemia' without haematological confirmation, and
many patients are diagnosed as having 'hypoglycaemia' and given
all manner of curious remedies without the biochemical confirmation of a low blood glucose having been made. One cause of
reactive hypoglycaemia is of particular interest in the diabetic
context. Around the time of appearance of late-onset diabetes
some patients experience erratic pancreatic function. The failing
beta cell – probably as a result of either a defective glucoreceptor or
impaired insulin release (Chapter 4) – may deliver insulin rather
too late in relation to the glucose load and such patients may
experience hypoglycaemic symptoms 2 or 3 hours after a meal,
especially when exercise diverts energy from the brain. The main
causes of hypoglycaemia are listed in Table 18.1.

Whatever the cause, the clinical features of hypoglycaemia
embrace a variable mix of two main elements:

cerebral dysfunction, and
autonomic symptoms associated with the mobilisation of anti-
insulin hormones especially adrenal catecholamine release.

The symptoms experienced by individual patients are quite
variable and especially dependent upon the rate of onset or the
severity of the hypoglycaemia: thus it is of value to distinguish
between acute, sub-acute and chronic hypoglycaemia.

Acute hypoglycaemia

Acute hypoglycaemic symptoms are usually experienced when the
blood glucose falls rapidly over the course of 30 minutes or less. In
the insulin-dependent diabetic, it is not the actual level of blood

Table 18.1   Causes of hypoglycaemia

FASTING HYPOGLYCAEMIA

1 Inappropriate insulin	(a) Mismanaged diabetic, extra exercise or late for meals
	(b) Insulinoma
	(c) Islet hyperplasia, pluriglandular syndrome
2 Tumours mimicking insulin	(a) Fibrosarcoma
	(b) Gastric carcinoma
3 Liver disease (see Chapter 19)	(a) Cirrhosis
	(b) Hepatitis
4 Inborn errors of metabolism	(a) Glycogen storage diseases
	(b) Fructose-intolerance: fructose 1–6 diphosphate aldolase deficiency
5 Endocrinopathy: increased sensitivity to insulin	(a) Hypopituitarism (plus post-hypophysectomy)
	(b) Addison's disease (see Chapter 19)
6 Hypoglycaemia of childhood	(a) Leucine sensitivity
	(b) Idiopathic ketotic hypoglycaemia
7 Drugs	B$_2$ receptor blockade (see Chapter 20), alcohol

REACTIVE HYPOGLYCAEMIA

1 Post-gastrectomy
2 Early stage of maturity onset diabetes
3 Inborn errors of metabolism (see 4 above)
4 Drugs: alcohol, aspirin, paracetamol

glucose coincident with the symptoms but the rate of fall which stimulates the neuroglycopenic features. The diabetic may experience symptoms if the blood glucose falls acutely from 16·0 to 4·0 mmol/l (290 to 72 mg/100 ml), whereas in the non-diabetic the blood glucose is usually 2·0 mmol/l (36 mg/100 ml) or less when symptoms occur. The signs and symptoms in the insulin-dependent diabetic usually conform to a pattern recognised by and unique to the individual patient. In general, however, acute neuroglycopenia starts with a vague sense of unreality, anxiety or frank panic. As autonomic defence mechanisms are mobilised, the side effects of the catecholamine response are evident with palpitations going on to tachycardia, facial flushing, shaking, sweating and intense hunger. The features may be brief if the autonomic response raises the blood glucose sufficiently to re-establish normal cerebral function, or the symptoms may rapidly be aborted by taking oral glucose. Diabetics with autonomic neuropathy (Chapter 16, p.206) or those taking certain beta-adrenergic blockers (Chapter 20, p.240) may not experience the autonomic warning symptoms in time to take emergency action; some diabetics, or patients having an insulinoma, may go on to lose consciousness. EEG changes will be evident during the attack but revert completely and quickly as the blood glucose rises. Especially in the elderly, hypoglycaemia may induce a transient hemiparesis: although the clinical features usually resolve quickly, they may persist for 2 or 3 hours after the acute episode of neuroglycopenia.

Subacute hypoglycaemia

When the blood glucose falls more gradually the features of activation of the autonomic system – sweating, tachycardia, etc. – are absent. Behaviour becomes abnormal, often resembling alco-holic intoxication, although negativism rather than aggression is more common, and reduction in spontaneous activity going on to sleepiness is characteristic. Although needing food the patient is often not hungry and, unfortunately, he may suffer frank nausea or anorexia.

Chronic hypoglycaemia

Chronic hypoglycaemia is the least common form of neuroglyco-penia and is almost always due to insulinoma, but may occur in a diabetic who unwittingly continues to take excessive insulin. The features are insidious: indeed, the absence of either acute or sub-acute hypoglycaemia may lead to the diagnosis being overlooked. Personality change, defective memory, paranoid psychosis, or frank dementia may occur. The course is usually progressive, or sometimes episodes of more acute hypoglycaemia may bring the correct diagnosis to light, when the blood glucose will be chronically low.

Hypoglycaemia in infants and children

Convulsions are unusual in adults, except in those having latent epilepsy or brain damage from previous hypoglycaemia, but are common in children. Apart from this, youngsters when hypoglycaemic become listless, irritable and clumsy and may have a transient inco-ordination of eye movements; in some a vacant stare or tiredness may be the clue.

Diagnosis of hypoglycaemia

Measurement of the blood glucose using a glucose-specific method (the glucose-oxidase-enzymatic method), from a blood sample obtained while the patient experiences symptoms, will establish that the clinical features are hypoglycaemic in origin. The insulin-dependent diabetic will often describe clear-cut symptoms coincident with extra exercise or when late for meals. In such circumstances it is perfectly reasonable to assume that the features are hypoglycaemic, but in the non-diabetic the diagnosis should not be made until there is biochemical confirmation. Having reached that point it is then necessary to investigate the underlying cause (see *investigation* below).

Even with diabetics, however, the diagnosis may not always be straightforward. Some diabetics become obsessed with obtaining negative urine tests or push their insulin doses up 'for kicks' and may try to conceal symptoms[5]. Others have curious changes of mood or behaviour, especially if sub-acutely hypoglycaemic, and in the absence of shaking, sweating or other features of a catecholamine release the diagnosis of hypoglycaemia may be overlooked. Hypoglycaemia in diabetics may have other implications:

Pregnancy: in early pregnancy the renal threshold may fall; patients adjusting insulin to urine tests may induce hypoglycaemia, being unaware that they are pregnant.

Diabetic nephropathy: impaired insulin clearance in diabetic renal disease (Chapter 14) may lead to falling insulin requirements and may present as unexplained hypoglycaemia.

Hypothyroidism or Addison's disease (Chapter 19, p. 232) should be excluded.

Some drugs (Chapter 20, p.240): beta-adrenergic blockers, salicylates, mono-amino oxidase inhibitors and alcohol may aggravate hypoglycaemia. Some drugs which interfere with the protein binding or handling of sulphonylureas may cause hypoglycaemia in those taking such oral agents.

Thus the recent drug history, renal function, liver function, the possibility of pregnancy in the young female, and endocrinopathy should be considered when unexplained hypoglycaemia occurs in diabetics.

Investigation of hypoglycaemia in the non-diabetic

As investigation is based upon the use of provocative tests and other procedures relevant to the presenting features, the investigation of fasting and reactive hypoglycaemia usually follows different lines.

Fasting hypoglycaemia   The simplest test is the *overnight fast*. Most patients with fasting hypoglycaemia will have a fasting blood glucose of 2·0 mmol/l (36 mg/100 ml) or less. Simultaneous measurement of plasma insulin will show whether insulin levels are appropriately low or inappropriately high; the latter is virtually diagnostic of insulinoma whilst low values are characteristic of the various other causes of fasting hypoglycaemia (Table 18.1).

Prolonged fast   When the overnight fast is normal and suspicion of insulinoma is still high, the prolonged fast is perhaps the best way of excluding the possibility. The test should not be carried out, however, until an overnight fast has been normal on two or more occasions; fasting may then be prolonged, if necessary up to 72 hours or until the patient experiences hypoglycaemic symptoms, when blood should be obtained and both glucose and insulin estimated.

Insulin tolerance test (insulin-induced hypoglycaemia test)   Ideally suited to assessing the pituitary-adrenal axis and therefore appropriate to investigation of hypoglycaemia due to pituitary or adrenal failure, the test can also be used in suspected insulinoma if *C-peptide* assay is included. For safety, an indwelling venous cannula should be inserted and glucose given immediately after obtaining blood if the patient becomes hypoglycaemic during the test. Fasting blood glucose and plasma cortisol are measured before giving soluble insulin 0·1 units/kg body weight (up to a maximum of 8 units) by intravenous injection. Blood samples for glucose and cortisol (plus C-peptide in insulinoma) are obtained at 20, 40, 60 and 90 minutes after insulin and if the glucose falls below 2·0 mmol/l (36 mg/100 ml) patients with pituitary or adrenal insufficiency will not show the usual rise in plasma cortisol of at least 275 nmol/l (10 µg/100 ml). Clearly in insulin-induced hypoglycaemia, insulin secretion should be absent: thus, measurable C-peptide would be evidence of inappropriate insulin secretion characteristic of insulinoma.

Intravenous glucagon test   Patients having an insulinoma will have an excessive release of insulin in response to glucagon (1 mg intravenously).

Many other provocative tests, for example, the tolbutamide and leucine tests, have now lost favour.

When inappropriate insulin secretion characteristic of insulinoma is demonstrated, *coelic axis arteriography* may help the surgeon to localise a pancreatic tumour.

Reactive hypoglycaemia   *The five-hour oral glucose tolerance test* is the ideal test in reactive hypoglycaemia. Blood samples are obtained before and at 30-minute intervals after 100 g glucose is given as Lucozade (470 ml) or Hycal. In reactive hypoglycaemia the blood glucose should fall below 2 mmol/l (36 mg/100 ml) and if this occurs it is also useful to measure plasma cortisol in the pre-nadir and subsequent samples. In symptomatic reactive hypoglycaemia the plasma cortisol should rise by at least 275 nmol/l (10 μg/100 ml) whereas this does not occur in disorders of the pituitary-adrenal axis. Measurement of plasma insulin is usually of little value in this test. However, gut hormone enthusiasts and those able to measure glucagon or other pancreatic peptides can have a lot of fun with the procedure.

Management of hypoglycaemia

In diabetics   Education in the principles of self-regulation (Chapter 10) is the basis of prevention in the insulin-dependent diabetic. Contrary to widespread belief, good control of hyperglycaemia need not imply increased risk of hypoglycaemia. Symptomatic trouble is much more likely in those experiencing wide and erratic swings in blood glucose, which may be better eliminated by a change in insulin regime or dietary modification.

In those whose acute attack cannot be aborted by oral glucose, glucagon 1·0 mg intramuscularly is often effective in restless patients; otherwise 25 g glucose given intravenously as 50% dextrose will awaken cerebral function sufficiently for them to take a further 25–50 g carbohydrate by mouth to prevent relapse. In those having taken a massive overdose of insulin (or been given insulin in error in the belief that unconsciousness is due to diabetic coma – Chapter 7) a dextrose infusion should maintain the blood glucose above 6·0 mmol/l (110 mg/100 ml), possibly supplemented by intravenous mannitol and hydrocortisone to counter cerebral oedema. Moreover, hydrocortisone will stimulate the mobilisation of glucose. Hypoglycaemia induced by sulphonylureas in the elderly may also require treatment by intravenous 5% dextrose infusion for 24 hours or more, until cerebral function returns.

Insulinoma   Having demonstrated fasting hypoglycaemia and inappropriate insulinism, and identified an abnormal circulation characteristic of a tumour by coeliac axis arteriography, surgical enucleation of a benign adenoma under intravenous dextrose infusion will bring complete relief. Radical excision may be necessary in malignant tumours which have already metastasised, removing as many secondaries as possible since they are usually slow-growing lesions. If hypoglycaemia due to malignant insulinoma is not controlled by surgery, oral diazoxide (Eudemine) is effective or, occasionally, the beta cytotoxic agent streptozotocin may be given. Diazoxide is a thiazide-related antihypertensive and anti-hypoglycaemic agent, the efficacy of which can be increased (and side effects diminished) by adding chlorothiazide (Saluric); glucagon may be used additionally to abort hypoglycaemic episodes.

Reactive hypoglycaemia   Dietary modification is the basis of management. Peaks of post-prandial hyperglycaemia may be prevented by reducing the refined carbohydrate (sugar) in main meals and by substituting increased dietary fibre (Chapter 9, p.116), while small carbohydrate snacks should be given between meals especially when symptoms or increased exercise are anticipated. The problem often involves modification of alcohol intake.

Conclusion

Despite a recent vast increase in our knowledge of blood glucose homeostasis and a rapidly expanding literature concerning gut and pancreatic hormones, we remain remarkably ignorant about glucose entry into the brain. We have to admit that the levels of blood glucose at which brain function becomes erratic are quite variable. Knowledge that the brain needs glucose to function normally should not be construed, however, as an excuse for the habit of constantly dipping into sugar goodies, nor as an argument against dieting in the over-fuelled. It is only when insulin is around in excess that dangerous hypoglycaemia occurs. Insulin-dependent diabetics have an excuse for taking sugar (occasionally) but even they should not make the possible risk of hypoglycaemia an excuse for regularly pinching the sugar. Glucose transport in the brain is not as vulnerable as some people would have us believe.

Further Reading

1 Cahill G.F. & Soeldner J.S. (1974) A non-editorial on non-hypoglycaemia. *New Engl. J. Med.*, **291**, 905–906
2 Marks V. (1974) The investigation of hypoglycaemia. *Br. J. hosp. Med.*, **11**, 731–743
3 Marks V. (1976) Diagnosis of hypoglycaemia. *Medicine, the Monthly Add-on Series*, **14**, 627
4 Marks V. (1976) Hypoglycaemia. *Medicine, the Monthly Add-on Series*, **14**, 646–651
5 Editorial (1978) Factitious hypoglycaemia. *Lancet*, **i**, 1293

CHAPTER 19

Diabetes Secondary to Other Disease

Ever since Oskar Minkowski's unfortunate dog developed diabetes (Chapter 2, p.14) the researcher has known that pancreatic removal or destruction causes diabetes in the experimental animal. Similarly in man, pancreatic disease or disorders in other systems having a direct bearing on carbohydrate metabolism may lead to *secondary diabetes*. Thus endocrinopathies associated with excess production of growth hormone, cortisol, epinehprine and glucagon are potentially diabetogenic, chronic liver disease adversely affects glucose tolerance, while haemochromatosis is doubly harmful as a consequence of both liver and pancreatic iron deposition. Especially in late-onset diabetes it is always wise to be on the lookout for these secondary forms of the disorder, particularly since in many cases diagnosis and treatment of the primary condition may ameliorate the diabetes. When a cure is not possible, as in carcinoma of the pancreas, the diabetes at least acts as a marker to alert the doctor to more serious underlying pathology.

Diabetes secondary to pancreatic disease

Acute pancreatitis Acute haemorrhagic pancreatitis with fat necrosis is frequently associated with transitory hyperglycaemia. The degree of hyperglycaemia often parallels the course of the disease and although it usually returns to normal after the episode, in some cases more permanent diabetes may remain. The combination of acute pancreatitis with severe diabetic metabolic decompensation – often taking the form of hyperosmolar coma (Chapter 7, p.99) – carries a poor prognosis.

Chronic pancreatitis Chronic pancreatitis, especially when accompanied by calcification, is associated with diabetes in 80% of cases (remember Thomas Cawley's patient, Chapter 2, p.13); overall, 20–40% of cases having chronic pancreatitis develop glucose intolerance. The diagnosis should always be considered when the onset of diabetes is associated with upper abdominal pain, and particularly if there is a history of such predisposing factors as gallbladder disease or alcoholism.

Carcinoma of the pancreas Although diabetes is believed frequently to be associated with carcinoma of the tail of the pancreas where the islets are most numerous, carcinoma of the head may also have this association either because pancreatic duct pressure is altered or through involvement of the autonomic nervous system. Even in the absence of pain, carcinoma of the pancreas should always be considered in the late-onset diabetic who is underweight or fails to gain weight with control of the diabetes. Obstructive jaundice may be the first clue. Whereas surgery may relieve jaundice, partial or complete pancreatectomy leaves the patient insulin-dependent.

Glucagonoma Glucagon-secreting pancreatic tumours have been recognised in recent years. The patient usually presents with angular stomatitis; painful glossitis, weight loss, normochromic normocytic anaemia, and relatively mild diabetes; skin lesions taking the form of 'necrotic migratory erythema' are a feature which helps the well-informed to make a spot diagnosis. Excessive pancreatic glucagon stimulates glycogenolysis and hepatic gluconeogenesis from amino acids yet despite dramatically high glucagon values on immunoassay the glucose intolerance is not severe. Glucagon presumably causes the low plasma-amino acid concentration, the protein wasting and mucocutaneous lesions. The pancreatic alpha-cell tumour is usually a benign adenoma and therefore surgical cure can be expected provided that the patient is carefully prepared for operation.

Liver disease

Although the liver lies at the centre of carbohydrate metabolism, neither are its ordinary biochemical functions, as routinely tested, affected by diabetes nor is it subject to the serious long-term diabetic complications. However, in newly-diagnosed or poorly-controlled diabetics the liver may be enlarged, soft on palpation, and show fatty infiltration on histological examination of biopsy tissue; these changes regress as the diabetes is brought under control. As a consequence of chronic excessive insulin dosage some diabetics develop hepatic glycogen infiltration, a feature which may be associated with the Somogyi effect (Chapter 10, p.132). Non-diabetic patients having chronic liver disease tend to show abnormal glucose tolerance, although the relationship between hepatic disease and the tendency to diabetes is complex. In liver disease there is a poor uptake of glucose after meals and impaired glucose release during fasting; thus, on testing glucose tolerance, fasting hypoglycaemia gives way to hyperglycaemia following the glucose challenge. Insulin secretion is normal or increased and may be augmented by the liver's impaired ability to break down insulin (normal breakdown occurs in hepatic microsomes under the influence of glutathione-insulin-transhydrogenase which splits the hormone into its A and B chains). In chronic liver disease resistance to the peripheral action of insulin, potassium depletion and altered glucagon secretion may all adversely affect carbohydrate and fat metabolism.

Haemochromatosis

In this inborn error of metabolism lifelong increased absorption of iron gives rise to the so-called bronzed diabetes which develops as a consequence of iron deposition and damage especially in the liver parenchyma and pancreas. Transport iron is normally tightly bound within molecules of transferrin, but in haemochromatosis, however, circulating transferrin is completely saturated and absorbed iron passing into the portal blood may not be so firmly bound to protein. Thus, free iron will reach and damage liver parenchyma and, as cirrhosis supervenes, vascular shunts will open to allow unbound iron to reach the pancreas, heart, testes and other tissues. Inheritance is probably polygenic but shows significant association with the histocompatibility antigens A3 and B14 (therefore differing from juvenile-onset diabetes). The severity of the clinical features relates to factors affecting iron balance, with alcohol intake both increasing absorption and aggravating liver damage, and menstruation having a protective effect through iron loss. The disorder is more common in males, but except in known relatives of haemochromatotics, is rarely diagnosed before the age of 40 years and, as demonstrated in the case of Mr. Ironside (Chapter 3, p.35), diagnosis is often difficult in the early stages. Besides measurement of unsaturated iron-binding capacity or saturation of transferrin, liver biopsy provides accurate confirmation of the diagnosis and evidence of the degree of liver damage; between 30 and 80% of patients develop diabetes mellitus and often require insulin therapy.

Repeated venesection arrests and partially reverses haemochromatosis and, in particular, may improve the glucose intolerance.

However, treatment has no effect on testicular atrophy, arthropathy or portal hypertension, and hepatoma remains a common cause of death.

Diabetes and endocrine disease

Thyrotoxicosis Glucose intolerance in hyperthyroidism is commonly characterised by a high glycaemic peak during the first hour of the glucose tolerance test. The diabetogenic tendency is a consequence of stimulation of glycogenolysis and gluconeogenesis by thyroid hormone, although accelerated insulin catabolism and insulin resistance due to lipolysis may also play a part. In most cases the diabetes improves with treatment of the thyrotoxicosis.

Cushing's syndrome Disorders associated with sustained excess of circulating free cortisol (or the use of corticosteroid drugs, Chapter 20, p.239) frequently cause glucose intolerance due to stimulation of lipolysis and gluconeogenesis. Although obesity, diabetes mellitus and hypertension often coexist and lead to a suspicion of Cushing's syndrome, especially if the patient has a Cushinoid appearance, the disorder is extremely rare (one or two cases per million population per annum) and can be excluded most easily by measurement of the urinary free cortisol. Cushing's syndrome is confirmed by high ACTH values in pituitary-dependent disease or the ectopic ACTH syndrome, and by low ACTH values and impaired response to metyrapone stimulation in adrenal tumours. The associated diabetes usually disappears on effective treatment of the hypercorticism. As patients with pituitary-dependent Cushing's disease are in poor condition for adrenalectomy due to weakness and potassium depletion, pre-operative inhibition of cortisol synthesis with metyrapone and aminoglutethimide is advisable. Thereafter, treatment should be directed at the pituitary gland to prevent Nelson's syndrome (high ACTH values, skin pigmentation and pituitary tumour, often of a locally malignant type), but if future fertility is important it may be deferred, with regular surveillance maintained to exclude the syndrome.

Acromegaly The skeletal overgrowth, especially that affecting the vault and supraorbital ridges of the skull, the lower jaw, vertebrae, hands and feet, and the exaggerated skin folds may develop so slowly and insidiously that neither the patient nor his close relatives are aware of any abnormality. The diagnosis is often made by chance when the patient attends hospital for some other reason, or when in some cases the patient complains of headache (associated with stretching of the dura) or presents with hypertension, cardiac failure associated with acromegalic cardiomyopathy, or with glycosuria. Old photographs help to assess the duration of the disorder. The true incidence of diabetes mellitus consequent upon acromegaly is variably quoted. As in other endocrinopathies, the distinction between abnormal glucose tolerance and frank diabetes mellitus is not always made; approximately 25% of acromegalics have abnormal glucose tolerance whilst only half this number will develop clinical diabetes mellitus. The mean interval between the onset of acromegaly and the appearance of diabetes is about ten years. The disorder is usually mild but may become insulin-dependent, and some cases are difficult to control until the growth hormone levels are reduced. Despite the relationship between growth hormone and diabetic complications (Chapters 13; 14; 15), retinopathy is an unusual feature in acromegalics with diabetes. Acromegalics having visual field defects are usually treated by frontal craniotomy or through the sphenoidal sinus, while those without visual field defects are still better treated by transphenoidal hypophysectomy than by conventional high-voltage irradiation. The treatment of acromegaly with bromocriptine (Parlodel) now gives favourable results either alone or in combination with surgery. Bromocriptine relieves the headache and hypertension, significantly improves glucose tolerance and oral hypoglycaemic agents or insulin dosage may usually be reduced or withdrawn.

Hyperaldosteronism Glucose intolerance in primary hyperaldosteronism is thought to be related to the associated potassium depletion. Frank diabetes is rare, and surgical treatment usually results in an improved glucose tolerance.

Phaeochromocytoma Diabetes may be associated with the epinephrine-secreting variety of phaeochromocytoma as a consequence of the effect of excess catecholamines on glycogenolysis and lipolysis, as well as the inhibition of insulin secretion. Again, the glucose intolerance improves following surgery.

Endocrine hypofunction

Because of the relationship between autoimmunity and some cases of diabetes (Chapter 4, p.44), hypothyroidism and adrenocortical insufficiency (Addison's Disease) are commonly associated with diabetes. Whereas in both disorders there is usually a tendency to hypoglycaemia, treatment may cause deterioration in diabetic control or bring diabetes to light in the previously undiagnosed case. Occasionally, however, insulin resistance occurs in hypothyroidism, when the known diabetic may present with a significant paradoxical deterioration in control coincident with the onset of the disorder.

Further Reading

1 Editorial (1977) Carcinoma of the pancreas. *Br. med. J.*, **ii**, 1497–1498
2 Editorial (1977) Treatment of idiopathic haemochromatosis. *Lancet*, **i**, 291–292
3 Editorial (1977) Idiopathic haemochromatosis. *Br. med. J.*, **ii**, 1242
4 Havard C.W.H. (1977) Assessment of thyroid function during treatment of hyper- and hypothyroidism. In *Clinical Medicine and Therapeutics* (Ed. P. Richards & H. Mather) Oxford: Blackwell Scientific Publications, 170–177
5 Editorial (1977) Pituitary-dependent Cushing's Disease. *Br. med. J.*, **i**, 1049
6 Jenkins J.S. (1977) Practical assessment of hypothalamic, pituitary and adrenal function. In *Clinical Medicine and Therapeutics* (Ed. P. Richards & H. Mather) Oxford: Blackwell Scientific Publications, 178–188
7 Wass J.A.H., Thorner M.O. & Besser G.M. (1977) Therapeutic potential of bromocriptine. In *Clinical Medicine and Therapeutics* (Ed. P. Richards & H. Mather) Oxford: Blackwell Scientific Publications, 189–197
8 Mallinson C.N., Bloom S.R., Warin A.P. & Salmon, P.R. (1974) A glucagonoma syndrome. *Lancet*, **ii**, 1
9 Bloom S.R. (1975) Glucagon. *Br. J. hosp. Med.*, **13**, 150–160

CHAPTER 20

Diabetes and Other Disorders

With particular reference to Surgery, Infection, Drugs, Vascular Disease, Skin Conditions *and* Psychiatric Disorders

Diabetics have no special immunity to other disorders. On the contrary, there is an increased risk of degenerative vascular disease (Chapter 13), some have an increased tendency to autoimmune disorders (Chapter 4, p.44) and in general infections are more troublesome and difficult to eradicate.

Diabetes also has a special relationship to other disease because any illness, accident, and surgical or emotional trauma will, by stimulating the hormones of stress, antagonise insulin, favour lipolysis and drive the patient towards hyperglycaemia, gluco-neogenesis and possibly ketoacidosis (Fig. 20.1). As a result of this special relationship in which insulin and other hormones play key rôles, we can make the following observations:

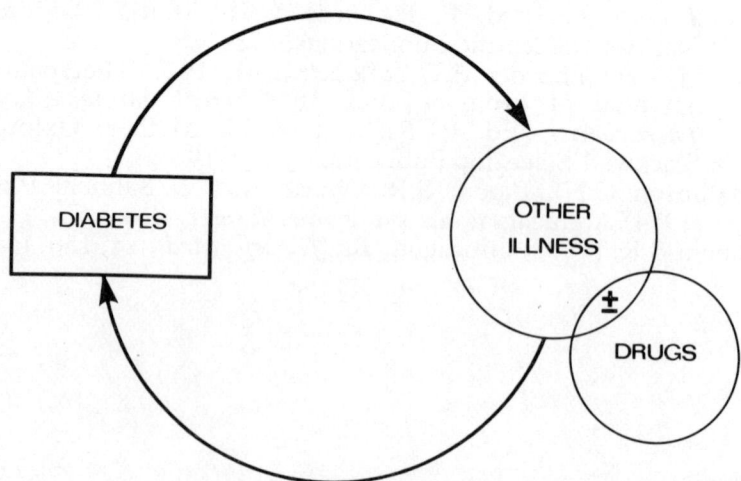

Fig. 20.1 The interrelationship between diabetes, illness and treatment with diabetogenic (+) or hypoglycaemic (−) drugs

1 any illness may bring to light diabetes in the previously undiagnosed patient;
2 any illness may upset the previously stable diabetic; and
3 drugs, intravenous nutrition and other medications which affect glucose metabolism may be diabetogenic (or hypoglycaemic) and upset diabetic control.

It follows that the cardiologist, the surgeon, the rheumatologist (or any other ologist) may suddenly find that he has a diabetic on his hands and likewise those caring for diabetics may be faced with all manner of additional problems. Successful treatment depends upon a good understanding of the particular disorder, how it relates to the carbohydrate metabolism of the diabetic patient and also upon a good relationship between disciplines. Corticosteroids and the stress of surgery are diabetogenic, yet neither should be withheld from the diabetic in situations where they are of proven value. When of doubtful benefit, however, the risks must be carefully weighed, particularly in the diabetic with other complications. For instance, the orthopaedic surgeon, doing a good line in hip replacement, may spoil a splendid series (or reputation) by operating on a diabetic without taking account of lower limb neuropathy or an elevated blood urea. In general, more thought must be given to several aspects which may have a bearing both on the outcome of surgery or the management of any other debilitating illness. For example:

1 diabetics withstand fasting badly and are more in need of careful intravenous therapy;
2 the osmotic diuresis of uncontrolled diabetes may lead even the mild diabetic into a hyperosmolar state when unable to drink;
3 trauma may drive the diabetic into ketoacidosis;
4 shock may induce lactic acidosis;
5 dehydration and hyperosmolality will lead to a hypercoaguable state with added risk of venous thrombosis and other complications;
6 in poorly-controlled diabetes infection is difficult to eradicate because of impaired phagocytosis, decreased chemotaxis and altered response to phytohaemagglutination; and
7 degenerative vascular disease, renal involvement and neuropathy may all affect the outcome.

Although these considerations apply to major illness or surgery even relative minor ailments may upset the diabetic. Whereas in an influenza epidemic the majority can take to their beds for 48 hours and eat nothing, the insulin-dependent diabetic may be driven into ketoacidosis if fuel and fluid intake are not maintained. Many an elderly diabetic will blame the sugar in his cough bottle for the deterioration shown by his urine tests, when more often than not the stress of infection is the real cause of the trouble, and in the female the menstrual periods are a common cause of erratic diabetic control.

Many of the factors applicable to diabetics undergoing surgery are also relevant in other serious illnesses or to their intensive care.

Surgical management

Elective surgery The diabetic should be admitted well in advance of operation (preferably two or three days) so that the following assessments can be made:

> diabetic control, and evidence of vascular or neurological complications: ECG, urea, electrolytes, in addition to a full clinical examination and the usual routines relevant to the particular procedure.

Diabetics, however mild, are best taken through surgery on an intravenous régime based upon dextrose and insulin, which has the advantage of preventing lipolysis, maintaining relatively normal blood glucose values and being suited to any unforeseen emergencies. Otherwise an overnight fast, followed by the stress of surgery may leave the patient with little metabolic reserve to cope with post-anaesthetic nausea, vomiting or other sequelae. The aim should be to maintain the blood glucose in the 6·0 to 12·0 mmol/l (108–216 mg/100 ml) range; this can be achieved by using 5% dextrose (100 ml per hour) with insulin added to the intravenous régime (see Chapter 7). Provided that the insulin is added to the infusion as each bottle comes into use, the problem of its absorption to glass or plastic is minimal and certainly no greater than the vagaries of release from subcutaneous injection sites in its routine use; an infusion pump or paediatric giving-set can be used if preferred. The test of any system lies in the blood glucose value. Most patients require insulin in approximately the same amounts as their normal daily requirements; thus those usually having 60 units daily might have five 500 ml bottles of 5% dextrose with 12 units of short-acting insulin in each bottle. Patients who usually take purified porcine insulin (Chapter 10, p.134) should have short-acting porcine preparations (Actrapid, Novo or Neutral, Nordisk). The régime can be started in the late evening of the pre-operative day, and since the 5 g dextrose per hour is in excess of normal overnight refuelling the intravenous insulin is appropriate even though insulin routinely given on the pre-operative day may still be effective. For those unable to feed post-operatively the régime can be continued as necessary; otherwise, subcutaneous insulin is given as usual on the first post-operative day and the infusion discontinued.

Perfect metabolic control might be achieved with the *artificial pancreas* (a servo-controlled intravenous infusion of insulin/ glucose at rates computed from on-line measurements of the blood glucose concentration). Short of this ideal, those patients in good control pre-operatively can be maintained on the above régime adjusted according to fasting and subsequent 4-hourly blood glucose estimations on the day of operation. With a continuous infusion the blood glucose remains remarkably constant and only minor adjustment of the insulin dose (upwards or downwards by 2–4 units per 500 ml dextrose) are required. Saline or potassium chloride can be added as necessary according to routine surgical practice and electrolyte values. Those patients who are normally controlled by oral hypoglycaemic agents usually require 1–2 units of insulin per hour with the dextrose infusion. Mild diabetics controlled by diet alone, and expected to eat normally on the evening following operation, need not have the intravenous régime, although even they when undergoing a particularly stressful procedure will always do better on it.

Emergency surgery Whereas emergency surgery can also be managed on the above régime, correction of

> diabetic control,
> ketoacidosis,
> lactic acidosis, and
> hyperosmolality,

may be necessary as a matter of urgency. The patient should be assessed with acidosis and hydration in mind; measurement of urea, electrolytes and blood gas analysis is essential; treatment with fluid, electrolyte and insulin should follow the principles outlined in Chapter 7. When is it safe to operate? Provided that the patient is well hydrated, waiting until the blood glucose is in the 6·0 to 12·0 mmol/l (108–216 mg/100 ml) range is unnecessary. On the other hand, acidosis must be corrected. If the patient is significantly hyperglycaemic at the outset, effective correction usually produces a fall in blood glucose at the rate of 5·0 mmol/l (90 mg/100 ml) per hour. Thus if the initial glucose value were

30.0 mmol/l (540 mg/100 ml), the surgeon might be advised that pre-operative treatment for three hours would be necessary to bring the blood glucose below 15·0 mmol/l (270 mg/100 ml). Thereafter, the intravenous régime for elective surgery could be followed.

Infection

Post-operative sepsis (or any other infection in the non-surgical patient) can temporarily profoundly affect the diabetic, particularly because the hormones of stress antagonise insulin through lipolysis, gluconeogenesis and ketogenesis. The principles of management are two-fold: bring the diabetes under control, and treat the infection along the usual lines.

Remember that ketoacidosis may cause leucocytosis (Chapter 7, p.94) and that vasodilation of acidosis may prevent pyrexia. Thus in the diabetic leucocytosis may not mean infection and absence of temperature may also be misleading. If dehydrated, hyperosmolar, acidotic or unable to take sufficient fluid and calories orally, an intravenous régime of dextrose and insulin should be used to tide the patient through the acute phase of the illness.

Whether the incidence of infection is greater in diabetes than in other conditions is difficult to evaluate. The relationship previously mentioned between infection, stress and upset diabetic control brings infection in diabetics more frequently to medical attention but, nevertheless, it is always wise to be alert to occult tuberculosis, pyelonephritis (Chapter 14, p.182) and other forms of infection.

Drugs and diabetes

Some chemical agents have a powerful cytotoxic effect on the pancreatic beta cells; thus, streptozotocin and alloxan can be used to make the experimental animal diabetic. Also, several drugs in common use have a variable effect upon carbohydrate metabolism, some antagonising insulin or the oral hypoglycaemic agents, while others are mildly hypoglycaemic. And some are downright misleading: for example, salicylates are marginally hypoglycaemic but can give false-positive results with the Clinitest (Chapter 5, p.65), when patient and doctor may be misled into thinking that the drug is causing hyperglycaemia when the reverse may be the case.

Drugs causing hyperglycaemia

Corticosteroids All corticosteroids raise the blood glucose by stimulating gluconeogenesis and as the renal threshold to glucose is simultaneously lowered (Chapter 10, p.131), there may be an increase in glycosuria and diabetic symptoms disproportionate to the effect on the blood glucose. When corticosteroids are used in emergency, any effect on diabetic control can be countered by increasing the dose of insulin. In chronic use it is often wise slightly to reduce the dietary intake to prevent excessive weight gain.

Oral contraceptives The diabetogenic action is due to oestrogen rather than to progesterone and since the newer preparations contain lower doses of oestrogen the effect, which is similar to that of corticosteroids, is minimal. There is no contra-indication to the use of the contraceptive pill, so far as its effect on glucose tolerance is concerned, by the diabetic who can, if necessary, be advised about adjusting the insulin dose. But remember Sally (Chapter 3) who had gestational diabetes: in such cases the diabetogenic effect of the pill might induce frank diabetes. Whether diabetics over the age of 30 years should have the pill in view of the increased risk of vascular disease and hypertension is another consideration.

Diuretics All the thiazides may be diabetogenic, possibly related to their potassium-depleting effect. However, diazoxide (Eudemine), although not a diuretic but pharmacologically related to the thiazides, has the most powerful effect on pancreatic function; thus, in addition to its hypotensive effect, diazoxide is used in the management of certain forms of hypoglycaemia (Chapter 18). Frusemide (Lasix), ethacrynic acid (Edecrin) and chlorthalidone (Hygroton) have less effect upon tolerance, while the potassium-sparing diuretics – amiloride (Midamor), triamterene (Dytac) and spironolactone (Aldactone) – are not known to be diabetogenic: these last are, therefore, the better choice for diabetic patients.

Salbutamol (Ventolin) Used in chronic chest disease but also to diminish uterine contraction in premature labour (Chapter 12), salbutamol may increase insulin requirements (in some patients, significantly) due to its effect on increased FFA levels[6].

Isoniazide and *phenytoin* may occasionally impair glucose tolerance.

Drugs causing hypoglycaemia

Beta-adrenoreceptor blocking drugs may aggravate insulin-induced hypoglycaemia, partly due to interference with adrenaline-mediated hepatic glycogenolysis. Since this involves the hepatic beta$_2$ type of receptor, the so-called 'cardioselective' beta$_1$-blocking preparations, for example, atenolol (Tenormin) or acebutolol (Sectral), should be safer for insulin-dependent diabetics than propanolol (Inderal) or oxprenolol (Trasicor) which are less cardioselective. These beta-blockers also interfere with hypoglycaemic awareness. However, in treating the mild non-insulin-dependent patient having hypertension or angina (see below), beta-blockers may cause a small rise in blood glucose[7].

Alcohol Insulin-dependent diabetics should be cautious lest excess consumption of alcohol induces hypoglycaemia by interfering with hepatic glucose release. Diabetics are normally advised to avoid carbohydrate-containing alcoholic drinks but when drinking and missing meals (Chapter 18) these would be safer, or an extra snack could also be taken.

Salicylates, when taken in large doses, are mildly hypoglycaemic yet simultaneously give false-positive results with the Clinitest, but not with the glucose-specific Clinistix. An occasional aspirin can be ignored.

Monoamine oxidase inhibitors marginally enhance the effect of insulin and oral hypoglycaemic agents.

Drugs which potentiate the hypoglycaemic effect of sulphonylureas Several drugs will tend marginally to enhance the hypoglycaemic effect of the sulphonylureas either by interference with protein binding or by inhibition of metabolism: these include sulphonamides, salicylates, phenylbutazone, oxyphenbutazone, monoamine oxidase inhibitors, cyclophosphamide, chloramphenicol and tetracycline. Because these drugs are usually prescribed during illness likely to raise the blood glucose through stress, hypoglycaemia is rarely of clinical significance. On the other hand clofibrate (Atromid-S) often used chronically in diabetes (Chapter 6) may diminish the need for sulphonylureas.

Vascular disease

The pathogenesis of atheroma and degenerative vascular disease in relation to diabetes has been discussed in Chapter 13. In general, the management is based on the same principles as in the non-diabetic, but some aspects of particular significance in diabetes are worth noting.

Myocardial infarction The prognosis for recovery is rather worse, especially in diabetic females, than in the general population. Although silent infarction is said to be commoner in diabetics, accurate evaluation is difficult. Nevertheless, cardiac denervation due to autonomic neuropathy has been reported in diabetics dying of myocardial infarction.

Cardiac failure Mild cardiac failure is common in elderly diabetics. Whether diabetic cardiomyopathy is a definite entity is uncertain, although small-blood-vessel disease may affect myocardial function (Chapter 13, p.172). The treatment of cardiac failure should be along the usual lines, although when using diuretics it is probably better, where there is a choice, to use the potassium-sparing preparations (see above).

Hypertension Arteriosclerotic hypertension is common in diabetics and as it is a potential risk factor for atheroma and retinopathy this is an added reason for controlling the blood pressure. Beta-adrenergic blocking drugs, especially if not beta$_1$ cardioselective, must be used with caution in insulin-dependent diabetics as must thiazide diuretics in mild diabetics. In view of the underlying tendency to renal involvement in the long-standing insulin-dependent diabetic, spironolactone or a combination of beta$_1$ selective blockade plus potassium-sparing diuretics is suitable in mild-to-moderate hypertension. More severe hypertension must be treated on its merits, although diazoxide (Eudemine) has a marked effect on pancreatic function (Chapter 18, p.226), and should be avoided.

Non-cardiac oedema Following a period of poor diabetic control corrected by insulin or other therapy, diabetics may develop fluid retention with ankle, or more generalised, oedema as its main feature. Remember that in the osmotic diuresis of uncontrolled diabetes, the coincident sodium loss will lead to a tendency to *hyponatraemia* because thirsty patients drink water rather than brine (Sodium, Chapter 7, p.89). Improved control stops the salt loss and may unmask fluid retention in patients with an underlying defect in sodium excretion. Patients with mild cardiac disease, females prone to pre-menstrual fluid retention or others with impaired renal osmoregulation are most likely to be affected. The features are usually temporary and respond to diuretics, but if such treatment has to be continued for more than a few weeks, fuller investigation of renal function, including osmoregulation, is advisable because underlying diabetic nephropathy (Chapter 14) and autonomic neuropathy (Chapter 16) may be responsible.

Skin conditions in diabetes

Infections

Boils and carbuncles   Because hyperglycaemia predisposes to pyogenic infections, especially those caused by staphylococci, skin sepsis is frequently found in the newly diagnosed or poorly controlled diabetic.

Moniliasis   *Candida albicans* thrives on moist areas of skin, particularly the intertrigenous areas below the breasts, the axillae, the vagina and around the anal region of obese females. Again, raised glucose levels favour the infection, which may also cause balanitis in men. There may be intense irritation in areas of redness, oedema or maceration of the skin which inappropriate treatment with corticosteroids or antibiotics may cause to increase. The diagnosis can be confirmed by microscopic examination of scrapings for mycelia. The features respond to control of the diabetes, although relief may be added by nystatin cream or pessaries.

Epidermophytosis   Athlete's foot is more common in poorly-controlled diabetics and the infection may spread to the groins as reddened, irritating moist areas.

Other skin conditions

Necrobiosis lipoidica diabeticorum   A relatively uncommon lesion which is seen most typically on the shins of the female patient, although it occurs occasionally on the upper limbs or trunk. The early lesions are elevated yellow-centred papules with reddened edges which gradually coalesce, their centres becoming atrophic and depressed rather than elevated. Telangiectasis or pigmented scarring may occur. The lesions are usually indolent, persistent, painless and more unsightly than of serious significance; ulceration or secondary infection is unusual. Histologically, the microcirculation of the skin is obliterated with disintegration of collagen fibres, but there is no structural relationship with the lesions of diabetic small-blood-vessel disease. The lesions may occur in non-diabetics, or may lead to the diagnosis of diabetes. No specific treatment other than protection of the shins from injury is necessary.

Eruptive xanthomata Seen also in non-diabetics with hyper-triglyceridaemia, the lesions are usually found in patients having lipid disorders and diabetes mellitus (Chapter 6, p.82). Eruptive papular xanthomata, consisting of sharply demarcated flat or nodular lesions, usually occur on the buttocks, thighs and back.

Tuberous xanthomata Occurring in similar circumstances to eruptive xanthomata, these lesions develop on the elbows, knees, hands and feet, sometimes reaching the size of a hen's egg, and form hemispherical projections which are pale yellow in colour.

Xanthelasma These raised yellow fatty deposits on the eyelids are usually of little significance, but since they can occur in hypercholesterolaemia (hyperbetalipoproteinaemia) which may be associated with diabetes, the blood lipids should be checked in any patient having either xanthomata or xanthelasma.

Vitiligo When a diabetic has vitiligo, the lesions should alert one to other autoimmune disorders associated with diabetes – thyroid disease, pernicious anaemia, Addison's disease and alopecia.

Drug rashes Extremely rare side-effect of sulphonylurea therapy.

Dupuytren's contractures These palmar lesions are said to be more common in diabetics, but whether they occur independently of diabetes associated with liver disease is uncertain.

Skin blisters Skin blisters similar to those seen in phenobarbitone overdosage may occasionally occur in diabetic coma.

Insulin injections Considering that diabetics give their own injections, often in circumstances of dubious hygiene, infection or abscesses at injection sites are remarkably uncommon (allergy, lipoatrophy and lipohypertrophy, see Chapter 10).

Psychiatric disorders

Depressive illness The stress of depressive illness may cause chronic deterioration in diabetic control until the disorder is diagnosed and effectively treated. Thus, patients normally controlled by diet or oral hypoglycaemic agents may require insulin temporarily.

Dementia, psychosis, personality disorders Chronic insulin overdosage (or the development of an islet cell adenoma in a diabetic) should always be considered and excluded when diabetics show personality change, psychosis or memory loss (Chapter 18, p.222).

Manipulative behaviour Remember Tom Brown's schooldays (Chapter 7, p.94). Unexplained ketoacidosis or other upsets in diabetic control for no apparent cause should be investigated from this point of view. The child psychiatrist experienced in the diabetic's problems will often uncover family or social pressures which, even if not eliminated, can through better understanding be dealt with more sympathetically by the diabetic specialist or the family doctor.

Further Reading

1 Walsh C.H. & Malins J.M. (1977) Menstruation and control of diabetes. *Br. med. J.*, **ii**, 177–179
2 Editorial (1977) Beta blockers for diabetics. *Lancet*, **i**, 843
3 Deacon S.P., Karunanayake A. & Barnett D. (1977) Acebutolol, atenolol, and propanolol and metabolic responses to acute hypoglycaemia in diabetics. *Br. med. J.*, **ii**, 1255–1257
4 Griffin J.P. (1974) Drug interactions with oral hypoglycaemic agents. *Prescriber's J.*, **14**, 103–106
5 Tansey M.J.B., Opic L.H. & Kennelly B.M. (1977) High mortality in obese women with acute myocardial infarction. *Br. med. J.*, **i**, 1624–1626
6 Fredholm B.B., Lunell N.O., Persson B. & Wager J. (1978) Actions of salbutamol in late pregnancy. *Diabetologia*, **14**, 235–242
7 Wright A.D., Barber S.G., Kendall M.J. & Poole P.H. (1979) Beta-adrenoceptor-blocking drugs and blood sugar control in diabetes mellitus. *Br. Med. J.*, **i**, 159–161

CHAPTER 21

The Natural History of Diabetes

Examination of the previously diagnosed or long-standing diabetic. Assessment of complications, control and prognosis

> . . . life is short, disgusting and painful, thirst unquenchable, death inevitable . . .
>
> Aretaeus the Cappadocian
> 2nd Century A.D.

Having encountered a catalogue of varied diabetic complications in the preceding chapters, the despairing reader may be excused for believing that nothing has changed and that despite the discovery of insulin, life for the diabetic is still too short, disgusting and painful. Yet many diabetics, nourished by injected insulin, enjoy forty or more years of relatively trouble-free times. Good diabetic control during pregnancy has significantly improved the maternal and fetal outcome. Perhaps a better awareness of the need for enhanced control throughout the duration of diabetes, and its achievement by multiple injections or improved insulin delivery systems monitored by blood glucose or other methods, will breed a new generation of diabetics enjoying brighter times than at present. Because of much individual variation, it is difficult to paint a natural history of diabetes in clear outline. Nevertheless, some observations may be useful, particularly for those assessing previously-diagnosed or long-standing patients who may have recently come under their care.

At the outset it is worth drawing a distinction between the juvenile-onset insulin-dependent diabetic and those who develop the disorder in later life (although the local football team, Chapter 3) reminds us that there are many other variations on these broad themes). Look at Figure 21.1; notice the difference between the abrupt onset of insulin-dependent diabetes compared with late-onset or milder diabetes. Also, whereas after diagnosis the blood glucose is brought into a range low enough to avert serious

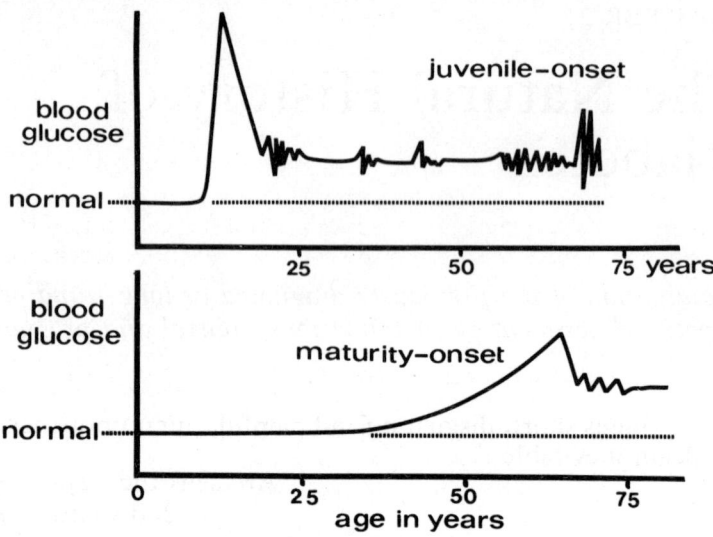

Fig. 21.1 Diagrammatic comparison of juvenile-onset and maturity-onset diabetes. Note the abrupt onset of the former and the gradual onset of the latter with, in both, failure of the blood glucose to return to the normal base-line

symptoms of thirst and polyuria, it is rarely brought fully back to the non-diabetic baseline. The more gradual onset of mild diabetes in middle life means that such patients may have lived through months or years of abnormal glucose tolerance; indeed, it is often some other illness which brings the diagnosis to light. Remember Jack Spratt (Chapter 3) whose diabetes was diagnosed at the time of a myocardial infarct, and Mr. Puff (Chapter 3) who had evidence of retinopathy and nephropathy at the time of diagnosis. About 10–15% of late onset diabetics will have retinopathy at the time of diagnosis, and 30% will have mild painless peripheral neuropathy.

In contrast, the juvenile-onset diabetic virtually never has evidence of specific diabetic complications at the time of diagnosis. Various factors discussed in earlier sections may affect the progress of complications:

blood glucose control and basement membrane thickening,
platelet adhesiveness,
fibrin deposition,
blood viscosity,
altered lipid metabolism,
hypertension,
altered hormone levels: growth hormone, catecholamines,

glucagon, etc,
diet, or
renal function.

but the outstanding influence upon the clinical appearance of complications is the *duration of diabetes*. In juvenile-onset diabetics, evidence of significant complications is unusual in the first 10 years of the disorder, yet after 20 years those totally free of complications are the exception. Thus, careful examination at regular intervals becomes increasingly important as time passes and is especially valuable from 10 years of diabetes onwards.

Assessment of diabetic complications

How should the patient be assessed? What do you think about the following?

fluorescein angiography of the retinae
renal biopsy
sural nerve biopsy
cardiac and coronary angiography
fasting blood lipids
24-hour metabolic profile of blood glucose, growth hormone, lactate, pyruvate, etc
blood viscosity at high and low shear rates
platelet adhesiveness and plasma beta-thromboglobulin estimation
motor nerve conduction velocity

'Actually doctor, I was thinking of going on holiday next week . . . do you think I'll be fit to go after all that? And if you find anything what can you do for me, doctor?' 'Oh!, well if we find something we'd then go on to test your baroreceptor response to . . .' Clearly there must be a compromise between enthusiastic endeavour and usefulness to the patient. Perhaps we might start more gently:

height and weight in relation to correct weight;
cardiovascular system and peripheral pulses;
blood pressure lying and standing;
palpate liver edge;
examine legs and feet for features of ischaemia, neuropathy or minor infection;
examine eyes, including opthalmoscopy of retinae;
urine sample for glucose, albumin and microscopy;
blood for urea, creatinine, electrolytes, haematological indices, ESR; and
chest x-ray, ECG.

This will involve having 20 minutes to spare, removing the patient's shoes, and the back-up of laboratory services. But it should suffice to establish a reasonable impression of where the patient stands in relation to the onset of complications. Additional investigations are usually indicated only if clinical examination reveals further specific problems, for example retinopathy, vascular disease and neuropathy.

Remember Peter (Chapter 3) diagnosed at the age of 12 years and now being examined at the age of 30 years after 18 years of trouble-free insulin-dependent diabetes. Suppose that we go through the simple routine and find that height, weight, blood pressure (standing and lying), peripheral nerves and pulses, urine and blood samples all normal, but we do find one or two scattered microaneurysms in one eye only? Provided that diabetic control is being maintained satisfactorily it would be reasonable to have a baseline assessment by an ophthalmologist at this stage and arrange for the eyes to be re-examined after 12 months.

Next, let us look at Tom Brown (Chapter 7, p.94) who, since his boisterous schooldays, has never taken his diabetes too seriously, is also aged 30 years and has been diabetic since the age of 10 years. In his case the fundi show more widespread microaneurysms and one or two areas of discreet new vessel formation, but the remainder of his examination is satisfactory with two exceptions: a trace of proteinuria and an ESR of 30 mm in the first hour. The well-established retinopathy, proteinuria and raised ESR are strongly suggestive of coincident diabetic nephropathy despite the still normal blood urea. Although there is no obvious evidence of peripheral neuropathy, Tom does admit to recent impotence, characteristic of early autonomic neuropathy. Tom is now in need of expert ophthalmology and although with light coagulation (Chapter 15, p.196) vision may be preserved, he is likely to develop increasing impediments in the next decade as he moves towards the late diabetic syndrome (p.251).

But if Peter enjoys a much longer period of well being than Tom, can the difference be attributed entirely to life-style and Peter's more careful diabetic self-regulation? Many diabetics, although insulin-dependent, can be shown by measurement of C-peptide (Chapter 4, p.48) to retain some residual pancreatic beta cell function. Perhaps if Peter has this advantage, his better diabetic control may be a consequence of some servo-assistance from his own pancreas helping exogenous insulin to maintain normal blood-glucose homeostasis. Although retention of some residual beta cell function is advantageous, there are probably many other factors quite apart from patient compliance, including anti-insulin antibodies, variation in nutrient absorption and fore-gut hormonal secretion, which may make control easier in some diabetics than in others.

Assessment of control in the juvenile-onset diabetic

Traditional methods of assessing diabetic control usually have been based upon random blood glucose estimation at out-patient review and home testing of urine glucose. Whereas these may be adequate for the mild diabetic whose blood glucose remains reasonably stable, they fail to reflect the wide fluctuations in glucose homeostasis which characterise insulin-dependent diabetes particularly in adolescence or early adult life. Such additional aspects as

> steady weight: correct for age, height and sex,
> enquiry about symptoms of uncontrolled diabetes, and
> freedom from hypoglycaemic attacks,

are even less satisfactory, being at best only crude indices of the quality of control or the need for reappraisal of insulin and dietary therapy. When diabetic control is poor, blood lipids and several other metabolic parameters inevitably will be abnormal, hence their measurement in the poorly controlled patient is of little value. Abnormal values in a well controlled diabetic may be a reflection of renal or other vascular complications.

Two recent developments have brought new precision to the assessment of control: measurement of haemoglobin A_1 (Hb A_{1c}) and home monitoring of *blood* glucose.

Measurement of haemoglobin A_1 When haemoglobin is separated on a cation exchange column, a small amount is seen as a fast-moving component which has been identified as the minor haemoglobin A_{1c} (Hb A_{1c} or fast Hb A_1). Although structurally similar to ordinary haemoglobin (Hb A), fast Hb A_1 differs in having one extra glucose molecule. Conversion of Hb A to fast Hb A_1 occurs in the red blood cells in the peripheral circulation during their life span. Hyperglycaemia will favour increased uptake of glucose so that Hb A_1 values in excess of the normal range (3–6%) reflect the degree of hyperglycaemia prevailing during the life cycle of the measured red cells (Fig. 21.2). In other words, measurement of fast Hb A_1 provides in one simple blood test an index of the integrated plasma glucose over an extended period of up to three months.

The glucose uptake in hyperglycaemia associated with increased

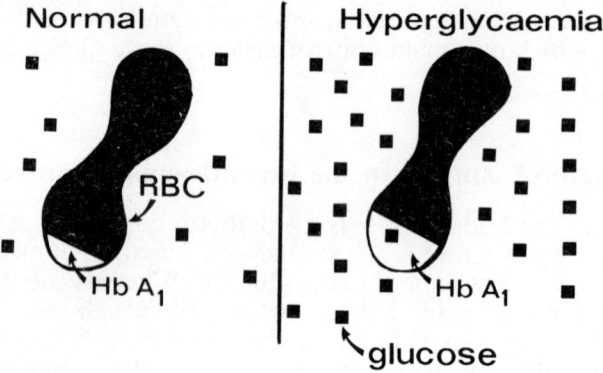

Fig. 21.2 Diagrammatic comparison of red blood cells circulating in plasma with normal and high glucose content. Greater conversion to fast haemoglobin A_1 (Hb A_{1C}) in hyperglycaemia

conversion to fast Hb A_1 is analogous to the capillary basement membrane changes (Chapter 14) – both processes are independent of insulin. Hence, measurement of fast Hb A_1 is not only a measure of control but also a mirror to the potentially serious consequence of poor control in other tissues. Not surprisingly, fast Hb A_1 is now as important to diabetic control as the bank rate is to the money market. Of course there are snags: the test only reflects intermittent or more constant *hyperglycaemia* and, like urine testing, it cannot register *hypoglycaemia*, nor can it be used in the day-to-day adjustment of control. There can also be another problem: any underlying haemolytic process, or the concomitant use of drugs which shorten the life span of red cells, may give falsely low values. Nevertheless, the test, which is well suited to the intermittent review of the diabetic clinic, has added a new dimension to the assessment of control.

Home monitoring of *blood* glucose (Chapter 10, p.129) provides patients with a means of insulin dose adjustment and assessment of control far more relevant to their usual activities than tests obtained in the artificial circumstances of the hospital ward or clinic. The striking advantage of this approach to self-regulation is the ability to avoid both hyperglycaemia and hypoglycaemia. Better control is achieved by redistributing the insulin doses rather than increasing their total. Most patients prefer the elimination of guesswork and do not find it irksome to prick their finger for the blood sample.

Avoid judging diabetic control on a random blood glucose value obtained at a single visit to the diabetic clinic. A patient may have a high value following nocturnal hypoglycaemia, needing less rather than more insulin (see Somogyi effect, Chapter 10). Recent well-being, weight trends, diet, insulin dose and usual activities at that time of day also should be taken into account.

The late diabetic syndrome

Knud Lundbaek, who in 1954 first established the concept of diabetic angiopathy – widespread vascular disease involving large, medium and small arteries besides the retinal and glomerular capillaries – in long-standing diabetics, has described the late diabetic syndrome as that stage at which patients show evidence of multisystem pathology. The trouble for the patient is not just that several essential functions are failing – sight, proprioception, renal function, peripheral perfusion and the like – but that there are also various adverse interactions. For example, non-diabetics with failing vision can compensate to some extent by touch and other forms of proprioception but diabetics lose sight and sense simultaneously and become all the more clumsy. Erratic swings in blood glucose – anything between 3·0 and 30·0 mmol/l (54–540 mg/100 ml) – in the course of a day are a consequence of variable gut motility of autonomic neuropathy affecting food absorption, the patient's diminished ability to exercise as usual and altered renal handling of insulin, besides other factors. Poor renal function, in addition to causing vague ill-health and normo-chromic anaemia, upsets free water clearance and creates other defects in the elaborate network of fluid regulation, resulting in hyponatraemia through failure to dilute the urine. Renal disease puts the resting blood pressure up and on standing autonomic neuropathy puts it down. Plasma lipids are in disarray. Platelets are aggregating, the blood is more viscous and fibrin is being deposited in glomerular basement membranes and elsewhere. Perhaps fortunately for patients at this stage, in addition to peripheral and autonomic neuropathy, diabetic encephalopathy clouds the awareness of the various impediments. There is an ever-present risk of pyelonephritis or other infection. This is not the time to consider pituitary ablation to save sight, nor to contemplate transplantation to save renal function. Even an attempt to salvage a pre-gangrenous foot by quick surgery may result in cardiac or respiratory arrest under anaesthesia as a consequence of auto-nomic neuropathy and vascular disease. Attempts to bring the diabetes under strict control, besides being too late, are often thwarted by dangerous hypoglycaemia. A failure to recover from cardiac arrest may be a blessing.

Natural history of maturity-onset diabetes

Although reminded of Mr. Puff (Chapter 3) who was in the late diabetic syndrome at the time of diagnosis, many elderly diabetics have minimal clinical evidence of specific diabetic complications. Vision is more likely to be affected by the refractive changes of age or by cataract rather than by retinopathy. The predominantly exudative retinopathy seen in late-onset diabetes (Chapter 15) can be arrested by clofibrate (Atromid-S) or photocoagulation, and more serious proliferative retinopathy affects but a few. Control of diabetes is relatively simple in that the vast majority of patients are responsive to diet and oral hypoglycaemic agents, and in those developing insulin-dependent diabetes around three-score years or more, control is aimed at relieving the thirst and polyuria rather than obtaining the blood glucose values expected in the young. In later life the natural history is more likely to be influenced by the following:

> other medical conditions, including *cancer*,
> degenerative vascular disease – cardiac, peripheral ischaemia, stroke, and
> deteriorating renal function.

Thus in assessing the elderly, even if the metabolic control of the diabetes is stable, these possibilities should always be kept in mind. And whenever a patient develops diabetes in later life, especially if underweight, the possibility of pancreatic or other neoplasia should be considered. Those whose diabetes appears stable on a simple drug régime may drift towards hypoglycaemia as the renal excretion of sulphonylureas and other drugs diminishes. Indeed, all drug therapy, particularly including the extensively-prescribed diuretics, requires revision as the years pass.

Despite all those aspects which need regular review, many patients who develop mild maturity-onset diabetes will remain entirely well, without evidence of either specific diabetic complications or of other disorders, living happily into ripe old age. Even so, ultimately a stroke or other insult may suddenly convert placid metabolic homeostasis into dangerous hyperglycaemia and a serious hyperosmolar state (Chapter 7).

Assessment of control in the maturity-onset diabetic

The same principles in terms of symptoms and weight trends as apply to insulin-dependent patients (see page 249) should be taken into account. However, since blood glucose values tend to be less variable from day to day in mild diabetes, results at clinic visits are an adequate reflection of the current state of control. Remember that the blood glucose rises slightly with age and that attempts to induce euglycaemia in *asymptomatic* elderly patients may not do their brains (or your reputation) any good.

Prognosis in diabetes

Precise figures are difficult to give, although Figure 21.3 shows the mortality in diabetes mellitus at different ages of onset. For the individual patient, the presence or absence of complications or other illness are the best guide to prognosis.

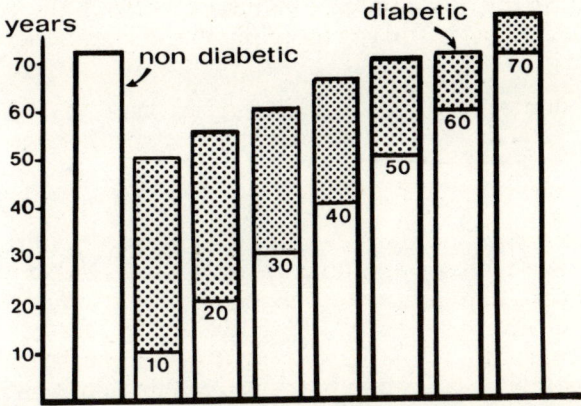

Fig. 21.3 Diagrammatic representation comparing life prognosis in the non-diabetic with those developing the disorder at 10, 20, 30 years etc. Diabetic period of life hatched. Note that those of onset in early years have a much poorer prognosis for life than those becoming diabetic in later years. Based on references 21.4, 21.5 and other data

Sadly, the insulin era has afforded ample opportunity to witness, but so far not to avert, many serious diabetic complications. Looked at one way, 40% of juvenile-onset diabetics survive for 40 years or more, but looked at another, 50% of those diagnosed in youth die by the age of 50 from nephropathy, cardiac disease or other complications[4,5]. We can only hope that the improved control now being achieved by many patients will change these appalling statistics in the same way that better control in pregnancy (Chapter 12) has improved fetal mortality.

Further Reading

1 Gabbay K.H. (1976) Glycosylated hemoglobin and diabetic control. *New Engl. J. Med.*, **295**, 443–444
2 Editorial (1978) Glycolysated haemoglobin and diabetic control. *Br. med. J.*, **i**, 1373–1374
3 Gonen B. & Rubenstein A.H. (1978) Haemoglobin A_1 and diabetes mellitus. *Diabetologia*, **15**, 1–8
4 Deckert T., Poulsen J.E. & Larsen M. (1978) Prognosis of diabetics with diabetes onset before the age of thirty-one. 1. Survival, causes of death and complications. *Diabetologia*, **14**, 363–370
5 Deckert T. *et al.* (1978). II. Factors influencing prognosis. *Diabetologia*, **14**, 371–378

CHAPTER 22

Diabetics at Risk in Society

Ignorance about diabetes breeds fear in all and sundry. From their different standpoints, parents, teachers, employers, insurance companies and even doctors regard diabetes as a risky business. Patients are often afraid about childbearing, recreation, food and travel; training colleges, employers, insurance companies and some doctors shy away from diabetics. One aim of this text has been to help doctors in making it easier for diabetics to lead normal lives and, at the same time, to encourage patients by giving them maximal assistance particularly in coping with the various impediments as far as is presently possible. This is not a novel approach. In 1934, Dr. R.D. Lawrence (Chapter 8) and others founded the British Diabetic Association, an organisation which year by year does more and more to foster these ideals by giving patients help and advice and encouraging research into the unsolved diabetic mysteries. Similar organisations are spread throughout the world, united under the banner of the International Diabetes Federation.

How should we approach the question of advising diabetics about employment, driving, travel and the like? The 19th century historian Walter Bagehot in his classic essay *The English Constitution* described the monarch as having 'The right to be consulted, the right to encourage, the right to warn', a triad which illuminates precisely the place of the doctor with regard to the diabetic's problems. The right to be consulted is usually in the patient's best interests, for otherwise an employer might discriminate against a diabetic on the grounds of the disorder when, in the patient's case, diabetes may be no impediment to the work in question. Doctors are often quick to place restraints upon their patients (diet, smoking and alcohol, for example). Equally, we should be prepared to encourage diabetics in seeking employment, in coping with foreign travel or in recreational activities, but we must also be prepared to warn those who develop serious complications against foolhardy pursuits.

Mankind has always faced a risky world. As some risks diminish – acute infections, for example – such others as road accidents increase. We constantly devise new ways of attempting to diminish certain risks. Thus, for the common good, society may place restrictions on individual liberty by legislating to limit the speed and the unroadworthiness of vehicles (and drivers) in the hope of reducing road accidents, or when some drivers are greater risks than others, insurance companies may modify the premium accordingly. Diabetics and their doctors must abide by the rules of the game and act within the law on all these aspects, and they must do so even if the law is foolish. Thus a few years ago when the Western World was enjoying the greatest explosion of overnutrition of all time, the non-sugar (slimming) sweetener cyclamate was banned in many Western countries on the grounds of a remote risk of cancer. Better to die of obesity (a risk well known to life assurers) said the legislators, as they unwittingly denied diabetics one of the palatable ways of adding sweetness to their dull diets. So far, governments have not been able to muster the same courage in facing the carcinogenic risks of cigarette smoking, yet on these and other aspects of everyday life diabetic patients will seek medical advice, whether or not covered by law. Although concerned here with broad principles, each problem must be judged on its merits. For example, James, the professional footballer (Chapters 3; 10) wants to go skin-diving. It sounds risky (skin-diving can be), but when the details are examined, we recall that we are dealing with a diabetic accustomed to regular energetic exercise. He will always be in the company of other experts and he is a good swimmer. The period of immersion can be defined clearly, so what is the risk? Hypoglycaemia? But if James takes less of the insulin which will be effective at the time of diving and extra insulin with a large meal when the dive is over, all should be well. On the other hand, Tom Brown (Chapters 7; 21), who has always been erratic and who has never really come to grips with the principles of diabetic self-regulation, should not even be allowed to go swimming on his own. Thus in terms of employment, driving, recreation and travel each case must be judged on its merits.

Adolescent risks

Adolescent diabetics are particularly vulnerable, not just on account of growing up in a society whose rules they seek to question or reject, but as they establish increasing independence from parental supervision, they are also at risk of drifting away from the supervision of the diabetic clinic. Childhood fears of injections are now behind them and they have usually fully mastered the principles of self-regulation with insulin. The confidence of youth, the pressures of school examinations or a new job causes them to default on follow-up. Often there is another reason: adolescents may resent sitting in a lengthy queue in an out-patient department, surrounded by the halt and the maimed, ultimately to have a brief interview with an inexperienced or harassed young doctor who seems to understand less about insulin-glucose homeostasis than the patients. Adolescents should be seen by the most experienced doctor available, not only to assess diabetic control, but also because they often have anxieties about the future, sex and contraception, and other problems which require a sympathetic hearing. A patient lost at this stage, when good diabetic control is of such importance to their future, may next be seen many years later (and often too late) because of one or more serious diabetic complications.

Other adolescents have a different problem. Unable properly to cope with life and diabetes, repeated hospital admissions in ketoacidosis are their muted cry for help. On each occasion, the duty doctor as he copes with the exciting fluid and electrolyte problem, identifies urinary infection, a sore throat or gastro-enteritis as the reason for the ketoacidosis. Valuable school-time is repeatedly lost, things get worse and worse and the real cause may still be overlooked. Remember Tom Brown's schooldays (Chapter 7). Ketoacidosis is defined as a medical emergency: true, but it is often a social problem in disguise. Such youngsters usually respond well to management by psychiatrists and social workers experienced in the problems of the adolescent, often thereafter becoming more conscientious in diabetic self-regulation than others.

Employment, driving, travel and recreation

With the exception of those situations where the patient might be a risk to himself or others, there should be no discrimination against diabetics. The insulin-dependent are usually barred from flying aircraft, active service in the armed forces or driving public service vehicles. The nub of the problem is the risk of hypoglycaemia. In decisions about employment, driving, travel or recreation, each case must be judged on individual aptitude in relation to the patient's understanding of diabetic self-regulation. Those patients adjusting their own dose on a two-injection four-insulin system (Chapter 10) are better able to adapt to changing working hours, intercontinental travel or unusual exercise in the context of sport or recreation. Some patients having difficulty in obtaining employ-ment can be helped in Britain by being registered as disabled, when medical social workers, in co-operation with the Department of Employment and Productivity, are then better able to find them suitable work.

Having the right to be consulted and to encourage patients in leading as normal and uninhibited a life as possible, the time will also come when the doctor must warn those with retinopathy or other impediments about giving up activities which might be made hazardous. This is particularly important with regard to driving and occupational risks.

Marriage, childbearing and family life

A better knowledge of the genetics of diabetes, in which family clustering affects the maturity-onset rather than the juvenile-onset diabetic, allows us to reassure the young insulin-dependent patient about marriage and the unlikelihood of their offspring becoming diabetic. Even when both parents are diabetic the chances are remote. The diabetic female should, however, be warned before pregnancy of the intensity of ante-natal care that she will require (Chapter 12) and, indeed, there is a strong case for planning each pregnancy so that diabetic control can be optimal from conception onwards to minimise the risk of fetal malformation (Chapter 12). Problems can arise when a diabetic with retinopathy or other complications plans to marry. The prognosis should be discussed with the prospective partner and the potential risks of childbearing explained if the patient is female. Because the presence of complications will also affect life prognosis, the adoption of children might be equally inadvisable.

Marriage problems can arise, particularly for the male diabetic who becomes impotent (Chapter 16). The patient may attempt to conceal the problem from his doctor. Sensible explanation of the underlying cause to both partners usually relieves the family tension.

The risks in diet, smoking and alcohol

Dietary intervention has always been so central to the management of diabetes that we have our patients virtually eating out of our hands. Inevitably we must be prepared for questions about diet and the risks of heart disease – a tricky subject, not to be taken lightly in diabetics especially because they are an identified risk group. Those who have read Chapter 9 will appreciate that this text is not yoked unquestioningly to the low-cholesterol, low-fat, polyunsaturated bandwagon which rolls blindly on as the panacea for heart disease. Instead, we would place greater emphasis on appreciation of the different fuel needs of the growing adolescent, the energetic, the idle and the overweight. The overfuelled and the lazy would do better to avoid cream and indulge less in the fatted calf, but the active and energetic, having a carbohydrate intake based upon generous amounts of daily bread, vegetables, fruit and fibre, would come to no harm by augmenting fat intake in response to the increased fuel requirements of exercise. There will always be obsessional patients who regard dietary rituals as an insurance policy and guarantee of good health. Without damping the ardour of such individuals it would not be prudent to give patients the impression that any particular dietary system will maintain clean coronary arteries. (If any reader knows of such a diet, we would be glad to hear of it; no prizes for effects on fasting blood lipids, it is healthy arteries that interest our patients!)

In contrast, health warnings about cigarette smoking should be emphasised to diabetics, especially with regard to advising adolescents against starting the habit. Here it is all gain; removal of a clearly identified coronary risk factor, a carcinogen and a drain on finances are all to the patients' advantage. Alcohol can be taken with good sense and in moderation, but always remember to stress the risks of hypoglycaemia in the insulin-dependent (Chapters 18 and 20). Diabetics should be strongly advised against drinking and driving. Many of the excess calories of the late-onset diabetic are alcoholic in origin, hence moderation or abstinence may have to be advised in the overweight.

Medical risks

Many diabetics have access to expert medical treatment, guidance and encouragement, but some are less fortunate. Although the difference is often attributed to the uneven spread of diabetic clinics, with centres of excellence separated by wide areas of neglect, perhaps the real fault lies with many medical schools which still give disproportionately scant attention to diabetes mellitus in the medical curriculum. It is easier for a camel to pass through the eye of a needle than it is for a student to get through a course in medicine without attending lectures in the fundamentals of biochemistry and intermediary metabolism. Yet knowledge of clinical diabetes is often an optional extra, acquired by chance encounter somewhere between ausculating the heart and palpating the spleen. This always seems a curious oversight, particularly as

the disorder provides the medical teacher with a unique opportunity of embracing – in a relatively common clinical entity – the
fundamentals of biochemistry, metabolism, pathology, genetics
and the like. Perhaps it is because diabetic problems carry us
quickly to the interface between disciplines, for instance, vessel
wall disease in the boundary between pathology and metabolism,
or retinopathy in the grey area between medicine and ophthalmology, that medical teachers stick to safer ground and their
students venture forth into the world unsure of clinical diabetes.
So long as the subject is neglected, some patients are going to get a
raw deal and may be more at risk than others.

Driving the message home

In an advancing world where high technology medicine has so
many exciting applications, patients are quick to learn of developments relevant to their own special problems. Worn down by
regular injections, diabetics have their hopes exalted by news of
'oral insulin', pancreatic islet cell transplantation or the 'artificial
pancreas'. Doctors must expect to be consulted about these
advances by eager patients. To date only the 'artificial pancreas' (a
servo-controlled intravenous insulin/glucose infusion at rates
computed from continuous blood glucose estimations) is oper-
ational for use with patients but involves tethering the diabetic to a
laboratory or a hospital bed. Skin-diving with the 'artificial
pancreas' is out. But just as divers have discovered new under-
water vistas with oxygen tanks on their backs, perhaps with further
development diabetics will reach new horizons using more portable systems. In the meantime we must encourage our patients to
use the presently available conventional systems to their best
advantage, and we must do this even though educating diabetics in
the principles of insulin self-regulation and adjusting some basic
rules in order to cope with work or travel is time consuming and,
by some standards, unrewarding.

We encourage our patients to make great sacrifices in order to
improve their diabetic control – why do this they might reasonably
ask? We must be prepared to warn them about the potential risks of
poor diabetic control. Not necessarily at the onset of diabetes, but
certainly once the insulin-dependent diabetic is well established in
controlling the disorder it is prudent to warn the patient about the
serious complications. The overwhelming evidence from diabetics
who have lost vision through retinopathy points to the fact that
they would have preferred to have had advance warning. Taking

patients into our confidence in order to encourage them towards maximal co-operation in terms of good blood glucose control seems, on the basis of currently available evidence, to be one of the better ways and perhaps ultimately the only way of minimising the risks of long-term complications. Earlier (in Chapter 8) the anology of teaching both driving and motor car maintenance was made with reference to learning how to control diabetes and to delay or prevent complications. In facing our responsibilities to our patients this seems an appropriate vehicle in which to drive the message home. And even if at the end of the day it becomes apparent that good diabetic control will not prevent *all* the various complications (nobody can yet be absolutely certain) at least those who fully understand how to regulate their disorder will have been able to go about their business or relaxation, making the most of life, without going in fear of diabetes.

Further Reading

1 Knibbs S. & Jackson J.G.L. (1975) Social and emotional complications of diabetes. In *Complications of Diabetes* (Ed. H. Keen & R.J. Jarrett) London: Edward Arnold, 265–277

For the patient

1 Bloom A. (1978) *Diabetes Explained*. Baltimore: University Park Press
2 Colwell A.R.J. (1978) *Understanding your Diabetes*. Springfield, Illinois: Charles C. Thomas
3 *The Diabetic Handbook*. London: British Diabetic Association

CHAPTER 23

Conclusion: Great Expectations . . .

Diabetes mellitus remains as much a challenge to the fundamental researcher as it does to those involved in diabetic care. We have attempted to weld the varied facets of the disorder into a cohesive story without peddling ideas which go against the grain of common knowledge, or common sense. Nevertheless, experts are bound to disagree with many of the views expressed in this text. We hope that those experiencing a rush of blood glucose to the head over any particular point of contention will appreciate, on reflection, that the aim throughout has been to stimulate an interest in the subject besides attempting to give practical advice to those dealing with the day-to-day problems of the diabetic patient. It is relatively easy to set down a catalogue of disconnected facts and conflicting ideas. We hope that we have provided a better insight by bringing the more controversial aspects into sharper relief.

Aetiology and diagnosis

The account of the metabolic disorder was built around the concept – so ably expressed by the founding father of diabetes, Aretaeus the Cappadocian – of the melting down of the flesh and limbs into the urine. Aretaeus can be excused for omitting insulin or the osmotic effects of glucose from his description of the disorder. Although unable to match the clarity of his style, today we see the function of insulin as the essential regulator of fuel storage and release. An abundance of insulin stimulates energy storage; insulin shortage starts the chain reaction of fat and protein melting, releasing the fuel and essential raw-materials for gluco-neogenesis and ketogenesis.

Many other attractive hormones jostle insulin for our attention. For example, the hormone of stress – catecholamines, cortisol, glucagon and growth hormone – frequently consort to oppose insulin. The digestive avenue of the fore-gut is also rich in exciting hormones which influence glucose uptake. Likewise, a variety of

interesting peptides besides glucagon are secreted in the pancreatic islets so close to the insulin-producing beta cell. Yet insulin
remains the Great Dictator. Only when insulin secretion is
impaired does the opposition gain the upper hand. And when the
beta cells fail, the injection of insulin reimposes control over the
metabolic chaos created in its absence. In severe diabetic emergencies, however, insulin alone is ineffective. Not so much because of
the anti-insulin hormones, but because the hyperglycaemia of
insulin lack may have such profound effects on electrolyte and
water balance that intravenous fluids are essential to restore
plasma volume and renal function. Indeed, realisation of this
fundamental aspect of hyperglycaemia allows us now to treat
diabetic emergencies with relatively small amounts of insulin
provided that intravenous fluids are used judiciously.

Until the precise functional significance of the other hormones is
more fully understood, it seems reasonable to continue to view
diabetes mellitus as an absolute or relative deficiency of insulin.
Inevitably, the pancreatic islets remain an intense focus of study
and in the next decade we can expect to learn much more about

> insulin molecular biology,
> genetic decoding of pre-proinsulin,
> regulation of insulin secretion, and
> abnormalities of insulin secretion in diabetes.

We can anticipate that much more will be discovered about the
peripheral action of insulin with particular reference to

> the physiology of insulin receptors,
> glucose transport, and
> the intracellular action of insulin on protein, carbohydrate
> and fat metabolism.

Despite having ascribed a central rôle to insulin, both in terms of
aetiology and treatment, no doubt there will be considerable spin-
off concerning the parts played by the opposing hormones,
especially those secreted by the remaining cells of the pancreatic
islets and the fore-gut[1].

Research in tissue transplantation, by widening our knowledge
of the histocompatibility antigen system (HLA), has clarified our
understanding of the genetics of diabetes. Juvenile-onset diabetes
(JOD) is genetically clearly distinguishable from maturity-onset
diabetes (MOD). Although about 80% of youngsters have no
family history of diabetes, many do have a preponderance of
certain histocompatibility antigens (B8, B15, B18, DW3, DW4,
DRW3 and DRW4). This implies that the inheritance of these

antigens creates a *susceptibility* to diabetes in youngsters. But some other stimulus is essential to launch the susceptible patient into clinical diabetes – is viral infection the missing link? Although the interface between the HLA system, genetic susceptibility and immunology is rapidly coming into clearer focus, we are not yet able to identify with certainty the stimulus which so suddenly and dramatically sets in motion the metabolic upset of juvenile-onset insulin-dependent diabetes. Prevention will depend upon its identification and the feasibility of defusing (immunising) those at risk[2].

The ability to detect islet cell antibodies (ICA) has also helped to illuminate the mysteries of insulin-dependent (Type I) diabetes. ICA appear to be markers for two distinct groups: juvenile-onset diabetes, and polyendocrine or auto-immune associated diabetes.

Although both groups are metabolically similar in terms of severity of diabetes and insulin dependence, ICA are only present at or around the time of diagnosis in the juvenile-onset and, as mentioned above, some other spark is essential to light up the diabetic features; in other words, ICA are usually detected only after the diabetes is clinically obvious. Polyendocrine diabetes, characteristically more common in females, and with onset more commonly in adult life, is often associated with other organ-specific antibodies. In these patients ICA can be detected before the clinical onset of diabetes and may remain permanently positive. Whether or not facilities are available for measuring ICA, it is always prudent to be alert to the possible development of hypothyroidism, Addison's disease or pernicious anaemia, especially in the female who develops insulin-dependent diabetes in adult life. Because ICA are found in both HLA-associated juvenile-onset diabetes and in the auto-immune related disorder it seems that altered immunity affecting the pancreatic beta cell is fundamental to insulin-dependent diabetes whether due to inheritance of HLA-associated immunodeficiency or autoimmunity. In other words, at least two patterns of altered immunity causing islet cell destruction (and ICA release) have been identified in insulin-dependent (Type I) diabetes. This is an area in which intense research directed towards prevention of insulin-dependent diabetes is sure to continue (Fig. 23.1)

The ability to type patients according to HLA status, and to measure ICA, may tempt some people to launch into clever new classifications of diabetes mellitus. But juvenile-onset and polyendocrine diabetes represent a tiny proportion of those who develop the disorder. Pending a universally-agreed classification, we preferred to wander off and select our football teams (Chapter

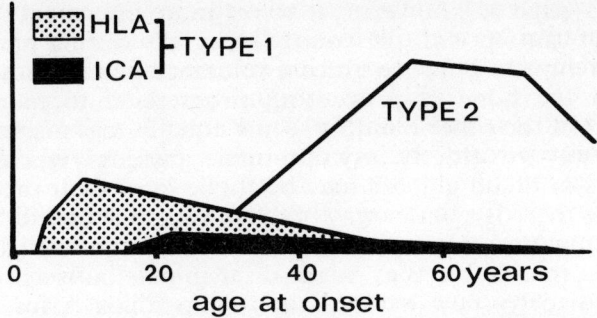

Fig. 23.1 Diagram of incidence of new cases of diabetes at different ages showing that the main peak of type 1 diabetes occurs in the HLA-associated juvenile-onset group, that the vast majority of new cases are non-insulin dependent (type 2) occurring in later life, while some of type 1 diabetes is associated with persistent islet cell antibodies (ICA) and occurs throughout adult life. Not to scale

3) in the hope of emphasising to the reader the broad panorama of disorders of glucose tolerance which masquerade under the banner of diabetes mellitus. The vast majority of those who develop diabetes do so in later life. Admittedly, maturity-onset diabetes clusters in some families, but until the phenotypes or genotypes of those at risk, and their relationship to obesity, hyper-lipidaemia, ageing or vascular disease, are better understood, we would prefer to stay with our football team. That motley collection should serve to emphasise that we still have much to learn about the long list of risk factors (liver and pancreatic disease, lipid disorders, abnormal nutrition, haemochromatosis, myocardial infarction, endocrino-pathy and so on) for diabetes mellitus.

The clinical detection and diagnosis of diabetes is easy insofar as urine and blood glucose estimation is simple and reliable. But there are still serious doubts about where normal glucose tolerance ends and diabetes begins. One way out of the difficulty is to classify patients into one of three groups: diabetic, borderline or doubtful, and normal. This makes sense to the epidemiologist who wishes to study the grey area between normality and diabetes. But it leaves patients who get caught in the middle ground without a satisfactory answer to a problem which may affect their employment or insurance prospects. Having submitted themselves to a GTT they expect a clear decision. Because blood glucose rises (like blood pressure) with age, we drew up arbitrary guide-lines (Chapter 5) which take age into account. We did not intend to imply that glucose tolerance deteriorates with age as sharply as indicated in

Table 5.2 (page 66); however, it seems more important to err on the side of caution with the young (especially during pregnancy) and to attempt to improve glucose tolerance by dietetic or other means in the hope of preventing progression to more florid diabetes. On the other hand, it seems equally reasonable to give more leeway to elderly asymptomatic patients where minor deviations in blood glucose may be the least of their problems.

Perhaps there is a better way of diagnosing diabetes. The belief that examination of capillary basement membrane thickness (BMT) in muscle biopsies might discriminate between diabetes and non-diabetes now looks slightly shop-soiled[3,4], for we now know that even with the most sophisticated methods of electron microscopy increased BMT can be detected only after prolonged hyperglycaemia. On the other hand, measurement of haemoglobin A_1 might become an alternative parameter of the glucose under-utilisation which is the essence of diabetes. This involves the patient in nothing more than a simple blood test while providing the doctor with a time-averaged integrated value reflecting the mean blood glucose over the preceding weeks.

The natural history of diabetes

The journey through glucose intolerance by way of insulin secretion or such fresh peaks of excitement as the association in juvenile-onset diabetes with certain histocompatibility antigens ultimately may seem immensely despairing when the end of the road is renal failure, blindness, lower limb trophic ulceration or death from a sudden heart attack. Yet much depends upon perspective. Nelson's great naval victories would have been an equally depressing catalogue of tragedies if history had been dependent upon the records of his naval surgeons and the details of injuries, battle scars and premature death amongst these illustrious men. What is the true perspective of diabetes today? Are more diabetic complications coming under scrutiny because we are more alert to such possibilities? Should we instead emulate Lord Nelson at the Battle of Copenhagen by putting the ophthalmoscope to our blind eye and ignore the early signs of retinopathy? That was a perhaps wholly reasonable attitude to strike so long as we remained powerless to respond to these tell-tale warning signals, but times have changed. Today we have the expertise to treat retinopathy and prolong reasonable vision, to prevent gangrene and at least to postpone some of the ultimate miseries. Indeed, it is more important than ever that we should examine our patients regularly for early evidence of:

retinopathy,
nephropathy,
peripheral and autonomic neuropathy,
lower limb trophic ulceration, and
hypertension and degenerative vascular disease.

Effective screening should diminish the chance of blindness or need for amputation and alert us to hypertension (one of the atheroma and retinopathy risk-factors amenable to treatment). The duration of diabetes remains the single most important factor affecting the likelihood of these specific complications becoming clinically evident, especially in patients with the juvenile-onset insulin-dependent disorder, and as the years pass it becomes increasingly prudent to be watchful for early tell-tale signs. On the other hand, those developing diabetes in later life may have one or more of these complications at the time of diagnosis.

Yet there is another aspect which should not be overlooked. Forget not that the vast majority of diabetics, even though initially severely distressed by thirst and polyuria, thereafter remain symptom-free by dietary manipulation with or without the judicious prescription of oral hypoglycaemic agents. Only a small proportion of these patients ever develop clinically-significant complications. Remember also that in later life diabetes may develop secondarily to some other seriously life-threatening disease when the aim should simply be to avoid the osmotic diuresis and symptoms of uncontrolled diabetes and where the question of diabetic complications may never arise. For these patients, therefore, diabetes is relatively benign.

But many diabetics, especially those developing the disorder in youth or in their prime, do not have the same life expectancy as non-diabetics. What more can we do to prevent the onset of specific diabetic complications? Here we return to the core question: does poor diabetic control accelerate the patient to the junkyard?

The case for improved diabetic control

Today we have reached the stage where the finger of accusation can be pointed, with virtual certainty, at hyperglycaemia. Biochemical studies have shown that the fundamental lesion in glomerular capillaries – basement membrane thickening – results from increased incorporation of carbohydrate into its glycoprotein structure as a direct consequence of hyperglycaemia. This lesion causes altered membrane porosity and is the forerunner of fibrin deposition and the more florid features of renal damage. Despite the fact that hyperglycaemia seems as corrosive to our patients' capillaries as salt is to the undersides of our motor cars, doubts remain. Some of the main arguments of the disbelievers embrace the following:

> other factors may be involved,
> apparently well-controlled diabetics develop complications, and
> as yet unidentified genetic influences may be present.

Let us look at these points in turn.

1   Almost certainly there *are* other factors. For example, growth hormone is known to influence basement membrane thickening and diabetic retinopathy, but it does not cause the characteristic diabetic lesion (in man or the experimental animal) in the absence of hyperglycaemia. And it is worth remembering that erratic diabetic control is a stimulus to growth hormone secretion. Without the sweet soil of hyperglycaemia, growth hormone – or other additional factors – cannot propagate diabetic micro-angiopathy.

2   Diabetic complications are quite frequently found in apparently well-controlled diabetics, but can we be sure that any patient is well controlled? It is now appreciated that many of the problems which caused high fetal mortality in diabetic pregnancies can be virtually eliminated by keeping the blood glucose close to the normal range. During pregnancy the diabetic patient has an added incentive to co-operate closely with treatment, but it has to be admitted that such degrees of good control are rarely achieved or maintained at other times.

3   The main support for an underlying genetic cause came from examination of muscle biopsies which apparently showed abnormal thickening of the capillary membrane at the time of diagnosis of diabetes, yet other careful workers have been unable to confirm these findings. As discussed on page 266 this digression into muscle has only proved that examining muscle capillaries is a poor substitute for renal glomeruli which show no evidence of basement membrane disease before the diagnosis of diabetes. Despite the suggestion that basement membrane thickening may be genetically determined, the lesion can be reproduced easily in the experimental animal made hyperglycaemic. Furthermore, the extent of the lesion correlates with the degree of hyperglycaemia

maintained over an extended period of time. Nevertheless, now that examination of the HLA system has added a new precision to the genetics of diabetes perhaps one or more of the HLA haplotypes will be found to be associated with an enhanced risk of diabetic complications. This seems unlikely, however, because most of the clinical and histological features of the complications are shared by juvenile- and maturity-onset diabetics and have been found in those with diabetes secondary to other disease.

Definite proof that small blood vessel disease can be prevented in diabetic patients by maintaining a normal blood glucose is lacking because normoglycaemia cannot be sustained over the years of a diabetic lifetime with currently available methods of treatment. But in a random allocation prospective trial comparing the effect of single daily injections of long-acting insulin with multiple daily injections, it has been shown that after four years, patients having multiple injections were better controlled and showed fewer retinal microaneurysms[5].

Whether improved control will diminish the diabetic's chances of developing atheroma remains much less clear. Indeed, the risk factors for atheroma in the diabetic are poorly understood. However, both hyperglycaemia on the one hand and hyperinsulinism on the other can be shown to have adverse effects on vessel wall metabolism (Chapter 13). Thus there are at least theoretical grounds for believing that good control (avoidance of wide swings in the blood glucose) might be less atherogenic. But vascular thrombosis also involves subtle upsets in platelet behaviour, fibrinogen/fibrin homeostasis and blood viscosity, all of which can be found to be abnormal in diabetes especially when it is poorly controlled and renal function becomes impaired. Thus, diabetic control may influence atheroma and other large vessel disease but proof is lacking.

Although the relationship between control and chronic diabetic peripheral and autonomic neuropathy remains uncertain, poor control may well be related to acute painful neuropathies both by diverting glucose into the sorbitol-fructose pathway and by modifying the water content of peripheral nerve tissue.

Poor diabetic control may not be at the root of all evil, but the onus now lies heavily upon those who believe that diabetic complications arise independently of blood glucose homeostasis to prove their case. Nor should they be allowed to use the argument of risks of hypoglycaemia to deflect those who are able to achieve better control from continuing to do so.

New methods of achieving better control

Increasing awareness of the potential hazards of poor control has stimulated a search for better alternatives to conventional therapy. Although research into islet cell transplantation is progressing energetically with laboratory animals, there is no immediate hope of replacing the failing human pancreas with islets nurtured or stored in tissue culture. On the other hand, the 'artificial pancreas' (a servo-controlled intravenous insulin/glucose infusion at rates computed from continuous blood glucose estimations) is available and can be used to maintain perfect control during intercurrent illness, at surgery, or in the labour suite[6]. But it does involve tethering the patient to bulky equipment and up to now has had no place in routine diabetic care. Other continuous subcutaneous delivery systems, which involve slinging a small infusion pump to the waist, have been developed to infuse insulin steadily with programmed or manual speedup at mealtimes[7,8]. Even without the blood glucose feedback of the 'artificial pancreas', good diabetic control has been demonstrated in the short term[9,10]. But they are still more restrictive on patient activity, especially for the sporting youngster, than conventional injections. Nevertheless, there is ample scope for the bioengineer, or any reader with an inventive turn of mind.

Increasing the fibre content of the diet, by reducing the marked upsurge in blood glucose following meals, can improve control both in the mild diabetic whose pancreas responds sluggishly to feeding and in the insulin-dependent patient whose sub-cutaneously-injected hormone cannot mimic the brisk insulin release enjoyed by the non-diabetic.

The use of highly purified insulins which are only weakly immunogenic, have no magic potential to improve control by comparison with conventional insulins. Nevertheless in 'brittle' diabetes or in those receiving in excess of 100 units of conventional insulin daily, where large amounts of insulin antibodies are found, conversion to purified insulin usually improves diabetic control presumably because the antibodies have contributed to the brittle state or poor blood glucose homeostasis.

In discussing insulin therapy (Chapter 10), the analogy was made of the trials and tribulations of the golf course. Insulin therapy is not an exact science, but now that we have the technology to allow patients to measure their own blood glucose and adjust insulin dosage frequently under home conditions rather than occasionally in the artificial circumstances of the diabetic clinic or hospital, there is at least the *prospect* of improved diabetic control. Patients learn at first hand the effects of feeding and exercise upon blood glucose homeostasis and can, with practice, as in golf, aim to improve their handicap. The imperative need now is to put these better methods of management to the test by assessing carefully whether they prevent or delay the onset of diabetic complications. Just as home monitoring of blood glucose has brought a new precision to the day to day adjustment of insulin dosage, measurement of haemoglobin A_1 in the out-patient clinic has enhanced our ability to assess control between clinic visits (Chapter 21, p.249).

It is always easier to identify the problem than to guarantee its elimination, but those responsible for diabetic care will surely admit that many patients have been denied the opportunity of even elementary guidance in the principles of self-regulation which, when sensibly interpreted and applied, can improve diabetic control. Too often, improved control is equated with a heightened risk of hypoglycaemia. This can be a problem when attempting to manage diabetics with single daily injections of long-acting insulin, but a twice-daily four-insulin system can create an insulin profile remarkably close to the physiological norm, avoiding extremes of hyper- and hypoglycaemia.

It would be too much to expect better diabetic control to be easily extended to all patients. It may never be possible to purge diabetics of all their handicaps: sanitation has not eliminated infection – but should not be abandoned on this account!

Other developments

Despite uncertainties about diabetic control and its achievement, there are many aspects of diabetic care which are constantly being improved and which are of proven value to the patient. Amongst the credits are:

> oral hypoglycaemic agents;
> highly-purified insulins;
> care in pregnancy;
> emergency care and surgery;
> treatment of acute metabolic decompensation;
> ophthalmology; and
> foot care and prevention of ulceration in those having peripheral neuropathy.

Oral hypoglycaemic agents, whether used temporarily, intermittently or permanently are a boon to countless diabetics. With the exception of the potential of the biguanides to aggravate lactic acidosis in some unsuitable patients, they are remarkably free of side effects. Anxiety about the risk of atherogenesis, especially in the case of sulphonylureas, which followed in the wake of the UGDP studies (Chapter 13, p.169), should at least caution us not to prescribe oral agents unnecessarily nor to use them as a substitute for sensible dieting. Whatever the fears of atherogenesis, however, those who develop diabetes in old age – often thin and undernourished – should not be subjected to insulin injections if a sulphonylurea will impose placid control over the distressing symptoms of hyperglycaemia.

The newer purified insulins are of proven benefit in patients having insulin allergy or lipoatrophy at injection sites and in those with insulin resistance. All youngsters, and especially females, should have purified insulin so that they can wear a bathing costume without embarrassment. The 'purer is better' ideology, however, does not mean that these will prevent or diminish diabetic complications, but if their use gives improved control so much the better.

The outlook for the pregnant diabetic, both in terms of maternal and fetal mortality, has improved enormously so that where there is first class diabetic and obstetric care, fetal mortality has fallen towards 4%. The only blemish, and a cause for increasing concern, is the threefold excess of congenital defects compared with the general population. Nevertheless, the realisation that hyperglycaemia creates a totally unsuitable environment in which to nurture a fetus, also raises the possibility that better control from conception might diminish the risk of congenital defects.

Better understanding of the water and electrolyte imbalances associated with severe insulin lack and hyperglycaemia have steadily improved the outcome in acute metabolic decompensation. All these patients tend to be hyperosmolar, although some are more hyperosmolar than others. The diuresis of hyperglycaemia creates a tendency to *hypernatraemia* which the patient corrects by drinking water rather than brine, but drowsiness or other intercurrent illness may blunt the thirst: drinking stops yet diuresis does not. Then hypernatraemia and serious hyperosmolar coma may overtake the patient.

A greater awareness of the difference between mild ketonuria and severe ketonaemia by checking for *plasma* as well as urinary ketones, and more energetic therapy for the potassium losses have both helped. As a consequence, the place of insulin has been relegated to a low-key, low-dosage profile whilst restoration of both plasma volume and osmolality is the urgent problem. Much has yet to be learned, however, about movements of such other ions as magnesium, management of the hypercoagulable state and the use of dichloracetate in lactic acidosis. Meantime, a greater awareness of the latter (severe acidosis *without* excess plasma ketones) and prompt treatment with bicarbonate, will save lives.

The strides made in eye treatment have not always been matched by our ability to get the patient to the ophthalmologist. Whatever schemes are devised to help patients it would seem prudent to warn those at risk (especially the insulin-dependent of more than 10 years' standing) to seek advice should there be any change in eyesight, however slight. The eye specialist expert in diabetic management has several ways of arresting deterioration in, or improving vision:

light and laser coagulation;
clofibrate and anti-platelet agents;
pituitary ablation;
urokinase injections;
vitrectomy; and
low-vision acuity aids.

These advances are no substitute, however, for careful surveillance of patients at risk by those responsible for diabetic care. Similarly, education in foot care and the provision of chiropody services are the surest ways for diabetics to keep ten toes.

The recent rapid increase in knowledge about diabetic autonomic neuropathy, although not equalled by much improvement in treatment or in our ability to prevent the pain or parasthesiae of peripheral neuropathy, has at least helped us in advising patients how to cope with the distressing symptoms.

Perhaps there will be better ways of dealing with diabetics and their problems; the researcher must certainly be given every encouragement. In the meantime, guiding the patient in the pathways of metabolic righteousness – avoiding the peaks of hyperglycaemia or the pitfalls of hypoglycaemia – is the essential aim. Instead of putting the telescope to the eye of faith in the hope of seeing an over-optimistic tomorrow, we might more appropriately re-interpret Lord Nelson's most famous battle signal 'England expects . . .' into 'Diabetics expect that we will do our best for them.' The disorder remains an outstanding opportunity for those involved in diabetic care – researchers, health educationists, nutritionists, chiropodists, nurses and the various branches of the medical profession – to respond to the challenge.

Further Reading

1 Bloom S.R. (1979) Alimentary hormones. *Medicine, the Monthly Add-on Journal, 3rd Series*, **15**, 733–736

2 Rotter J.I. & Rimoin D.L. (1979) Diabetes mellitus: the search for genetic markers. *Diabetes Care*, **2**, 215–226

3 Gundersen H.J.G., Osterby R. & Lundbaek K. (1978). The basement membrane controversy. *Diabetologia*, **15**, 361–364

4 Siperstein M.D. & Feingold K.R. (1978) Hyperglycaemia and diabetic microangiopathy. *Diabetologia*, **15**, 365–368

5 Tchobroutsky G. (1978) Relationship of diabetic control to development of microvascular complications. *Diabetologia*, **15**, 143–152

6 Nattrass M., Alberti K.G.M.M.M., Dennis K.S., Gillibrand P.N., Letchworth A.T. & Buckle A.J.L. (1978) A glucose-controlled insulin infusion system for diabetic women during labour. *Br. med. J.*, **ii**, 599–602

7 Editorial (1979) New insulin-delivery systems for diabetics. *Lancet*, **i**, 1275–1277

8 Arky R.A. (1979) The engineering of blood sugar. *New Engl. J. Med.*, **300**, 618–619

9 Pickup J.C., Keen H., Parson J.A., Alberti K.G.M.M. & Rowe A.J. (1979) Continuous subcutaneous infusion: improved blood-glucose and intermediary-metabolite control in diabetes. *Lancet*, **i.**, 1255–1257

10 Tamboralane W.V., Sherwin R.S., Genel M. & Felig P. (1979) Restoration of normal lipid and amino-acid metabolism in diabetic patients treated with a portable infusion pump. *Lancet*, **i**, 1258–1261

Average Weights: Males and Females

Height in shoes; weight in light indoor clothing. Based upon Metropolitan Life Insurance data, USA and Canada, 1959. Ideally, patients should keep their weight down to the average for their height in the 20–24 age band

Males

HEIGHT		WEIGHT															
		15–16 years		17–19 years		20–24 years		25–29 years		30–39 years		40–49 years		50–59 years		60–69 years	
metre	ft/in	kg	lb	kg	lb	kg	lb	kg	lb	kg	lb	kg	lb	kg	lb	kg	lb
1.52	5.0	44.5	98	51.3	113	55.3	122	58.1	128	59.4	131	60.8	134	61.7	136	60.3	133
1.55	5.1	46.3	102	52.6	116	56.7	125	59.4	131	60.8	134	62.7	137	63	139	61.7	136
1.58	5.2	48.5	107	54	119	58.1	128	60.8	134	62.1	137	63.5	140	64.4	142	63	139
1.60	5.3	50.8	112	55.8	123	59.9	132	62.6	138	64	141	65.3	144	65.8	145	64.4	142
1.63	5.4	53.1	117	57.6	127	61.7	136	64	141	65.8	145	67.1	148	67.6	149	66.2	146
1.65	5.5	55.3	122	59.4	131	63	139	65.3	144	67.6	149	68.9	152	69.4	153	68	150
1.68	5.6	57.6	127	61.2	135	64.4	142	67.1	148	69.4	153	70.8	156	71.2	157	69.9	154
1.70	5.7	59.9	132	63	139	65.8	145	68.5	151	71.2	157	73	161	73.5	162	72.1	159
1.73	5.8	62.1	137	64.9	143	67.6	149	70.3	155	73	161	74.8	165	75.3	166	73.9	163
1.75	5.9	64.4	142	66.7	147	69.4	153	72.1	159	74.8	165	76.7	169	77.1	170	76.2	168
1.78	5.10	66.2	146	68.5	151	71.2	157	73.9	163	77.1	170	78.9	174	79.4	175	78.5	173
1.80	5.11	68.0	150	70.3	155	73	161	75.8	167	78.9	174	80.8	178	81.6	180	80.5	178
1.83	6.0	69.9	154	72.6	160	75.3	166	78	172	81.2	179	83	183	83.9	185	83	183
1.85	6.1	72.1	159	74.4	164	77.1	170	80.3	177	83	183	84.8	187	85.7	189	85.3	188
1.88	6.2	74.4	164	76.2	168	78.9	174	82.6	182	85.3	188	87.1	192	88	194	87.5	193
1.91	6.3	76.9	169	78	172	80.8	178	84.4	186	87.5	193	89.4	197	90.3	199	89.8	198

Females

HEIGHT		WEIGHT															
		15–16 years		17–19 years		20–24 years		25–29 years		30–39 years		40–49 years		50–59 years		60–69 years	
metre	ft/in	kg	lb	kg	lb	kg	lb	kg	lb	kg	lb	kg	lb	kg	lb	kg	lb
1.47	4.10	44	97	44.9	99	46.3	102	48.5	107	52.2	115	55.3	122	56.7	125	57.6	127
1.50	4.11	45.5	100	46.3	102	47.6	105	49.9	110	53.1	117	56.2	124	57.6	127	58.5	129
1.52	5.00	46.7	103	47.6	105	49	108	51.3	113	54.4	120	57.6	127	59	130	59.4	131
1.55	5.1	48.5	107	49.4	109	50.8	112	52.6	116	55.8	123	59	130	60.3	133	60.8	134
1.58	5.2	50.3	111	51.3	113	52.2	115	54	119	57.2	126	60.3	133	61.7	136	62.1	137
1.60	5.3	51.7	114	52.6	116	53.5	118	55.3	122	58.5	129	61.7	136	63.5	140	64	141
1.63	5.4	53.1	117	54.4	120	54.9	121	56.7	125	59.9	132	63.5	140	65.3	144	65.8	145
1.65	5.5	54.9	121	56.2	124	56.7	125	58.5	129	61.1	135	64.8	143	67	148	67.6	149
1.68	5.6	56.1	125	57.6	127	58.5	129	60.3	133	63	139	66.7	147	68.9	152	69.4	153
1.70	5.7	58.1	128	59	130	59.9	132	61.7	136	64.4	142	68.5	151	70.8	156	71.2	157
1.73	5.8	59.9	132	60.8	134	61.7	136	63.5	140	66.2	146	70.3	155	72.6	160	73	161
1.75	5.9	61.7	136	62.5	138	63.5	140	65.3	144	68	150	72.1	159	74.4	164	74.8	165
1.78	5.10	—	—	64.4	142	65.3	144	67.1	148	69.9	154	74.4	164	76.7	169	—	—
1.80	5.11	—	—	66.7	147	67.6	149	69.4	153	72.1	159	76.7	169	78.9	174	—	—
1.83	6.0	—	—	68.9	152	69.9	154	71.7	158	74.4	164	78.9	174	81.6	180	—	—

APPENDIX 2

Simple Carbohydrate Restricted Diet

The None, Some, as-Much-as-You-Like Diet

This diet can be used *safely* by any patient from diagnosis until he is more carefully assessed by a dietician. It makes a useful basis for the diet in the elderly. No weighing is necessary.

---

1   **Cut out completely – NONE**

SUGAR-CONTAINING FOODS
Sugar, glucose, jam, marmalade, honey, syrup, sweets, chocolates, treacle, buns, cakes, sweet biscuits, chocolate biscuits, pastry, pies, *tinned fruit*, grapes, *lemonade, glucose drinks*, beer, stout, sweet wines, sweet sherry.

---

2   **Take in moderation – SOME**

STARCHES – CONTAIN SOME SUGAR
Bread, rolls, scones, porridge, peas, potatoes, plain biscuits, pudding cereals, breakfast cereals, thick soup, plain ice-cream, fruit (except grapes), fruit juice, dry wine, dry sherry, light beer.

FATS
Butter, margarine, cream.

---

3   **Take as desired – AS MUCH AS YOU LIKE**

PROTEIN AND NON-FATTENING FOODS
Meat, fish, cheese, eggs, vegetables (except peas and potatoes), clear soup, Oxo, Bovril, Marmite, tea and coffee (milk from allowance, no sugar).

Do not exceed one pint of milk daily

Use diabetic jams or diabetic drinks which do not contain sugar. Saccharine for sweetening.

Carbohydrate Exchange List

Each of the following contains about 10 g carbohydrate, ie. 1 portion (or exchange) of carbohydrate.

	ounces	*grams*
Cereal Foods		
All-bran – 3 level tablespoons	$\frac{2}{3}$	20
Breakfast Cereals		
Cornflakes – 3 heaped tablespoons	$\frac{1}{2}$	15
Rice Krispies – 3 heaped tablespoons	$\frac{1}{2}$	15
Shredded Wheat – 1 biscuit	$\frac{1}{2}$	15
Weetabix – 1 biscuit	$\frac{1}{2}$	15
Biscuits		
Tea biscuits – 2 biscuits	$\frac{1}{2}$	15
Cream crackers – 2 biscuits	$\frac{1}{2}$	15
Digestive – 2 small/1 large biscuit	$\frac{1}{2}$	15
Abernethy – 1 biscuit	$\frac{1}{2}$	15
Bread	$\frac{2}{3}$	20
Pudding Cereals		
Custard powder ⎫		
Cornflour ⎪ 2 heaped teaspoons	$\frac{1}{3}$	10
Rice, sago ⎬		
Semolina, tapioca ⎭		
Chappati made from wheat starch	$\frac{1}{2}$	15
Cornmeal and oatmeal – 1 level tablespoon	$\frac{1}{2}$	15
Flour – 1 level tablespoon	$\frac{1}{2}$	15
Pasta (before cooking) – 1 heaped tablespoon	$\frac{1}{2}$	15
Porridge (cooked) – 4 level tablespoons	4	120
Rice (boiled) – 1 heaped tablespoon	1	30
Ryvita – $1\frac{1}{2}$ biscuits	$\frac{1}{2}$	15
Vitawheat – 2 biscuits	$\frac{1}{2}$	15
Milk		
Milk (fresh) – $\frac{1}{3}$pint	7	210
Milk (evaporated, unsweetened) – 6 tablespoons	3	90

	ounces	*grams*

Fruit

(Stewed fruit should be cooked without sugar, but may be sweetened with saccharine afterwards)

	ounces	grams
Apples (raw with skin and core) – 1 medium	4	120
(baked with skin) – 1 medium	4	120
(stewed) – 6 tablespoons	5	150
Banana (ripe without skin) – 1 small	2	60
Cherries (raw with stone) – 20	4	120
Currants (dried) – 1 level tablespoon	$\frac{1}{2}$	15
Damsons (stewed with stones) – 10	5	150
Dates (with stones) – 2	$\frac{2}{3}$	20
Figs (dried stewed) – 1	$1\frac{1}{2}$	45
Grapes (whole) – 10	2	60
Greengages (stewed with stones) – 4	4	120
Nectarines (with stones) – 2	3	90
Oranges (without peel) – 1 medium	4	120
Orange juice (fresh or tinned, unsweetened) – 8 tablespoons	4	120
Peaches (fresh with stones) – 1 medium	4	120
(dried, stewed) – 2 halves	2	60
Pears (raw with skin and core) – 1 medium	4	120
(stewed) – $2\frac{1}{2}$ halves	5	150
Pineapple juice (tinned, unsweetened) – 6 tablespoons	3	90
Plums (raw with stones) – 3 large	4	120
(stewed with stones) – 5 medium	8	240
Prunes (stewed with stones) – 4 medium	2	60
Raisins (dried) – 1 level tablespoon	$\frac{1}{2}$	15
Raspberries (raw or stewed) – 6 level tablespoons	6	180
Strawberries (fresh, ripe) – 15	6	180
Sultanas (dried) – 1 level tablespoon	$\frac{1}{2}$	15
Tangerines (without peel) – 2	4	120

Vegetables

	ounces	grams
Beans (baked, tinned) – 2 level tablespoons	2	60
(broad, tinned/boiled) – 2 level tablespoons	5	150
(butter, boiled) – 2 level tablespoons	2	60
(Haricot, boiled) – 2 level tablespoons	2	60
Parsnips (boiled) – 2 heaped tablespoons	3	90
Peas (fresh or frozen, boiled) – 4 heaped tablespoons	4	120
(tinned) – 2 heaped tablespoons	2	60

	ounces	*grams*
Potatoes (boiled) – 1 size of hen's egg	2	60
(chipped) – 4 large chips	1	30
(crisps) – 1 packet	$\frac{3}{4}$	25
(mashed) – 1 heaped tablespoon	2	60
(roast) – 1 small	$1\frac{1}{2}$	45
Sweet corn (tinned) – 2 level tablespoons	$1\frac{1}{2}$	45

Beverages

Bengers food, Bournvita, Ovaltine, Horlicks – 2 heaped teaspoons	$\frac{1}{2}$	15
Cocoa powder – 5 heaped teaspoons	$\frac{1}{2}$	15
Coca-cola or Pepsi-Cola	3	90
Beer	1 pint	600 ml
Lager	1 pint	600 ml
Cider (bottled, sweet)	$\frac{1}{2}$ pint	300 ml
Stout (bottled)	$\frac{1}{2}$ pint	300 ml

Desserts

Ice cream (plain) – 1 small brickette	2	60
Jelly (after preparation)	2	60
Yoghurt (plain) – 1 carton	6	180
(fruit) – $\frac{1}{2}$ carton	2	60

APPENDIX 4

High-fibre Carbohydrate Exchanges

The carbohydrate in the diabetic diet should come from sources with a high-fibre content. The best sources are *wholemeal bread* and *flour, bran, fruit* and *vegetables*. Each of the following portions contains 10 grams of *Carbohydrate* = 1 *Exchange*

Wholemeal bread	—	1 small slice
Allinsons bread	—	1 slice
All-Bran	—	3 level tablespoons
Shredded Wheat	—	1 biscuit
Weetabix	—	1 biscuit
Puffed Wheat	—	4 level tablespoons
Porridge (cooked)	—	4 level tablespoons
Ryvita	—	$1\frac{1}{2}$ biscuits
Vitawheat	—	2 biscuits
Broad beans	—	2 level tablespoons
Butter beans	—	2 level tablespoons
Haricot beans	—	2 level tablespoons
Baked beans	—	2 level tablespoons
Peas, tinned	—	2 heaped tablespoons
Peas, fresh or frozen	—	4 heaped tablespoons
Apple	—	1 medium
Damsons (stewed)	—	10
Figs (stewed)	—	1
Plums (stewed)	—	5 medium
Plums (raw)	—	3 large
Prunes (stewed)	—	4 medium
Raspberries	—	6 level tablespoons
Salted peanuts	—	4 oz packet

'Diabetic' Foods and Drinks

Most *'diabetic' foods* are sweetened with *sorbitol* or *fructose* instead of *sucrose*. They contain as much energy as the ordinary equivalent. THEY ARE FATTENING. For the child wanting a substitute for sweets or candies an *apple* or other fruit is a better alternative.

Diabetic foodstuff	Suitability for slimmers	General remarks
Jams, marmalade and preserves	NO	An acceptable substitute
Chocolate	NO	High in saturated fat; poor flavour
Sweets or candies	NO	Should not be encouraged; better to have fruit instead
Biscuits and cake	NO	Carbohydrate reduced; a small portion of the real thing would be better
Tinned fruit in water	YES	Insipid
Tinned fruit in syrup	NO	Expensive
Drinks: squashes	YES	Should be recommended to all diabetics
Beer	NO	More expensive: *high alcohol content*

APPENDIX 6

Diet in Illness or Emergencies

The insulin-dependent diabetic needs a regular intake of carbohydrate to prevent ketoacidosis (20 g carbohydrate every 3–4 hours). The following is a list of suitable alternatives to ordinary meals. If the patient is unable to take a light diet, has significant ketonuria or is vomiting, intravenous fluids are indicated.

	10 grams of carbohydrate or 1 Exchange		*20 grams of carbohydrate or 2 Exchanges*	
	fl oz	ml	fl oz	ml
Lucozade	2	60	4	120
Coca-Cola	3	90	6	180
Milk	7	200	14	400
Condensed milk	$\frac{2}{3}$	20	$1\frac{1}{3}$	40
Ribena	$\frac{2}{3}$	20	$1\frac{1}{3}$	40
Orange juice (fresh or tinned unsweetened)	4	120	8	240
	oz	g	oz	g
Complan powder	$\frac{2}{3}$	20	$1\frac{1}{3}$	40
Benger's Food	$\frac{1}{2}$	15	1	30
Bournvita, Horlicks, Ovaltine	$\frac{1}{2}$	15	1	30
Ice-cream	2	60	4	120
Yoghurt, plain	6	180	12	360
Yoghurt, fruit	2	60	4	120

Index